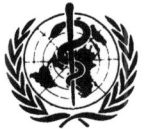

WORLD HEALTH ORGANIZATION

INTERNATIONAL AGENCY FOR RESEARCH ON CANCER

IARC MONOGRAPHS
ON THE
EVALUATION OF CARCINOGENIC RISKS TO HUMANS

Occupational Exposures to Mists and Vapours from Strong Inorganic Acids; and Other Industrial Chemicals

VOLUME 54

This publication represents the views and expert opinions
of an IARC Working Group on the
Evaluation of Carcinogenic Risks to Humans,
which met in Lyon,

15–22 October 1991

1992

IARC MONOGRAPHS

In 1969, the International Agency for Research on Cancer (IARC) initiated a programme on the evaluation of the carcinogenic risk of chemicals to humans involving the production of critically evaluated monographs on individual chemicals. In 1980 and 1986, the programme was expanded to include the evaluation of the carcinogenic risk associated with exposures to complex mixtures and other agents.

The objective of the programme is to elaborate and publish in the form of monographs critical reviews of data on carcinogenicity for agents to which humans are known to be exposed, and on specific exposure situations; to evaluate these data in terms of human risk with the help of international working groups of experts in chemical carcinogenesis and related fields; and to indicate where additional research efforts are needed.

This project is supported by PHS Grant No. 2UO1CA33193-10 awarded by the US National Cancer Institute, Department of Health and Human Services. Additional support has been provided since 1986 by the Commission of the European Communities.

©International Agency for Research on Cancer 1992

ISBN 92 832 1254-1

ISSN 0250-9555

All rights reserved. Application for rights of reproduction or translation, in part or *in toto*, should be made to the International Agency for Research on Cancer.

Distributed for the International Agency for Research on Cancer
by the Secretariat of the World Health Organization

PRINTED IN THE UK

CONTENTS

NOTE TO THE READER 5

LIST OF PARTICIPANTS 7

PREAMBLE
    Background 13
    Objective and Scope 13
    Selection of Topics for Monographs 14
    Data for Monographs 15
    The Working Group 15
    Working Procedures 15
    Exposure Data 16
    Evidence for Carcinogenicity in Humans 17
    Studies of Cancer in Experimental Animals 21
    Other Relevant Data 23
    Summary of Data Reported 24
    Evaluation 26
    References 30

GENERAL REMARKS 33

THE MONOGRAPHS
    Occupational exposures to mists and vapours from sulfuric acid and other strong
        inorganic acids 41
        Annex: Chemical and physical properties and uses of sulfuric acid and
        sulfur trioxide 121
    Sulfur dioxide and some sulfites, bisulfites and metabisulfites 131
    Hydrochloric acid 189
    Diethyl sulfate 213
    Diisopropyl sulfate 229
    1,3-Butadiene 237

SUMMARY OF FINAL EVALUATIONS 287

APPENDIX 1. SUMMARY TABLES OF GENETIC AND RELATED EFFECTS . 291

APPENDIX 2. ACTIVITY PROFILES FOR GENETIC AND RELATED
    EFFECTS 299

CUMULATIVE INDEX TO THE *MONOGRAPHS* SERIES 311

NOTE TO THE READER

The term 'carcinogenic risk' in the *IARC Monographs* series is taken to mean the probability that exposure to an agent will lead to cancer in humans.

Inclusion of an agent in the *Monographs* does not imply that it is a carcinogen, only that the published data have been examined. Equally, the fact that an agent has not yet been evaluated in a monograph does not mean that it is not carcinogenic.

The evaluations of carcinogenic risk are made by international working groups of independent scientists and are qualitative in nature. No recommendation is given for regulation or legislation.

Anyone who is aware of published data that may alter the evaluation of the carcinogenic risk of an agent to humans is encouraged to make this information available to the Unit of Carcinogen Identification and Evaluation, International Agency for Research on Cancer, 150 cours Albert Thomas, 69372 Lyon Cedex 08, France, in order that the agent may be considered for re-evaluation by a future Working Group.

Although every effort is made to prepare the monographs as accurately as possible, mistakes may occur. Readers are requested to communicate any errors to the Unit of Carcinogen Identification and Evaluation, so that corrections can be reported in future volumes.

IARC WORKING GROUP ON THE EVALUATION OF CARCINOGENIC RISKS TO HUMANS: OCCUPATIONAL EXPOSURES TO MISTS AND VAPOURS FROM STRONG INORGANIC ACIDS; AND OTHER INDUSTRIAL CHEMICALS

Lyon, 15–22 October 1991

LIST OF PARTICIPANTS

Members

H.M. Bolt, Institute for Occupational Physiology at the University of Dortmund, Ardeystrasse 67, 4600 Dortmund 1, Germany

V.J. Feron, Department of Biological Toxicology, TNO Toxicology and Nutrition Institute, PO Box 360, 3700 AJ Zeist, The Netherlands

F. Forastiere, Epidemiological Unit, Latium Regional Health Authority, via Santa Costanza 53, 00198 Rome, Italy

C. Garner, University of York, Jack Birch Unit of Environmental Carcinogenesis, Department of Biology, Heslington, York Y01 5DD, United Kingdom

M. Gérin, University of Montréal, Department of Occupational and Environmental Health, Faculty of Medicine, CP 6128, Station A, Montréal, Quebec H3C 3J7, Canada

B. Goldstein, Environmental and Occupational Health Sciences Institute, 675 Hoes Lane, Piscataway, NJ 08854-5635, USA

M. Hayashi, Division of Mutagenesis, Biological Safety Research Center, National Institute of Hygienic Sciences, 1-18-1 Kami Yooga, Setagaya-ku, Tokyo 158, Japan

U. Heinrich, Fraunhofer Institute of Toxicology and Aerosol Research, Nikolai Fuchs Strasse 1, 3000 Hanover 61, Germany

T. Kauppinen, Institute of Occupational Health, Topeliuksenkatu 41 a A, 00250 Helsinki, Finland

R.J. Kavlock, Developmental Toxicology Division (MD-71), Health Effects Research Laboratory, US Environmental Protection Agency, Research Triangle Park, NC 27711, USA

K.A. L'Abbé, Department of Preventive Medicine and Biostatistics, McMurrich Building, 4th Floor, Faculty of Medicine, University of Toronto, Toronto, Ontario, Canada M5S 1A8

G. Matanoski, Johns Hopkins University, 624 North Broadway, Room 280, Baltimore, MD 21205, USA (*Chairperson*)

R. Melnick, National Institute of Environmental Health Sciences, PO Box 12233, Research Triangle Park, NC 27709, USA

G. Nordberg, Department of Environmental Medicine, University of Umeå, 90 187 Umeå, Sweden

G. Pershagen, Institute of Environmental Medicine, Karolinska Institute, Box 60208, 104 01 Stockholm, Sweden

T. Sanner, Laboratory for Environmental and Occupational Cancer, Institute for Cancer Research, Montebello, 0310 Oslo 3, Norway (*Vice-Chairperson*)

C.L. Soskolne, 13-103 Clinical Sciences Building, Department of Health Services Administration and Community Medicine, Faculty of Medicine, University of Alberta, Edmonton, Alberta, Canada T6G 2G3

V. Turusov, Laboratory of Carcinogenic Substances, All-Union Cancer Research Centre, Kashirskoye Shosse 24, Moscow 115478, Russia

M.A. Waters, National Institute for Occupational Safety and Health, 4676 Columbia Parkway, R-14, Cincinnati, OH 45226-1998, USA

Representative and observers[1]

Representative of the National Cancer Institute

E.F. Heineman, Environmental Epidemiology Branch, Epidemiology and Biostatistics Program, National Cancer Institute, Executive Plaza North, Room 418, 6130 Executive Boulevard, Rockville, MD 20892, USA

Representative of ILSI Risk Science Institute

S. Olin, International Life Sciences Institute, Risk Science Institute, 1126 Sixteenth Street NW, Washington DC 20036, USA

Electric Power Research Institute

R.E. Wyzga, Electric Power Research Institute, 3412 Hillview Avenue, PO Box 10412, Palo Alto, CA 94303, USA

European Chemical Industry, Ecology and Toxicology Centre

G. Paddle, Imperial Chemical Industries, plc, Alderley Park, Macclesfield, Cheshire SK10 4TJ, United Kingdom

International Institute of Synthetic Rubber Producers

J.F. Acquavella, Monsanto Co.–A2SL, 800 North Lindbergh Boulevard, St Louis, MO 63167, USA

---

[1]Unable to attend, M. De Smedt, Industrial Medicine and Hygiene Unit, Health and Safety Directorate, Commission of the European Community, Bâtiment Jean Monnet, 2920 Luxembourg, Grand Duchy of Luxembourg

PARTICIPANTS

Secretariat

P. Boffetta, Unit of Analytical Epidemiology
E. Cardis, Director's Office
M. Friesen, Unit of Environmental Carcinogenesis and Host Factors
M.-J. Ghess, Unit of Carcinogen Identification and Evaluation
M. Gilbert, International Programme on Chemical Safety, World Health Organization, 1211 Geneva 27, Switzerland
E. Heseltine, Lajarthe, 24290 St Léon-sur-Vézère, France
M. Kogevinas, Unit of Analytical Epidemiology
V. Krutovskikh, Unit of Multistage Carcinogenesis
E. Matos, Unit of Carcinogen Identification and Evaluation
D. McGregor, Unit of Carcinogen Identification and Evaluation
D. Mietton, Unit of Carcinogen Identification and Evaluation
H. Møller, Unit of Carcinogen Identification and Evaluation
H. Nakazawa, Unit of Multistage Carcinogenesis
C. Partensky, Unit of Carcinogen Identification and Evaluation
I. Peterschmitt, Unit of Carcinogen Identification and Evaluation, Geneva
R. Saracci, Unit of Analytical Epidemiology
D. Shuker, Unit of Environmental Carcinogenesis and Host Factors
L. Tomatis, Director
H. Vainio, Chief, Unit of Carcinogen Identification and Evaluation
J. Wilbourn, Unit of Carcinogen Identification and Evaluation

Secretarial assistance

J. Cazeaux
M. Lézère
S. Reynaud

PREAMBLE

IARC MONOGRAPHS PROGRAMME ON THE EVALUATION OF CARCINOGENIC RISKS TO HUMANS[1]

PREAMBLE

1. BACKGROUND

In 1969, the International Agency for Research on Cancer (IARC) initiated a programme to evaluate the carcinogenic risk of chemicals to humans and to produce monographs on individual chemicals. The *Monographs* programme has since been expanded to include consideration of exposures to complex mixtures of chemicals (which occur, for example, in some occupations and as a result of human habits) and of exposures to other agents, such as radiation and viruses. With Supplement 6 (IARC, 1987a), the title of the series was modified from *IARC Monographs on the Evaluation of the Carcinogenic Risk of Chemicals to Humans* to *IARC Monographs on the Evaluation of Carcinogenic Risks to Humans*, in order to reflect the widened scope of the programme.

The criteria established in 1971 to evaluate carcinogenic risk to humans were adopted by the working groups whose deliberations resulted in the first 16 volumes of the *IARC Monographs* series. Those criteria were subsequently updated by further ad-hoc working groups (IARC, 1977, 1978, 1979, 1982, 1983, 1987b, 1988, 1991a; Vainio *et al.*, 1992).

2. OBJECTIVE AND SCOPE

The objective of the programme is to prepare, with the help of international working groups of experts, and to publish in the form of monographs, critical reviews and evaluations of evidence on the carcinogenicity of a wide range of human exposures. The *Monographs* may also indicate where additional research efforts are needed.

The *Monographs* represent the first step in carcinogenic risk assessment, which involves examination of all relevant information in order to assess the strength of the available evidence that certain exposures could alter the incidence of cancer in humans. The second step is quantitative risk estimation. Detailed, quantitative evaluations of epidemiological data may be made in the *Monographs*, but without extrapolation beyond the range of the data

---

[1] This project is supported by PHS Grant No. 2 UO1 CA33193-10 awarded by the US National Cancer Institute, Department of Health and Human Services. Since 1986, the programme has also been supported by the Commission of the European Communities.

available. Quantitative extrapolation from experimental data to the human situation is not undertaken.

The term 'carcinogen' is used in these monographs to denote an exposure that is capable of increasing the incidence of malignant neoplasms; the induction of benign neoplasms may in some circumstances (see p. 22) contribute to the judgement that the exposure is carcinogenic. The terms 'neoplasm' and 'tumour' are used interchangeably.

Some epidemiological and experimental studies indicate that different agents may act at different stages in the carcinogenic process, and several different mechanisms may be involved. The aim of the *Monographs* has been, from their inception, to evaluate evidence of carcinogenicity at any stage in the carcinogenesis process, independently of the underlying mechanisms. Information on mechanisms may, however, be used in making the overall evaluation (IARC, 1991a; Vainio *et al.*, 1992; see also pp. 28-29).

The *Monographs* may assist national and international authorities in making risk assessments and in formulating decisions concerning any necessary preventive measures. The evaluations of IARC working groups are scientific, qualitative judgements about the evidence for or against carcinogenicity provided by the available data. These evaluations represent only one part of the body of information on which regulatory measures may be based. Other components of regulatory decisions may vary from one situation to another and from country to country, responding to different socioeconomic and national priorities. **Therefore, no recommendation is given with regard to regulation or legislation, which are the responsibility of individual governments and/or other international organizations.**

The *IARC Monographs* are recognized as an authoritative source of information on the carcinogenicity of a wide range of human exposures. A users' survey, made in 1988, indicated that the *Monographs* are consulted by various agencies in 57 countries. Each volume is generally printed in 4000 copies for distribution to governments, regulatory bodies and interested scientists. The *Monographs* are also available *via* the Distribution and Sales Service of the World Health Organization.

3. SELECTION OF TOPICS FOR MONOGRAPHS

Topics are selected on the basis of two main criteria: (a) there is evidence of human exposure, and (b) there is some evidence or suspicion of carcinogenicity. The term 'agent' is used to include individual chemical compounds, groups of related chemical compounds, physical agents (such as radiation) and biological factors (such as viruses). Exposures to mixtures of agents may occur in occupational exposures and as a result of personal and cultural habits (like smoking and dietary practices). Chemical analogues and compounds with biological or physical characteristics similar to those of suspected carcinogens may also be considered, even in the absence of data on a possible carcinogenic effect in humans or experimental animals.

The scientific literature is surveyed for published data relevant to an assessment of carcinogenicity. The IARC surveys of chemicals being tested for carcinogenicity (IARC, 1973-1990) and directories of on-going research in cancer epidemiology (IARC, 1976-1989/90) often indicate those exposures that may be scheduled for future meetings. Ad-hoc working groups convened by IARC in 1984, 1989 and 1991 gave recommendations as to which agents should be evaluated in the *IARC Monographs* series (IARC, 1984, 1989, 1991b).

As significant new data on subjects on which monographs have already been prepared become available, re-evaluations are made at subsequent meetings, and revised monographs are published.

4. DATA FOR MONOGRAPHS

The *Monographs* do not necessarily cite all the literature concerning the subject of an evaluation. Only those data considered by the Working Group to be relevant to making the evaluation are included.

With regard to biological and epidemiological data, only reports that have been published or accepted for publication in the openly available scientific literature are reviewed by the working groups. In certain instances, government agency reports that have undergone peer review and are widely available are considered. Exceptions may be made on an ad-hoc basis to include unpublished reports that are in their final form and publicly available, if their inclusion is considered pertinent to making a final evaluation (see pp. 26 *et seq.*). In the sections on chemical and physical properties, on analysis, on production and use and on occurrence, unpublished sources of information may be used.

5. THE WORKING GROUP

Reviews and evaluations are formulated by a working group of experts. The tasks of the group are: (i) to ascertain that all appropriate data have been collected; (ii) to select the data relevant for the evaluation on the basis of scientific merit; (iii) to prepare accurate summaries of the data to enable the reader to follow the reasoning of the Working Group; (iv) to evaluate the results of experimental and epidemiological studies on cancer; (v) to evaluate data relevant to the understanding of mechanism of action; and (vi) to make an overall evaluation of the carcinogenicity of the exposure to humans.

Working Group participants who contributed to the considerations and evaluations within a particular volume are listed, with their addresses, at the beginning of each publication. Each participant who is a member of a working group serves as an individual scientist and not as a representative of any organization, government or industry. In addition, nominees of national and international agencies and industrial associations may be invited as observers.

6. WORKING PROCEDURES

Approximately one year in advance of a meeting of a working group, the topics of the monographs are announced and participants are selected by IARC staff in consultation with other experts. Subsequently, relevant biological and epidemiological data are collected by IARC from recognized sources of information on carcinogenesis, including data storage and retrieval systems such as BIOSIS, Chemical Abstracts, CANCERLIT, MEDLINE and TOXLINE—including EMIC and ETIC for data on genetic and related effects and teratogenicity, respectively.

For chemicals and some complex mixtures, the major collection of data and the preparation of first drafts of the sections on chemical and physical properties, on analysis, on production and use and on occurrence are carried out under a separate contract funded by the US National Cancer Institute. Representatives from industrial associations may assist in the preparation of sections on production and use. Information on production and trade is obtained from governmental and trade publications and, in some cases, by direct contact with industries. Separate production data on some agents may not be available because their publication could disclose confidential information. Information on uses may be obtained from published sources but is often complemented by direct contact with manufacturers. Efforts are made to supplement this information with data from other national and international sources.

Six months before the meeting, the material obtained is sent to meeting participants, or is used by IARC staff, to prepare sections for the first drafts of monographs. The first drafts are compiled by IARC staff and sent, prior to the meeting, to all participants of the Working Group for review.

The Working Group meets in Lyon for seven to eight days to discuss and finalize the texts of the monographs and to formulate the evaluations. After the meeting, the master copy of each monograph is verified by consulting the original literature, edited and prepared for publication. The aim is to publish monographs within nine months of the Working Group meeting.

The available studies are summarized by the Working Group, with particular regard to the qualitative aspects discussed below. In general, numerical findings are indicated as they appear in the original report; units are converted when necessary for easier comparison. The Working Group may conduct additional analyses of the published data and use them in their assessment of the evidence; the results of such supplementary analyses are given in square brackets. When an important aspect of a study, directly impinging on its interpretation, should be brought to the attention of the reader, a comment is given in square brackets.

7. EXPOSURE DATA

Sections that indicate the extent of past and present human exposure, the sources of exposure, the people most likely to be exposed and the factors that contribute to the exposure are included at the beginning of each monograph.

Most monographs on individual chemicals, groups of chemicals or complex mixtures include sections on chemical and physical data, on analysis, on production and use and on occurrence. In monographs on, for example, physical agents, biological factors, occupational exposures and cultural habits, other sections may be included, such as: historical perspectives, description of an industry or habit, chemistry of the complex mixture or taxonomy.

For chemical exposures, the Chemical Abstracts Services Registry Number, the latest Chemical Abstracts Primary Name and the IUPAC Systematic Name are recorded; other synonyms are given, but the list is not necessarily comprehensive. For biological agents, taxonomy and structure are described, and the degree of variability is given, when applicable.

Information on chemical and physical properties and, in particular, data relevant to identification, occurrence and biological activity are included. For biological agents, mode of replication, life cycle, target cells, persistence and latency, host response and description of nonmalignant disease caused by them are given. A description of technical products of chemicals includes trades names, relevant specifications and available information on composition and impurities. Some of the trade names given may be those of mixtures in which the agent being evaluated is only one of the ingredients.

The purpose of the section on analysis is to give the reader an overview of current methods, with emphasis on those widely used for regulatory purposes. Methods for monitoring human exposure are also given, when available. No critical evaluation or recommendation of any of the methods is meant or implied. The IARC publishes a series of volumes, *Environmental Carcinogens: Methods of Analysis and Exposure Measurement* (IARC, 1978–91), that describe validated methods for analysing a wide variety of chemicals and mixtures. For biological agents, methods of detection and exposure assessment are described, including their sensitivity, specificity and reproducibility.

The dates of first synthesis and of first commercial production of a chemical or mixture are provided; for agents which do not occur naturally, this information may allow a reasonable estimate to be made of the date before which no human exposure to the agent could have occurred. The dates of first reported occurrence of an exposure are also provided. In addition, methods of synthesis used in past and present commercial production and different methods of production which may give rise to different impurities are described.

Data on production, international trade and uses are obtained for representative regions, which usually include Europe, Japan and the USA. It should not, however, be inferred that those areas or nations are necessarily the sole or major sources or users of the agent. Some identified uses may not be current or major applications, and the coverage is not necessarily comprehensive. In the case of drugs, mention of their therapeutic uses does not necessarily represent current practice nor does it imply judgement as to their therapeutic efficacy.

Information on the occurrence of an agent or mixture in the environment is obtained from data derived from the monitoring and surveillance of levels in occupational environments, air, water, soil, foods and animal and human tissues. When available, data on the generation, persistence and bioaccumulation of the agent are also included. In the case of mixtures, industries, occupations or processes, information is given about all agents present. For processes, industries and occupations, a historical description is also given, noting variations in chemical composition, physical properties and levels of occupational exposure with time. For biological agents, the epidemiology of infection is described.

Statements concerning regulations and guidelines (e.g., pesticide registrations, maximal levels permitted in foods, occupational exposure limits) are included for some countries as indications of potential exposures, but they may not reflect the most recent situation, since such limits are continuously reviewed and modified. The absence of information on regulatory status for a country should not be taken to imply that that country does not have regulations with regard to the exposure. For biological agents, legislation and control, including vaccines and therapy, are described.

8. EVIDENCE FOR CARCINOGENICITY IN HUMANS

(a) *Types of studies considered*

Three types of epidemiological studies of cancer contribute to the assessment of carcinogenicity in humans—cohort studies, case-control studies and correlation studies. Rarely, results from randomized trials may be available. Case reports of cancer in humans may also be reviewed.

Cohort and case-control studies relate individual exposures under study to the occurrence of cancer in individuals and provide an estimate of relative risk (ratio of incidence in those exposed to incidence in those not exposed) as the main measure of association.

In correlation studies, the units of investigation are usually whole populations (e.g., in particular geographical areas or at particular times), and cancer frequency is related to a summary measure of the exposure of the population to the agent, mixture or exposure circumstance under study. Because individual exposure is not documented, however, a causal relationship is less easy to infer from correlation studies than from cohort and case-control studies. Case reports generally arise from a suspicion, based on clinical experience, that the concurrence of two events—that is, a particular exposure and occurrence of a cancer—has happened rather more frequently than would be expected by chance. Case reports usually lack complete ascertainment of cases in any population, definition or enumeration of the population at risk and estimation of the expected number of cases in the absence of exposure. The uncertainties surrounding interpretation of case reports and correlation studies make them inadequate, except in rare instances, to form the sole basis for inferring a causal relationship. When taken together with case-control and cohort studies, however, relevant case reports or correlation studies may add materially to the judgement that a causal relationship is present.

Epidemiological studies of benign neoplasms, presumed preneoplastic lesions and other endpoints thought to be relevant to cancer are also reviewed by working groups. They may, in some instances, strengthen inferences drawn from studies of cancer itself.

(b) Quality of studies considered

The *Monographs* are not intended to summarize all published studies. Those that are judged to be inadequate or irrelevant to the evaluation are generally omitted. They may be mentioned briefly, particularly when the information is considered to be a useful supplement to that in other reports or when they provide the only data available. Their inclusion does not imply acceptance of the adequacy of the study design or of the analysis and interpretation of the results, and limitations are clearly outlined in square brackets at the end of the study description.

It is necessary to take into account the possible roles of bias, confounding and chance in the interpretation of epidemiological studies. By 'bias' is meant the operation of factors in study design or execution that lead erroneously to a stronger or weaker association than in fact exists between disease and an agent, mixture or exposure circumstance. By 'confounding' is meant a situation in which the relationship with disease is made to appear stronger or to appear weaker than it truly is as a result of an association between the apparent causal factor and another factor that is associated with either an increase or decrease in the incidence of the disease. In evaluating the extent to which these factors have been minimized in an individual study, working groups consider a number of aspects of design and analysis as described in the report of the study. Most of these considerations apply equally to case-control, cohort and correlation studies. Lack of clarity of any of these aspects in the reporting of a study can decrease its credibility and the weight given to it in the final evaluation of the exposure.

Firstly, the study population, disease (or diseases) and exposure should have been well defined by the authors. Cases of disease in the study population should have been identified in a way that was independent of the exposure of interest, and exposure should have been assessed in a way that was not related to disease status.

Secondly, the authors should have taken account in the study design and analysis of other variables that can influence the risk of disease and may have been related to the exposure of interest. Potential confounding by such variables should have been dealt with either in the design of the study, such as by matching, or in the analysis, by statistical adjustment. In cohort studies, comparisons with local rates of disease may be more appropriate than those with national rates. Internal comparisons of disease frequency among individuals at different levels of exposure should also have been made in the study.

Thirdly, the authors should have reported the basic data on which the conclusions are founded, even if sophisticated statistical analyses were employed. At the very least, they should have given the numbers of exposed and unexposed cases and controls in a case-control study and the numbers of cases observed and expected in a cohort study. Further tabulations by time since exposure began and other temporal factors are also important. In a cohort study, data on all cancer sites and all causes of death should have been given, to reveal the possibility of reporting bias. In a case-control study, the effects of investigated factors other than the exposure of interest should have been reported.

Finally, the statistical methods used to obtain estimates of relative risk, absolute rates of cancer, confidence intervals and significance tests, and to adjust for confounding should have been clearly stated by the authors. The methods used should preferably have been the generally accepted techniques that have been refined since the mid-1970s. These methods have been reviewed for case-control studies (Breslow & Day, 1980) and for cohort studies (Breslow & Day, 1987).

(c) Inferences about mechanism of action

Detailed analyses of both relative and absolute risks in relation to temporal variables, such as age at first exposure, time since first exposure, duration of exposure, cumulative exposure and time since exposure ceased, are reviewed and summarized when available. The analysis of temporal relationships can be useful in formulating models of carcinogenesis. In particular, such analyses may suggest whether a carcinogen acts early or late in the process of carcinogenesis, although at best they allow only indirect inferences about the mechanism of action. Special attention is given to measurements of biological markers of carcinogen exposure or action, such as DNA or protein adducts, as well as markers of early steps in the carcinogenic process, such as proto-oncogene mutation, when these are incorporated into epidemiological studies focused on cancer incidence or mortality. Such measurements may allow inferences to be made about putative mechanisms of action (IARC, 1991a; Vainio *et al.*, 1992).

(d) Criteria for causality

After the quality of individual epidemiological studies of cancer has been summarized and assessed, a judgement is made concerning the strength of evidence that the agent, mixture or exposure circumstance in question is carcinogenic for humans. In making their judgement, the Working Group considers several criteria for causality. A strong association (i.e., a large relative risk) is more likely to indicate causality than a weak association, although it is recognized that relative risks of small magnitude do not imply lack of causality and may be important if the disease is common. Associations that are replicated in several studies of the same design or using different epidemiological approaches or under different circumstances of exposure are more likely to represent a causal relationship than isolated observations from single studies. If there are inconsistent results among investigations, possible reasons are sought (such as differences in amount of exposure), and results of studies judged to be of high quality are given more weight than those from studies judged to be methodologically less sound. When suspicion of carcinogenicity arises largely from a single study, these data are not combined with those from later studies in any subsequent reassessment of the strength of the evidence.

If the risk of the disease in question increases with the amount of exposure, this is considered to be a strong indication of causality, although absence of a graded response is not necessarily evidence against a causal relationship. Demonstration of a decline in risk after cessation of or reduction in exposure in individuals or in whole populations also supports a causal interpretation of the findings.

Although a carcinogen may act upon more than one target, the specificity of an association (i.e., an increased occurrence of cancer at one anatomical site or of one morphological type) adds plausibility to a causal relationship, particularly when excess cancer occurrence is limited to one morphological type within the same organ.

Although rarely available, results from randomized trials showing different rates among exposed and unexposed individuals provide particularly strong evidence for causality.

When several epidemiological studies show little or no indication of an association between an exposure and cancer, the judgement may be made that, in the aggregate, they show evidence of lack of carcinogenicity. Such a judgement requires first of all that the studies giving rise to it meet, to a sufficient degree, the standards of design and analysis described above. Specifically, the possibility that bias, confounding or misclassification of exposure or outcome could explain the observed results should be considered and excluded with reasonable certainty. In addition, all studies that are judged to be methodologically sound should be consistent with a relative risk of unity for any observed level of exposure and, when considered together, should provide a pooled estimate of relative risk which is at or near unity and has a narrow confidence interval, due to sufficient population size. Moreover, no individual study nor the pooled results of all the studies should show any consistent tendency for relative risk of cancer to increase with increasing level of exposure. It is important to note that evidence of lack of carcinogenicity obtained in this way from several epidemiological studies can apply only to the type(s) of cancer studied and to dose levels and intervals between first exposure and observation of disease that are the same as or less than those observed in all the studies. Experience with human cancer indicates that, in some cases, the period from first exposure to the development of clinical cancer is seldom less than 20 years; latent periods substantially shorter than 30 years cannot provide evidence for lack of carcinogenicity.

9. STUDIES OF CANCER IN EXPERIMENTAL ANIMALS

For several agents (e.g., aflatoxins, 4-aminobiphenyl, bis(chloromethyl)ether, diethylstilboestrol, melphalan, 8-methoxypsoralen (methoxsalen) plus ultra-violet radiation, mustard gas and vinyl chloride), evidence of carcinogenicity in experimental animals preceded evidence obtained from epidemiological studies or case reports. Information compiled from the first 41 volumes of the *IARC Monographs* (Wilbourn *et al.*, 1986) shows that, of the 44 agents and mixtures for which there is *sufficient* or *limited evidence* of carcinogenicity to humans (see p. 26), all 37 that have been tested adequately produce cancer in at least one animal species. Although this association cannot establish that all agents and mixtures that cause cancer in experimental animals also cause cancer in humans, nevertheless, **in the absence of adequate data on humans, it is biologically plausible and prudent to regard agents and mixtures for which there is sufficient evidence (see p. 27) of carcinogenicity in experimental animals as if they presented a carcinogenic risk to humans.** The possibility that a given agent may cause cancer through a species-specific mechanism which does not operate in humans, see p. 28, should also be taken into consideration.

The nature and extent of impurities or contaminants present in the chemical or mixture being evaluated are given when available. Animal strain, sex, numbers per group, age at start of treatment and survival are reported.

Other types of studies summarized include: experiments in which the agent or mixture was administered in conjunction with known carcinogens or factors that modify carcinogenic effects; studies in which the endpoint was not cancer but a defined precancerous lesion; and experiments on the carcinogenicity of known metabolites and derivatives.

For experimental studies of mixtures, consideration is given to the possibility of changes in the physicochemical properties of the test substance during collection, storage, extraction, concentration and delivery. Chemical and toxicological interactions of the components of mixtures may result in nonlinear dose-response relationships.

An assessment is made as to the relevance to human exposure of samples tested in experimental systems, which may involve consideration of: (i) physical and chemical characteristics, (ii) constituent substances that indicate the presence of a class of substances, (iii) the results of tests for genetic and related effects, including genetic activity profiles, DNA adduct profiles, proto-oncogene mutation and expression and suppressor gene inactivation. The relevance of results obtained with viral strains analogous to that being evaluated in the monograph must also be considered.

(a) Qualitative aspects

An assessment of carcinogenicity involves several considerations of qualitative importance, including (i) the experimental conditions under which the test was performed, including route and schedule of exposure, species, strain, sex, age, duration of follow-up; (ii) the consistency of the results, for example, across species and target organ(s); (iii) the spectrum of neoplastic response, from preneoplastic lesions and benign tumours to malignant neoplasms; and (iv) the possible role of modifying factors.

As mentioned earlier (p. 15), the *Monographs* are not intended to summarize all published studies. Those studies in experimental animals that are inadequate (e.g., too short a duration, too few animals, poor survival; see below) or are judged irrelevant to the evaluation are generally omitted. Guidelines for conducting adequate long-term carcinogenicity experiments have been outlined (e.g., Montesano et al., 1986).

Considerations of importance to the Working Group in the interpretation and evaluation of a particular study include: (i) how clearly the agent was defined and, in the case of mixtures, how adequately the sample characterization was reported; (ii) whether the dose was adequately monitored, particularly in inhalation experiments; (iii) whether the doses and duration of treatment were appropriate and whether the survival of treated animals was similar to that of controls; (iv) whether there were adequate numbers of animals per group; (v) whether animals of both sexes were used; (vi) whether animals were allocated randomly to groups; (vii) whether the duration of observation was adequate; and (viii) whether the data were adequately reported. If available, recent data on the incidence of specific tumours in historical controls, as well as in concurrent controls, should be taken into account in the evaluation of tumour response.

When benign tumours occur together with and originate from the same cell type in an organ or tissue as malignant tumours in a particular study and appear to represent a stage in the progression to malignancy, it may be valid to combine them in assessing tumour incidence (Huff et al., 1989). The occurrence of lesions presumed to be preneoplastic may in certain instances aid in assessing the biological plausibility of any neoplastic response observed. If an agent or mixture induces only benign neoplasms that appear to be endpoints that do not readily undergo transition to malignancy, it should nevertheless be suspected of being a carcinogen and it requires further investigation.

(b) *Quantitative aspects*

The probability that tumours will occur may depend on the species, sex, strain and age of the animal, the dose of the carcinogen and the route and length of exposure. Evidence of an increased incidence of neoplasms with increased level of exposure strengthens the inference of a causal association between the exposure and the development of neoplasms.

The form of the dose-response relationship can vary widely, depending on the particular agent under study and the target organ. Since many chemicals require metabolic activation before being converted into their reactive intermediates, both metabolic and pharmacokinetic aspects are important in determining the dose-response pattern. Saturation of steps such as absorption, activation, inactivation and elimination may produce nonlinearity in the dose-response relationship, as could saturation of processes such as DNA repair (Hoel et al., 1983; Gart et al., 1986).

(c) *Statistical analysis of long-term experiments in animals*

Factors considered by the Working Group include the adequacy of the information given for each treatment group: (i) the number of animals studied and the number examined histologically, (ii) the number of animals with a given tumour type and (iii) length of survival. The statistical methods used should be clearly stated and should be the generally accepted techniques refined for this purpose (Peto et al., 1980; Gart et al., 1986). When there is no difference in survival between control and treatment groups, the Working Group usually compares the proportions of animals developing each tumour type in each of the groups. Otherwise, consideration is given as to whether or not appropriate adjustments have been made for differences in survival. These adjustments can include: comparisons of the proportions of tumour-bearing animals among the effective number of animals (alive at the time the first tumour is discovered), in the case where most differences in survival occur before tumours appear; life-table methods, when tumours are visible or when they may be considered 'fatal' because mortality rapidly follows tumour development; and the Mantel-Haenszel test or logistic regression, when occult tumours do not affect the animals' risk of dying but are 'incidental' findings at autopsy.

In practice, classifying tumours as fatal or incidental may be difficult. Several survival-adjusted methods have been developed that do not require this distinction (Gart *et al.*, 1986), although they have not been fully evaluated.

10. OTHER RELEVANT DATA

(a) Absorption, distribution, metabolism and excretion

Concise information is given on absorption, distribution (including placental transfer) and excretion in both humans and experimental animals. Kinetic factors that may affect the dose-reponse relationship, such as saturation of uptake, protein binding, metabolic activation, detoxification and DNA repair processes, are mentioned. Studies that indicate the metabolic fate of the agent in humans and in experimental animals are summarized briefly, and comparisons of data from humans and animals are made when possible. Comparative information on the relationship between exposure and the dose that reaches the target site may be of particular importance for extrapolation between species.

(b) Toxic effects

Data are given on acute and chronic toxic effects (other than cancer), such as organ toxicity, increased cell proliferation, immunotoxicity and endocrine effects. The presence and toxicological significance of cellular receptors is described.

(c) Reproductive and developmental effects

Effects on reproduction, teratogenicity, feto- and embryotoxicity are also summarized briefly.

(d) Genetic and related effects

Tests of genetic and related effects are described in view of the relevance of gene mutation and chromosomal damage to carcinogenesis (Vainio *et al.*, 1992).

The adequacy of the reporting of sample characterization is considered and, where necessary, commented upon; with regard to complex mixtures, such comments should be similar to those described for animal carcinogenicity tests on p. 21. The available data are interpreted critically by phylogenetic group according to the endpoints detected, which may include DNA damage, gene mutation, sister chromatid exchange, micronucleus formation, chromosomal aberrations, aneuploidy and cell transformation. The concentrations employed are given, and mention is made of whether use of an exogenous metabolic system affected the test result. These data are given as listings of test systems, data and references; bar graphs (activity profiles) and corresponding summary tables with detailed information on the preparation of the profiles are given in appendices (Waters *et al.*, 1987).

Positive results in tests using prokaryotes, lower eukaryotes, plants, insects and cultured mammalian cells suggest that genetic and related effects could occur in mammals. Results from such tests may also give information about the types of genetic effect produced and about the involvement of metabolic activation. Some endpoints described are clearly genetic in nature (e.g., gene mutations and chromosomal aberrations), while others are to a greater or lesser degree associated with genetic effects (e.g., unscheduled DNA synthesis). In-vitro tests for tumour-promoting activity and for cell transformation may be sensitive to changes that are not necessarily the result of genetic alterations but that may have specific relevance to the process of carcinogenesis. A critical appraisal of these tests has been published (Montesano et al., 1986).

Genetic or other activity manifest in experimental mammals and humans is regarded as being of greater relevance than that in other organisms. The demonstration that an agent or mixture can induce gene and chromosomal mutations in whole mammals indicates that it may have carcinogenic activity, although this activity may not be detectably expressed in any or all species. Relative potency in tests for mutagenicity and related effects is not a reliable indicator of carcinogenic potency. Negative results in tests for mutagenicity in selected tissues from animals treated *in vivo* provide less weight, partly because they do not exclude the possibility of an effect in tissues other than those examined. Moreover, negative results in short-term tests with genetic endpoints cannot be considered to provide evidence to rule out carcinogenicity of agents or mixtures that act through other mechanisms (e.g., receptor-mediated effects, cellular toxicity with regenerative proliferation, peroxisome proliferation) (Vainio *et al.*, 1992). Factors that may lead to misleading results in short-term tests have been discussed in detail elsewhere (Montesano *et al.*, 1986).

When available, data relevant to mechanisms of carcinogenesis that do not involve structural changes at the level of the gene are also described.

The adequacy of epidemiological studies of reproductive outcome and genetic and related effects in humans is evaluated by the same criteria as are applied to epidemiological studies of cancer.

(e) Structure-activity considerations

This section describes structure-activity relationships that may be relevant to an evaluation of the carcinogenicity of an agent.

11. SUMMARY OF DATA REPORTED

In this section, the relevant epidemiological and experimental data are summarized. Only reports, other than in abstract form, that meet the criteria outlined on p. 15 are considered for evaluating carcinogenicity. Inadequate studies are generally not summarized: such studies are usually identified by a square-bracketed comment in the preceding text.

(a) Exposures

Human exposure is summarized on the basis of elements such as production, use, occurrence in the environment and determinations in human tissues and body fluids. Quantitative data are given when available.

(b) Carcinogenicity in humans

Results of epidemiological studies that are considered to be pertinent to an assessment of human carcinogenicity are summarized. When relevant, case reports and correlation studies are also summarized.

(c) Carcinogenicity in experimental animals

Data relevant to an evaluation of carcinogenicity in animals are summarized. For each animal species and route of administration, it is stated whether an increased incidence of neoplasms or preoplastic lesions was observed, and the tumour sites are indicated. If the agent or mixture produced tumours after prenatal exposure or in single-dose experiments, this is also indicated. Negative findings are also summarized. Dose-response and other quantitative data may be given when available.

(d) Other data relevant to an evaluation of carcinogenicity and its mechanisms

Data on biological effects in humans that are of particular relevance are summarized. These may include toxicological, kinetic and metabolic considerations and evidence of DNA binding, persistence of DNA lesions or genetic damage in exposed humans. Toxicological information, such as that on cytotoxicity and regeneration, receptor binding and hormonal and immunological effects, and data on kinetics and metabolism in experimental animals are given when considered relevant to the possible mechanism of the carcinogenic action of the agent. The results of tests for genetic and related effects are summarized for whole mammals, cultured mammalian cells and nonmammalian systems.

When available, comparisons of such data for humans and for animals, and particularly animals that have developed cancer, are described.

Structure-activity relationships are mentioned when relevant.

For the agent, mixture or exposure circumstance being evaluated, the available data on endpoints or other phenomena relevant to mechanisms of carcinogenesis from studies in humans, experimental animals and tissue and cell test systems are summarized within one or more of the following descriptive dimensions:

(i) Evidence of genotoxicity (i.e., structural changes at the level of the gene): for example, structure-activity considerations, adduct formation, mutagenicity (effect on specific genes), chromosomal mutation/aneuploidy

(ii) Evidence of effects on the expression of relevant genes (i.e., functional changes at the intracellular level): for example, alterations to the structure or quantity of the product of a proto-oncogene or tumour suppressor gene, alterations to metabolic activation/-inactivation/DNA repair

(iii) Evidence of relevant effects on cell behaviour (i.e., morphological or behavioural changes at the cellular or tissue level): for example, induction of mitogenesis, compensatory cell proliferation, preoplasia and hyperplasia, survival of premalignant or malignant cells (immortalization, immunosuppression), effects on metastatic potential

(iv) Evidence from dose and time relationships of carcinogenic effects and interactions between agents: for example, early/late stage, as inferred from epidemiological studies; initiation/promotion/progression/malignant conversion, as defined in animal carcinogenicity experiments; toxicokinetics

These dimensions are not mutually exclusive, and an agent may fall within more than one of them. Thus, for example, the action of an agent on the expression of relevant genes could be summarized under both the first and second dimension, even if it were known with reasonable certainty that those effects resulted from genotoxicity.

12. EVALUATION

Evaluations of the strength of the evidence for carcinogenicity arising from human and experimental animal data are made, using standard terms.

It is recognized that the criteria for these evaluations, described below, cannot encompass all of the factors that may be relevant to an evaluation of carcinogenicity. In considering all of the relevant data, the Working Group may assign the agent, mixture or exposure circumstance to a higher or lower category than a strict interpretation of these criteria would indicate.

(a) *Degrees of evidence for carcinogenicity in humans and in experimental animals and supporting evidence*

These categories refer only to the strength of the evidence that an exposure is carcinogenic and not to the extent of its carcinogenic activity (potency) nor to the mechanisms involved. A classification may change as new information becomes available.

An evaluation of degree of evidence, whether for a single agent or a mixture, is limited to the materials tested, as defined physically, chemically or biologically. When the agents evaluated are considered by the Working Group to be sufficiently closely related, they may be grouped together for the purpose of a single evaluation of degree of evidence.

(i) *Carcinogenicity in humans*

The applicability of an evaluation of the carcinogenicity of a mixture, process, occupation or industry on the basis of evidence from epidemiological studies depends on the variability over time and place of the mixtures, processes, occupations and industries. The Working Group seeks to identify the specific exposure, process or activity which is considered most likely to be responsible for any excess risk. The evaluation is focused as narrowly as the available data on exposure and other aspects permit.

The evidence relevant to carcinogenicity from studies in humans is classified into one of the following categories:

Sufficient evidence of carcinogenicity: The Working Group considers that a causal relationship has been established between exposure to the agent, mixture or exposure circumstance and human cancer. That is, a positive relationship has been observed between the exposure and cancer in studies in which chance, bias and confounding could be ruled out with reasonable confidence.

Limited evidence of carcinogenicity: A positive association has been observed between exposure to the agent, mixture or exposure circumstance and cancer for which a causal interpretation is considered by the Working Group to be credible, but chance, bias or confounding could not be ruled out with reasonable confidence.

Inadequate evidence of carcinogenicity: The available studies are of insufficient quality, consistency or statistical power to permit a conclusion regarding the presence or absence of a causal association, or no data on cancer in humans are available.

Evidence suggesting lack of carcinogenicity: There are several adequate studies covering the full range of levels of exposure that human beings are known to encounter, which are mutually consistent in not showing a positive association between exposure to the agent, mixture or exposure circumstance and any studied cancer at any observed level of exposure. A conclusion of 'evidence suggesting lack of carcinogenicity' is inevitably limited to the cancer sites, conditions and levels of exposure and length of observation covered by the available studies. In addition, the possibility of a very small risk at the levels of exposure studied can never be excluded.

In some instances, the above categories may be used to classify the degree of evidence related to carcinogenicity in specific organs or tissues.

(ii) *Carcinogenicity in experimental animals*

The evidence relevant to carcinogenicity in experimental animals is classified into one of the following categories:

Sufficient evidence of carcinogenicity: The Working Group considers that a causal relationship has been established between the agent or mixture and an increased incidence of malignant neoplasms or of an appropriate combination of benign and malignant neoplasms in (a) two or more species of animals or (b) in two or more independent studies in one species carried out at different times or in different laboratories or under different protocols.

Exceptionally, a single study in one species might be considered to provide sufficient evidence of carcinogenicity when malignant neoplasms occur to an unusual degree with regard to incidence, site, type of tumour or age at onset.

Limited evidence of carcinogenicity: The data suggest a carcinogenic effect but are limited for making a definitive evaluation because, e.g., (a) the evidence of carcinogenicity is restricted to a single experiment; or (b) there are unresolved questions regarding the adequacy of the design, conduct or interpretation of the study; or (c) the agent or mixture increases the incidence only of benign neoplasms or lesions of uncertain neoplastic potential, or of certain neoplasms which may occur spontaneously in high incidences in certain strains.

Inadequate evidence of carcinogenicity: The studies cannot be interpreted as showing either the presence or absence of a carcinogenic effect because of major qualitative or quantitative limitations, or no data on cancer in experimental animals are available.

Evidence suggesting lack of carcinogenicity: Adequate studies involving at least two species are available which show that, within the limits of the tests used, the agent or mixture is not carcinogenic. A conclusion of evidence suggesting lack of carcinogenicity is inevitably limited to the species, tumour sites and levels of exposure studied.

(b) *Other data relevant to the evaluation of carcinogenicity*

Other evidence judged to be relevant to an evaluation of carcinogenicity and of sufficient importance to affect the overall evaluation is then described. This may include data on preneoplastic lesions, tumour pathology, genetic and related effects, structure-activity relationships, metabolism and pharmacokinetics, and physicochemical parameters.

Data relevant to mechanisms of the carcinogenic action are also evaluated. The strength of the evidence that any carcinogenic effect observed is due to a particular mechanism is assessed, using terms such as weak, moderate or strong. Then, the Working Group assesses if that particular mechanism is likely to be operative in humans. The strongest indications that a particular mechanism operates in humans come from data on humans or biological specimens obtained from exposed humans. The data may be considered to be especially relevant if they show that the agent in question has caused changes in exposed humans that are on the causal pathway to carcinogenesis. Such data may, however, never become available, because it is at least conceivable that certain compounds may be kept from human use solely on the basis of evidence of their toxicity and/or carcinogenicity in experimental systems.

For complex exposures, including occupational and industrial exposures, chemical composition and the potential contribution of carcinogens known to be present are considered by the Working Group in its overall evaluation of human carcinogenicity. The Working Group also determines the extent to which the materials tested in experimental systems are related to those to which humans are exposed.

(c) Overall evaluation

Finally, the body of evidence is considered as a whole, in order to reach an overall evaluation of the carcinogenicity to humans of an agent, mixture or circumstance of exposure.

An evaluation may be made for a group of chemical compounds that have been evaluated by the Working Group. In addition, when supporting data indicate that other, related compounds for which there is no direct evidence of capacity to induce cancer in humans or in animals may also be carcinogenic, a statement describing the rationale for this conclusion is added to the evaluation narrative; an additional evaluation may be made for this broader group of compounds if the strength of the evidence warrants it.

The agent, mixture or exposure circumstance is described according to the wording of one of the following categories, and the designated group is given. The categorization of an agent, mixture or exposure circumstance is a matter of scientific judgement, reflecting the strength of the evidence derived from studies in humans and in experimental animals and from other relevant data.

Group 1—The agent (mixture) is carcinogenic to humans.
The exposure circumstance entails exposures that are carcinogenic to humans.

This category is used when there is *sufficient evidence* of carcinogenicity in humans. Exceptionally, an agent (mixture) may be placed in this category when evidence in humans is less than sufficient but there is *sufficient evidence* of carcinogenicity in experimental animals and strong evidence in exposed humans that the agent (mixture) acts through a relevant mechanism of carcinogenicity.

Group 2

This category includes agents, mixtures and exposure circumstances for which, at one extreme, the degree of evidence of carcinogenicity in humans is almost sufficient, as well as those for which, at the other extreme, there are no human data but for which there is evidence of carcinogenicity in experimental animals. Agents, mixtures and exposure circumstances are assigned to either group 2A (probably carcinogenic to humans) or group 2B (possibly carcinogenic to humans) on the basis of epidemiological and experimental evidence of carcinogenicity and other relevant data.

Group 2A—The agent (mixture) is probably carcinogenic to humans.
The exposure circumstance entails exposures that are probably carcinogenic to humans.

This category is used when there is *limited evidence* of carcinogenicity in humans and *sufficient evidence* of carcinogenicity in experimental animals. In some cases, an agent (mixture) may be classified in this category when there is *inadequate evidence* of carcinogenicity in humans and *sufficient evidence* of carcinogenicity in experimental animals and strong evidence that the carcinogenesis is mediated by a mechanism that also operates in humans. Exceptionally, an agent, mixture or exposure circumstance may be classified in this category solely on the basis of *limited evidence* of carcinogenicity in humans.

Group 2B—The agent (mixture) is possibly carcinogenic to humans.
The exposure circumstance entails exposures that are possibly carcinogenic to humans.

This category is used for agents, mixtures and exposure circumstances for which there is *limited evidence* of carcinogenicity in humans and less than *sufficient evidence* of carcinogenicity in experimental animals. It may also be used when there is *inadequate evidence* of carcinogenicity in humans but there is *sufficient evidence* of carcinogenicity in experimental animals. In some instances, an agent, mixture or exposure circumstance for which there is *inadequate evidence* of carcinogenicity in humans but *limited evidence* of carcinogenicity in experimental animals together with supporting evidence from other relevant data may be placed in this group.

Group 3—The agent (mixture or exposure circumstance) is not classifiable as to its carcinogenicity to humans.

This category is used most commonly for agents, mixtures and exposure circumstances for which the evidence of carcinogenicity is inadequate in humans and inadequate or limited in experimental animals.

Exceptionally, agents (mixtures) for which the evidence of carcinogenicity is inadequate in humans but sufficient in experimental animals may be placed in this category when there is strong evidence that the mechanism of carcinogenicity in experimental animals does not operate in humans.

Agents, mixtures and exposure circumstances that do not fall into any other group are also placed in this category.

Group 4—The agent (mixture) is probably not carcinogenic to humans.

This category is used for agents or mixtures for which there is *evidence suggesting lack of carcinogenicity* in humans and in experimental animals. In some instances, agents or mixtures for which there is *inadequate evidence* of carcinogenicity in humans but *evidence suggesting lack of carcinogenicity* in experimental animals, consistently and strongly supported by a broad range of other relevant data, may be classified in this group.

References

Breslow, N.E. & Day, N.E. (1980) *Statistical Methods in Cancer Research*, Vol. 1, *The Analysis of Case-control Studies* (IARC Scientific Publications No. 32), Lyon, IARC

Breslow, N.E. & Day, N.E. (1987) *Statistical Methods in Cancer Research*, Vol. 2, *The Design and Analysis of Cohort Studies* (IARC Scientific Publications No. 82), Lyon, IARC

Gart, J.J., Krewski, D., Lee, P.N., Tarone, R.E. & Wahrendorf, J. (1986) *Statistical Methods in Cancer Research*, Vol.3, *The Design and Analysis of Long-term Animal Experiments* (IARC Scientific Publications No. 79), Lyon, IARC

Hoel, D.G., Kaplan, N.L. & Anderson, M.W. (1983) Implication of nonlinear kinetics on risk estimation in carcinogenesis. *Science*, 219, 1032–1037

Huff, J.E., Eustis, S.L. & Haseman, J.K. (1989) Occurrence and relevance of chemically induced benign neoplasms in long-term carcinogenicity studies. *Cancer Metastasis Rev.*, 8, 1–21

IARC (1973-1990) *Information Bulletin on the Survey of Chemicals Being Tested for Carcinogenicity/Directory of Agents Being Tested for Carcinogenicity*, Numbers 1-14, Lyon

    Number 1 (1973)   52 pages
    Number 2 (1973)   77 pages
    Number 3 (1974)   67 pages
    Number 4 (1974)   97 pages
    Number 5 (1975)   88 pages
    Number 6 (1976)   360 pages
    Number 7 (1978)   460 pages
    Number 8 (1979)   604 pages
    Number 9 (1981)   294 pages
    Number 10 (1983) 326 pages
    Number 11 (1984) 370 pages
    Number 12 (1986) 385 pages
    Number 13 (1988) 404 pages
    Number 14 (1990) 369 pages

IARC (1976–1989/90)

Directory of On-going Research in Cancer Epidemiology 1976. Edited by C.S. Muir & G. Wagner, Lyon

Directory of On-going Research in Cancer Epidemiology 1977 (IARC Scientific Publications No. 17). Edited by C.S. Muir & G. Wagner, Lyon

Directory of On-going Research in Cancer Epidemiology 1978 (IARC Scientific Publications No. 26). Edited by C.S. Muir & G. Wagner, Lyon

Directory of On-going Research in Cancer Epidemiology 1979 (IARC Scientific Publications No. 28). Edited by C.S. Muir & G. Wagner, Lyon

Directory of On-going Research in Cancer Epidemiology 1980 (IARC Scientific Publications No. 35). Edited by C.S. Muir & G. Wagner, Lyon

Directory of On-going Research in Cancer Epidemiology 1981 (IARC Scientific Publications No. 38). Edited by C.S. Muir & G. Wagner, Lyon

Directory of On-going Research in Cancer Epidemiology 1982 (IARC Scientific Publications No. 46). Edited by C.S. Muir & G. Wagner, Lyon

Directory of On-going Research in Cancer Epidemiology 1983 (IARC Scientific Publications No. 50). Edited by C.S. Muir & G. Wagner, Lyon

Directory of On-going Research in Cancer Epidemiology 1984 (IARC Scientific Publications No. 62). Edited by C.S. Muir & G. Wagner, Lyon

Directory of On-going Research in Cancer Epidemiology 1985 (IARC Scientific Publications No. 69). Edited by C.S. Muir & G. Wagner, Lyon

Directory of On-going Research in Cancer Epidemiology 1986 (IARC Scientific Publications No. 80). Edited by C.S. Muir & G. Wagner, Lyon

Directory of On-going Research in Cancer Epidemiology 1987 (IARC Scientific Publications No. 86). Edited by D.M. Parkin & J. Wahrendorf, Lyon

Directory of On-going Research in Cancer Epidemiology 1988 (IARC Scientific Publications No. 93). Edited by M. Coleman & J. Wahrendorf, Lyon

Directory of On-going Research in Cancer Epidemiology 1989/90 (IARC Scientific Publications No. 101). Edited by M. Coleman & J. Wahrendorf, Lyon

IARC (1977) *IARC Monographs Programme on the Evaluation of the Carcinogenic Risk of Chemicals to Humans. Preamble* (IARC intern. tech. Rep. No. 77/002), Lyon

IARC (1978) *Chemicals with Sufficient Evidence of Carcinogenicity in Experimental Animals*—IARC Monographs *Volumes 1-17* (IARC intern. tech. Rep. No. 78/003), Lyon

IARC (1978-1991) *Environmental Carcinogens. Methods of Analysis and Exposure Measurement*:

- Vol. 1. *Analysis of Volatile Nitrosamines in Food* (IARC Scientific Publications No. 18). Edited by R. Preussmann, M. Castegnaro, E.A. Walker & A.E. Wasserman (1978)
- Vol. 2. *Methods for the Measurement of Vinyl Chloride in Poly(vinyl chloride), Air, Water and Foodstuffs* (IARC Scientific Publications No. 22). Edited by D.C.M. Squirrell & W. Thain (1978)
- Vol. 3. *Analysis of Polycyclic Aromatic Hydrocarbons in Environmental Samples* (IARC Scientific Publications No. 29). Edited by M. Castegnaro, P. Bogovski, H. Kunte & E.A. Walker (1979)
- Vol. 4. *Some Aromatic Amines and Azo Dyes in the General and Industrial Environment* (IARC Scientific Publications No. 40). Edited by L. Fishbein, M. Castegnaro, I.K. O'Neill & H. Bartsch (1981)
- Vol. 5. *Some Mycotoxins* (IARC Scientific Publications No. 44). Edited by L. Stoloff, M. Castegnaro, P. Scott, I.K. O'Neill & H. Bartsch (1983)
- Vol. 6. *N-Nitroso Compounds* (IARC Scientific Publications No. 45). Edited by R. Preussmann, I.K. O'Neill, G. Eisenbrand, B. Spiegelhalder & H. Bartsch (1983)
- Vol. 7. *Some Volatile Halogenated Hydrocarbons* (IARC Scientific Publications No. 68). Edited by L. Fishbein & I.K. O'Neill (1985)
- Vol. 8. *Some Metals: As, Be, Cd, Cr, Ni, Pb, Se, Zn* (IARC Scientific Publications No. 71). Edited by I.K. O'Neill, P. Schuller & L. Fishbein (1986)
- Vol. 9. *Passive Smoking* (IARC Scientific Publications No. 81). Edited by I.K. O'Neill, K.D. Brunnemann, B. Dodet & D. Hoffmann (1987)
- Vol. 10. *Benzene and Alkylated Benzenes* (IARC Scientific Publications No. 85). Edited by L. Fishbein & I.K. O'Neill (1988)
- Vol. 11. *Polychlorinated Dioxins and Dibenzofurans* (IARC Scientific Publications No. 108). Edited by C. Rappe, H.R. Buser, B. Dodet & I.K. O'Neill (1991)

IARC (1979) *Criteria to Select Chemicals for IARC Monographs* (IARC intern. tech. Rep. No. 79/003), Lyon

IARC (1982) *IARC Monographs on the Evaluation of the Carcinogenic Risk of Chemicals to Humans*, Supplement 4, *Chemicals, Industrial Processes and Industries Associated with Cancer in Humans (IARC Monographs, Volumes 1 to 29)*, Lyon

IARC (1983) *Approaches to Classifying Chemical Carcinogens According to Mechanism of Action* (IARC intern. tech. Rep. No. 83/001), Lyon

IARC (1984) *Chemicals and Exposures to Complex Mixtures Recommended for Evaluation in* IARC Monographs *and Chemicals and Complex Mixtures Recommended for Long-term Carcinogenicity Testing* (IARC intern. tech. Rep. No. 84/002), Lyon

IARC (1987a) *IARC Monographs on the Evaluation of Carcinogenic Risks to Humans*, Supplement 6, *Genetic and Related Effects: An Updating of Selected* IARC Monographs *from Volumes 1 to 42*, Lyon

IARC (1987b) *IARC Monographs on the Evaluation of Carcinogenic Risks to Humans*, Supplement 7, *Overall Evaluations of Carcinogenicity: An Updating of* IARC Monographs *Volumes 1 to 42*, Lyon

IARC (1988) *Report of an IARC Working Group to Review the Approaches and Processes Used to Evaluate the Carcinogenicity of Mixtures and Groups of Chemicals* (IARC intern. tech. Rep. No. 88/002), Lyon

IARC (1989) *Chemicals, Groups of Chemicals, Mixtures and Exposure Circumstances to be Evaluated in Future IARC Monographs, Report of an ad hoc Working Group* (IARC intern. tech. Rep. No. 89/004), Lyon

IARC (1991a) *A Consensus Report of an* IARC Monographs *Working Group on the Use of Mechanims of Carcinogenesis in Risk Identification* (IARC intern. tech. Rep. No. 91/002), Lyon

IARC (1991b) *Report of an Ad-hoc* IARC Monographs *Advisory Group on Viruses and Other Biological Agents Such as Parasites* (IARC intern. tech. Rep. No. 91/001), Lyon

Montesano, R., Bartsch, H., Vainio, H., Wilbourn, J. & Yamasaki, H., eds (1986) *Long-term and Short-term Assays for Carcinogenesis—A Critical Appraisal* (IARC Scientific Publications No. 83), Lyon, IARC

Peto, R., Pike, M.C., Day, N.E., Gray, R.G., Lee, P.N., Parish, S., Peto, J., Richards, S. & Wahrendorf, J. (1980) Guidelines for simple, sensitive significance tests for carcinogenic effects in long-term animal experiments. In: *IARC Monographs on the Evaluation of the Carcinogenic Risk of Chemicals to Humans*, Supplement 2, *Long-term and Short-term Screening Assays for Carcinogens: A Critical Appraisal*, Lyon, pp. 311–426

Vainio, H., Magee, P., McGregor, D. & McMichael, A., eds (1992) *Mechanisms of Carcinogenesis in Risk Identification* (IARC Scientific Publications No. 116), Lyon, IARC (in press)

Waters, M.D., Stack, H.F., Brady, A.L., Lohman, P.H.M., Haroun, L. & Vainio, H. (1987) Apendix 1. Activity profiles for genetic and related tests. In: *IARC Monogarphs on the Evaluation of Carcinogenic Risks to Humans*, Suppl. 6, *Genetic and Related Effects: An Updating of Selected IARC Monographs from Volumes 1 to 42*, Lyon, IARC, pp. 687–696

Wilbourn, J., Haroun, L., Heseltine, E., Kaldor, J., Partensky, C. & Vainio, H. (1986) Response of experimental animals to human carcinogens: an analysis based upon the IARC Monographs Programme. *Carcinogenesis*, 7, 1853–1863

General Remarks on the Substances Considered

This fifty-fourth volume of *IARC Monographs* covers strong inorganic acids and some other industrial chemicals. Two of the agents were evaluated previously: diethyl sulfate (IARC, 1974, 1987) and 1,3-butadiene (IARC, 1986, 1987). Manufacture of isopropanol by the strong-acid process has already been evaluated as an exposure circumstance (IARC, 1977, 1987).

Selection of topics

Selection of strong inorganic acids as the main subject of this volume was prompted by the publication of several epidemiological studies that suggested that exposure by inhalation to mists and vapours of strong inorganic acids was associated with excess risk for laryngeal and other respiratory-tract cancers. These studies led to the hypothesis that acidity itself could exert a carcinogenic effect. The first monograph in this volume addresses that question and investigates the plausibility of the hypothesis by examining the evidence from studies of some of the many industries in which strong acids are used.

An acid may be defined as a substance with the potential to donate a hydrogen ion, although it may not exhibit its acidic properties in certain media (e.g., hydrochloric acid in pure benzene). In water, acids dissociate to varying degrees, donating their hydrogen ions to water molecules to produce the hydronium ion (H_3O^+) and the anion. The strength of an acid is usually measured by the pK_a value, which is the negative logarithm (to the base 10) of the acid ionization (dissociation) constant, K_a, for the reaction. The stronger the acid, the lower the pK_a value. Some acids, like sulfuric (H_2SO_4) and phosphoric (H_3PO_4), can donate more than one hydrogen ion; these acids have separate ionization constants for the loss of each hydrogen ion. A distinction must be made between a *solution of a strong acid* and a *strongly acidic solution*. A solution of a strong acid, for example, may be very dilute and not strongly acidic (pH close to neutrality, pH 7), and a weaker acid at a high concentration may give a highly acidic solution (low pH). In mechanistic terms, it remains to be established whether biological effects from strong inorganic acids are due to hydrogen ion concentration (which is not specific to the acid in question) or to the molecular species and its interactions in organisms.

The impact of inhaled acidic agents on the respiratory tract depends upon a number of interrelated factors. These include physicochemical characteristics, e.g., gas *versus* aerosol; particle size (small particles can penetrate deeper into the lung); water solubility (more soluble agents are more likely to be removed in the nose and mouth); free hydrogen ion concentration (more acidic agents have greater effects); and the buffering capacity of the overall airway and of the local deposition site. It is also conceivable that a specific anion can directly or indirectly modulate acute effects.

Given the general lack of information on the particle size of aerosols involved in occupational exposures to acids, it is difficult to identify their principal deposition site within the respiratory tract. Estimation of changes in the pH of the mucus is therefore problematic, as diffuse deposition would challenge the buffering capacity much less than would deposition of large particles at local sites.

It is difficult to separate the effects of pH and of changes in osmolarity since exposures to low pH may alter osmolarity by changing the concentrations of ionized and nonionized species and, thus, induce reactions that do not occur at neutral pH (Scott *et al.*, 1991). Data from assays for genotoxic activity *in vitro* suggest that eukaryotic cells are susceptible to genetic damage when the pH falls to about 6.5. Cells from the respiratory tract have not been examined in this respect. Mucus secretion may protect the cells of the airways from direct exposure to inhaled acidic mists, just as mucus plays an important role in protecting the gastric epithelium from its autosecreted hydrochloric acid. In considering whether pH itself induces genotoxic events *in vivo* in the respiratory system, comparison should be made with the human stomach, in which gastric juice may be at pH 1–2 under fasting or nocturnal conditions, and with the human urinary bladder, in which the pH of urine can range from < 5 to > 7 and normally averages 6.2. Furthermore, exposures to low pH *in vivo* differ from exposures *in vitro* in that *in vivo* only a portion of the cell surface is subjected to the adverse conditions, so that perturbation of intracellular homeostasis may be maintained more readily than *in vitro*.

The industries considered were selected because they involve particularly heavy use of inorganic acids: manufacture of isopropanol, synthetic ethanol, phosphate fertilizers, lead batteries, soap and detergents, sulfuric acid and nitric acid and those industries involving treatment of metals with acids. Because sulfuric acid is the principal strong inorganic acid used in these industries and is the acid on which most epidemiological data were available, it is discussed in detail in the monograph on occupational exposures to strong acid mists and in an appendix to that monograph. Sulfur trioxide is included in the same monograph because it is directly and rapidly converted to sulfuric acid when it comes into contact with water.

Sulfur dioxide is reviewed separately because it is a major contributor to atmospheric acidity and is an important industrial chemical. It dissolves slowly in water. Aqueous solutions of sulfur dioxide may contain bisulfites, sulfites and metabisulfites, depending on their acidity, temperature and ionic strength; sulfite and bisulfite are also metabolites of sulfur dioxide. Because of their close relationship with sulfur dioxide, some of these compounds are included in the monograph on this agent.

Hydrochloric acid is a strong inorganic acid which is formed when gaseous hydrogen chloride dissolves in water. Exposures may thus occur both to the gas and to hydrochloric acid mists. As it is also industrially important and data are available on cancer in experimental animals, this acid was considered in a separate monograph.

Diethyl sulfate and diisopropyl sulfate are relevant to an evaluation of the carcinogenicity of acids because they may occur simultaneously with sulfuric acid mists in the manufacture of isopropanol and synthetic ethanol. Monographs on these two substances are therefore included.

There is, inevitably, a great deal of overlap among these monographs. Exposures to acid mists and vapours occur in industries other than those described in the first monograph; these exposures are complex, and may be accompanied by exposures to known carcinogenic agents, such as nickel compounds (see IARC, 1990), chromium[VI] compounds (see IARC, 1990), inorganic arsenicals (see IARC, 1987), soots (see IARC, 1987), coal-tars (see IARC, 1987) and polycyclic aromatic hydrocarbons (see IARC, 1983). Epidemiological studies on nickel refining, other basic metals industries, chromate production, chromium plating and nickel plating were therefore considered to be uninformative for an evaluation of acids, and only passing reference is made to these studies. Some studies of copper smelter workers that specifically address exposure to sulfur dioxide are described in detail, however, in spite of the simultaneous occurrence of other suspect agents. The monographs do not emphasize studies of environmental exposures, which are usually at a much lower level than occupational exposures and for which causal relationships are more difficult to establish.

The final monograph in this volume is on 1,3-butadiene. It is included because an up-to-date evaluation of this very important monomer was clearly required and new data had become available since it was evaluated previously (IARC, 1987).

Issues in the evaluation of epidemiological studies of occupational exposure to mists and vapours from strong acids

(a) Site of cancer and mode of action

In the epidemiological studies reviewed, cancer of the upper respiratory system occurred frequently in association with occupational exposure to mists and vapours from strong acids, either alone or in addition to cancer of the lung. This finding is biologically plausible, given that the route of entry is inhalation. Inhalation of mists from strong acids could cause rapid local reactions; thus, the sites of primary response would be in the upper respiratory tract when the particles have an aerodynamic diameter[1] of 5–30 μm and in the tracheal, bronchial and bronchiolar regions when the particles are 1–5 μm.

These observations may be important for understanding the etiology of excess cancers in the upper airways, where cancer occurrence in association with industrial exposures is quite rare.

(b) Cancer incidence and mortality

Many of the available studies addressed cancer mortality rather than incidence. It is often the case that studies on incidence are not available, since in some areas of the world there is no system to ensure enumeration of all cancer cases. When the cancers observed are those for which survival after diagnosis is quite good, however, the true magnitude of an association between exposure and the cancer may be underestimated if only mortality is studied. For example, patients diagnosed with laryngeal or oropharyngeal cancer may live for a long time after treatment and may eventually die of another disease, so that their cause of death might not reflect the fact that they had had laryngeal or oropharyngeal cancer. Further,

---

[1] Aerodynamic diameter is a measure of particle size which takes into account both density and aerodynamic drag.

cancers at these sites frequently produce secondary lesions in the oropharyngeal region; these can obfuscate identification of the primary site, and death may be attributed to the secondary lesion. For these reasons, studies of cancer incidence are more sensitive for detecting any excess of upper respiratory cancer in association with occupational exposures than are mortality studies.

(c) *Life style factors*

Information on smoking habits is often not collected in epidemiological studies of occupational groups, mainly because of cost limitations. When the target site of interest is the lung and the magnitude of the excess cancer risk is small, the possibility must be entertained that the excess was due to a greater prevalence of smoking in the occupational group than among the reference population, and not to the occupational exposure. The same explanation can apply to a small excess risk for cancer of the larynx, since smoking is a major risk factor for this disease. In several of the studies examined, however, excesses of laryngeal cancer and not of cancer of the lung were seen in relation to occupational exposure. In these cases, the Working Group considered that smoking was not a major confounder, as the principal carcinogenic effect of smoking is on the lung. In some studies, the excesses are relatively large; in others, information on smoking was available and the excess risks persisted after adjustment for smoking. The latter studies were of greatest importance in evaluating the carcinogenic risk of occupational exposures to mists and vapours from strong acids.

(d) *Specification of exposure and dose-response*

Particularly in respect of the occupations considered in these monographs, it is difficult to specify the exposures of workers. The names of jobs and processes are usually the only available information for linking an individual to the exposure of interest. Furthermore, such linkage is done retrospectively and in the absence of industrial hygiene measurements. No process or job in any industry involves exposure to a single chemical, and exposures to chemicals within a single process or job may be so highly correlated that it is impossible to separate their effects in regard to cancer risks in epidemiological studies. In this situation, cancer risks must be examined across industries or even across processes to determine whether there are other situations in which only one of the chemicals is common and whether cancers at the same site are occurring in workers involved in these other processes. The presence of other known carcinogens within the industry must be reviewed to eliminate any confounding of the conclusions.

To determine that the evidence is sufficient to establish the carcinogenicity of an agent, observation of a dose- or exposure-response is helpful. In most situations, past exposures of workers were not measured, and processes, chemicals and levels of exposures have changed over time. Thus, exposures are based on estimates of the relative amounts of chemicals that are associated with jobs and processes, taking account of how these amounts vary over time. Such estimates are then tied to an individual's occupational history to give a proxy measure of cumulative dose. Despite the fact that this measure is only relative and gives a highly uncertain picture of true exposures over time, it may be a more reliable comparative measure of exposure between individuals than is the use of a few contemporary measures of the agents in the work environment. Estimates that include only selected jobs and a few values for each job can give little indication of the potential variability in exposure by job and may not represent past exposures within the industry.

Use of retrospective exposure scoring systems for estimating an exposure–response relationship is thus tenuous. Usually, no information on the appropriateness of the estimated relative ranks is available: a value of 10 may not actually represent an exposure that was 10 times one in the past; time spent in a job is used as an exposure score to estimate the incidence of cancer by 'dose'. It is not surprising that the results are most consistent when exposures are grouped categorically and cancer rates are determined on the basis of grouped data, although the sensitivity of a response based on a specific categorical grouping may be undefined.

References

IARC (1974) *IARC Monographs on the Evaluation of Carcinogenic Risk of Chemicals to Man*, Vol. 4, *Some Aromatic Amines, Hydrazine and Related Substances, N-Nitroso Compounds and Miscellaneous Alkylating Agents*, Lyon, pp. 277–281

IARC (1977) *IARC Monographs on the Evaluation of the Carcinogenic Risk of Chemicals to Man*, Vol. 15, *Some Fumigants, the Herbicides 2,4-D and 2,4,5-T, Chlorinated Dibenzodioxins and Miscellaneous Industrial Chemicals*, Lyon, pp. 223–243

IARC (1983) *IARC Monographs on the Evaluation of the Carcinogenic Risk of Chemicals to Humans*, Vol. 32, *Polynuclear Aromatic Compounds, Part 1, Chemical, Environmental and Experimental Data*, Lyon

IARC (1986) *IARC Monographs on the Evaluation of the Carcinogenic Risk of Chemicals to Humans*, Vol. 39, *Some Chemicals Used in Plastics and Elastomers*, Lyon, pp. 155–179

IARC (1987) *IARC Monographs on the Evaluation of Carcinogenic Risks to Humans*, Suppl. 7, *Overall Evaluations of Carcinogenicity: An Updating of* IARC Monographs *Volumes 1–42*, Lyon, pp. 100–106, 136–137, 175–176, 198, 229, 343–344

IARC (1990) *IARC Monographs on the Evaluation of Carcinogenic Risks to Humans*, Vol. 49, *Chromium, Nickel and Welding*, Lyon, pp. 49–256, 257–445

Scott, D., Galloway, S.M., Marshall, R.R., Ishidate, M., Jr, Brusick, D., Ashby, J. & Myhr, B.C. (1991) Genotoxicity under extreme culture conditions. A Report from ICPEMC Task Group 9. *Mutat. Res.*, **257**, 147–204

THE MONOGRAPHS

OCCUPATIONAL EXPOSURES TO MISTS AND VAPOURS FROM SULFURIC ACID AND OTHER STRONG INORGANIC ACIDS

1. Exposure Data

1.1 Introduction

Acidity has been defined in various ways. The Arrhenius concept (sometimes referred to as the aqueous concept) of acids and bases defines an acid as any substance that can increase the concentration of hydronium ion, H_3O^+, in aqueous solution. A somewhat more general approach, proposed independently in 1923 by the Danish chemist, J.N. Brønsted, and the British chemist, T.M. Lowry, defines an acid as a substance that can donate a proton (i.e., a hydrogen ion, H^+) to some other substance (Brady & Humiston, 1978).

The position of equilibrium in an acid–base reaction indicates the relative strengths of the acids and bases involved. Hydrogen chloride is a strong acid in water because the position of equilibrium in the ionization reaction lies far to the right [$HCl + H_2O \rightleftarrows H_3O^+ + Cl^-$]. Hydrogen fluoride, however, is said to be a weak acid because it is only very slightly dissociated in water (about 3% of a 1 M solution at room temperature). The strength of an acid is usually represented by the pK_a value, which is the negative logarithm (to the base 10) of the acid ionization (dissociation) constant, K_a, for the reaction in question. The stronger the acid, the lower the pK_a value; the weaker the acid, the higher the pK_a value. Some acids, like sulfuric (H_2SO_4) and phosphoric (H_3PO_4), can donate more than one proton; such acids have separate ionization constants for the loss of each proton.

Table 1 presents the dissociation constants and boiling-points for several acids; although the subject of this monograph is occupational exposure to strong inorganic acids, some organic acids are included in the table for comparison. The principal acids of interest for this monograph are sulfuric acid, hydrochloric acid, nitric acid and phosphoric acid. Exposure to chromic acid was evaluated previously (IARC, 1990).

Strong inorganic acids may be present in air in three different forms: mist, vapour and gas. The term 'mist' refers to a liquid aerosol formed by condensation of a vapour or atomization of a liquid (Hinds, 1985). A vapour is defined as the gaseous state of a substance which is a liquid or solid at normal temperature and pressure (Fowler & Fowler, 1964). Hydrochloric acid is a gas, which can also be present in workplace air as a mist when dissolved in water. Nitric, sulfuric and phosphoric acids are liquids that may be present in air as mists or vapours; they are, however, present primarily as mists because of their low volatility and their affinity for water. Sulfuric and nitric acids may further release sulfur trioxide vapours and gaseous nitrogen oxides, respectively, especially at high concentrations and elevated temperatures in the absence of atmospheric moisture (Sax & Lewis, 1987). The sampling

Table 1. Dissociation constants (pK_a) and boiling-points of some acids

Acid	pK_a[a]	Boiling-point (°C)
Hydrobromic acid	< 0	−67.0[b]
Hydrochloric acid	< 0	−84.9[b]
Chlorosulfonic acid	< 0	158[c]
Sulfuric acid	< 0 (step 1)[d] 1.92 (step 2)	315–338[c]
Methanesulfonic acid	< 0	200[c]
Ethanesulfonic acid	< 0	123 at 1 mm Hg [133.3 Pa]
Nitric acid	< 0	83[e]
Chromic acid (chromium trioxide)	0.74 (step 1) 6.49 (step 2)	Decomposes at 250 °C[e]
Perchloric acid	1.77	19 at 11 mm Hg [1467 Pa][e]
Phosphoric acid	2.12 (step 1) 7.21 (step 2) 12.67 (step 3)	261[f]
Chloroacetic acid	2.85	187.8[d]
Hydrofluoric acid	3.45	19.54[d]
Formic acid	3.75	100.7[d]

[a]From Guthrie (1978); Weast (1989). For acids with pK_a less than 0, there is no generally satisfactory way to measure the pK_a in aqueous solutions; reported pK_as were measured at 18–25 °C.
[b]From Weast (1989)
[c]From Sax & Lewis (1987)
[d]Step 1, release of first hydrogen; step 2, release of second hydrogen
[e]From Budavari (1989)
[f]From Hudson & Dolan (1982); Eller (1984)

techniques used traditionally do not allow differentiation between the liquid and gaseous forms of the acids nor determination of the distribution of particle sizes for the mists. Few data are available on particle size distribution of acid mists in the work environment.

The following section addresses several industries in which strong inorganic acids are manufactured or used in a manufacturing process and for which epidemiological studies were available. These are isopropanol manufacture, synthetic ethanol manufacture, pickling and other acid treatment of metals, sulfuric acid manufacture, soap and detergent manufacture, nitric acid manufacture, phosphate fertilizer manufacture and lead battery (accumulator) manufacture.

1.2 Description of the industries

1.2.1 *Isopropanol manufacture* (see also IARC, 1977, 1987)

Isopropanol is claimed by some to be the first petrochemical. During the latter part of the First World War, isopropanol was manufactured by the Ellis process which was quite similar to that used today. The basic chemistry of the process is the reaction of propylene with sulfuric acid to form isopropyl sulfates, which are then hydrolysed to isopropanol (Haberstroh & Collins, 1983a).

In the 'strong-acid process' (indirect hydration), propylene gas (C_3-feedstock, 40–60% propylene) and 88–93% sulfuric acid are fed to a reactor maintained at 25–30°C. The diisopropyl sulfate so formed is hydrolysed with hot water to give crude isopropanol, isopropyl ether and approximately 40% sulfuric acid. The aqueous alcohol is separated from the light, top-floating layer of isopropyl ether and isopropyl oil (largely polypropylenes composed of 3 and 4 propylene molecules, with less than 1% each of benzene (see IARC, 1987), toluene, alkyl benzenes, polyaromatics, hexane, heptane, acetone, ethanol, isopropanol and isopropyl ether) and is then refined by distillation. In the 'weak-acid process', propylene gas is fed continuously to a series of absorbers containing 60% sulfuric acid maintained at 60–65°C. This reaction produces diisopropyl sulfate, which is distilled and then hydrolysed to form crude isopropanol. This crude alcohol contains isopropyl ether, acetone, traces of methanol, water and oil (the composition of the oil produced in this process has not been reported). Refined isopropanol is obtained by distilling the crude alcohol in a series of columns and removing the impurities. Anhydrous isopropanol is made by breaking the alcohol–water azeotrope by introducing benzene. In the USA, the weak-acid process has replaced the older strong-acid process (Lynch et al., 1979; Papa, 1982; Teta et al., 1992). The reaction of propylene with sulfuric acid is a complex series of reactions in which water plays a major role in determining the concentration of the intermediate alkyl sulfates (Lynch et al., 1979). (See the monograph on diisopropyl sulfate, p. 229.)

Plants built in Europe use a direct hydration process in which propylene and water are reacted in the presence of a catalyst such as phosphoric acid on bentonite. One limitation of this route is that it requires a highly concentrated propylene feed rather than a dilute refinery stream (Papa, 1982).

Production of isopropanol in several countries is presented in Table 2.

Table 2. Trends in production of isopropanol in some countries (thousand tonnes)

Country	1980	1981	1982	1983	1984	1985	1986	1987	1988	1989	1990
Brazil	NR	NR	NR	6.7	6.8	6.3	6.0	4.5	5.4	NR	NR
Canada	72.2	73.3	67.2	63.3	62.9	NR	NR	NR	NR	NR	NR
China	NR	NR	NR	12.5	16.7	17.5	17.4	20.4	22.1	NR	NR
India	2.5	NR	2.6	2.9	2.8	NR	NR	NR	NR	NR	NR
Japan	NR	97.9	96.3	90.4	91.5	88.5	84.8	100.6	95.2	102.5	NR
Mexico	12.6	15.6	10.9	11.9	14.1	14.5	11.1	NR	NR	NR	NR
Spain	24.8	23.7	23.4	27.0	26.9	27.3	24.1	19.3	23.8	29.5	NR
USA	832.8	757.0	626.0	548.4	632.3	560.2	590.1	621.9	630.0	668.6	626.0

From Japan Chemical Week (1990); Anon. (1991); Dialog Information Services, (1991); NR, not reported

1.2.2 Synthetic ethanol manufacture

Ethanol has been made by fermentation processes throughout human history, and these processes still account for most of the ethanol produced worldwide. With the development of the petrochemical industry in the early twentieth century, however, processes were introduced for the production of synthetic ethanol from ethylene. The original esterification–hydrolysis process for synthetic ethanol has gradually been replaced by direct catalytic hydration of ethylene (Haberstroh & Collins, 1974, 1983b; Kosaric et al., 1987).

The esterification–hydrolysis process (indirect hydration process), first used commercially in 1930, is the older of the two ethylene-based routes and accounted for about 80% of production in the 1960s. This process takes place in two steps: ethylene is absorbed into 94–98% sulfuric acid at about 75 °C, producing a mixture of ethyl hydrogen sulfate and diethyl sulfate (see monograph, p. 213); this mixture is then diluted with water to produce ethanol. The overall yield is about 90% ethanol and 5–10% diethyl ether. The process can be modified to produce diethyl ether by increasing the residence time in the hydrolyser and then recycling the alcohol (Haberstroh & Collins, 1974; Kosaric et al., 1987). The reaction of ethylene with sulfuric acid is a complex series of reactions in which water plays a major role in determining the concentration of the intermediate alkyl sulfates (Lynch et al., 1979). (See the monograph on diethyl sulfate, p. 213.)

The direct hydration process, introduced in 1948, involves a water–ethylene reaction over a phosphoric acid (H_3PO_4) catalyst at about 250–300 °C and 6–8 MPa. The overall yield of ethanol is reported to be greater than 97%. This process has the advantages of higher yields, production of less diethyl ether as a by-product, lower plant maintenance costs, and elimination of the waste and pollution problems that characterized the esterification–hydrolysis route. Of the synthetic ethanol produced in 1970, 48% was made by direct hydration (Haberstroh & Collins, 1974, 1983b).

Several other methods for producing synthetic ethanol have been investigated, including homologation of methanol, carbonylation of methanol and methyl acetate, and catalytic conversion of synthesis gas (Kosaric et al., 1987).

Synthetic ethanol is purified in a simple three-column distillation unit. Recovery is 98%, and the high-grade product contains less than 20 mg/kg of total impurities. To produce anhydrous ethanol, the water–ethanol azeotrope obtained by distillation of the crude synthetic feedstock must be dehydrated. For economic reasons, large distilleries rely mostly on azeotropic distillation for ethanol dehydration. Benzene has been used as an azeotropic dehydrating (entraining) agent in many plants; cyclohexane and ethylene glycol have also been used. Some smaller plants use molecular sieve adsorption techniques to dry the ethanol azeotrope (Kosaric et al., 1987).

Worldwide production of synthetic ethanol in the early 1980s was estimated to be 2.3×10^9 litres/year, with western Europe accounting for 26.7%, North America for 38.6%, Asia (including the USSR) for 31.7%, and other countries (Japan, Israel, South Africa) for 3%. Most of the plants that produce synthetic ethanol are located in industrialized countries; the developing countries produce mainly fermentation ethanol. In the early 1980s in Canada, Germany, Italy and the United Kingdom, approximately 50% of the ethanol produced was by ethylene hydration; the corresponding figure for the USA was around 35% (Kosaric et al., 1987).

1.2.3 *Pickling and other acid treatment of metals*

Pickling is one of the most widely used industrial processes. It is used in small electroplating plants, in automobile manufacturing plants, in steel producing plants and in any plant where coatings are applied to a base metal. Pickling is a descaling process, in which oxides and scale are removed chemically from a metallic surface by immersion in a dilute inorganic acid (up to 25% acid), which is generally, but not exclusively, sulfuric or hydrochloric acid (see monograph, p. 189). While other descaling processes are in use, pickling is the most widely applied (Morse, 1983).

(a) Processes and acids

Although various kinds of pickling process are encountered under many different names, they can be classified into three general types: (i) stationary or vat pickling, (ii) batch pickling and (iii) continuous pickling. The degree of acid splashing, gas evolution and mist formation vary with the method employed. Stationary or vat pickling is used mostly within the electroplating industry, whereas batch and continuous pickling are generally used in large production industries. In vat pickling, the product is immersed in an acid solution and generally remains stationary, while the solution is kept in motion. In batch pickling, several pieces of the same product are immersed in the acid solution and are generally kept in motion. In continuous pickling, the product is usually a steel strip, which is uncoiled and passed in a horizontal or vertical direction through acid and water-rinse tanks or sprays (Morse, 1983).

Traditional acid pickling solutions are based on inhibited sulfuric, hydrochloric or phosphoric acids; nitric, hydrofluoric and chromic acids are used less frequently. The acids may be used separately, in combination or sequentially at various concentrations and temperatures, depending on the metal being treated, the degree and type of scale and the intended use of the treated metal surface. Schneberger (1981) reviewed typical processes for several categories of metal, including stainless-steel and high-nickel alloys, ferrous metals other than stainless-steel, cuprous metals (copper, brasses and bronzes), aluminium and its alloys, magnesium and zinc and galvanized steel.

Pickling underwent little technological change until fairly recently. In the steel industry, however, where sulfuric acid pickling was formerly used almost exclusively, there is now a trend toward hydrochloric acid pickling in continuous pickling lines. Choice of a particular type of pickling operation is chiefly dependent upon the product to be cleaned. For example, acid cleaning in batch electroplating plants and the pickling of steel bars and plates are generally done by the vat method. Some steel sheet and coils of steel rods and wire are cleaned by the batch method, whereas almost all steel strip is cleaned in high-speed (up to 300 m/min), continuous pickling lines (Morse, 1983).

In some stationary pickling lines, a separate alkaline vat is used to neutralize the acid; in most pickling lines in large production industries, however, water-rinse tanks remove the acid. The rate of pickling, and consequently of metal loss, is dependent on a number of factors, including: acid concentration, temperature of solution, time in bath, percentage of iron compounds in bath, inhibitors present and agitation of the solution. In any pickling process, descaling within a given time can be accomplished by using a high acid concentration at a low temperature or a low acid concentration at a high temperature (Morse, 1983). The major cause of escape of acid mist or vapour from acid tanks in pickling is the formation of hydrogen bubbles and steam which carry acid mist from the surface of the solution; the rate of gas formation depends on the factors above, which in turn affect the rate of pickling (Beaumont *et al.*, 1987).

(b) Pickling of stainless-steel

Pickling is used on a large scale in the manufacture of stainless-steel. The general sequence of operations involved in processing stainless-steel is: hot working, annealing, conditioning (mechanical or chemical), pickling, cold working, annealing, conditioning (chemical or electrolytic or salt bath), pickling, finishing. Some of the steps are repeated as often as necessary to bring the material to the desired thickness. Having been worked by hot or cold rolling, the steel is softened by annealing, during which process oxide forms. The steel is then conditioned for the pickling process, which is necessary to remove the oxide from the stainless-steel surface. In addition to removing this annealing scale, pickling also removes a very thin (1–5 μm) region depleted in chromium between the oxide and the bulk stainless-steel (Covino *et al.*, 1984).

Hot working is the process of mechanical deformation of a material at temperatures above its recrystallization temperature. Annealing is the process of maintaining metal at a specified temperature for a specific length of time and then gradually cooling it at a predetermined rate. This treatment removes the internal strains resulting from hot or cold rolling and eliminates distortions and imperfections; a stronger and more uniform metal results (Covino *et al.*, 1984).

Conditioning is a process used to prepare annealed metal for the pickling process. Its purpose is to alter the annealing scale in order to reduce the time, temperature and acid concentration used in the pickling process. Depending upon the nature of the oxide film, mechanical and/or chemical techniques are used. Abrasive blasting is one of the fastest conditioning techniques; chemical techniques include chemical conditioning, electrolytic acid conditioning, electrolytic neutral conditioning, and salt bath conditioning. Common chemical conditioning processes may involve the use of reducing (sulfuric and hydrochloric) or oxidizing (nitric) acids. There are three basic types of electrolytic conditioning: anodic, cathodic and alternating current; the most common acids associated with electrolytic conditioning are sulfuric and nitric acids. Electrolytic neutral conditioning is similar in mechanical design to electrolytic acid conditioning in that alternating cathodic and anodic electrodes are used to polarize the workpiece and induce oxidation and reduction of the surface scale; but this process involves a sodium sulfate solution instead of an acid. Salt bath treatments can be either reducing, oxidizing or electrolytic (Covino *et al.*, 1984).

The pickling of stainless-steels involves three distinct processes. The first is removal of thermally grown oxide scale to improve the appearance of the metal and to facilitate further cold working of the steel. The second process maximizes the resistance of the final steel product to corrosion by completely dissolving the chromium-depleted zone that is generally formed during short high-temperature anneals in oxidizing environments. The third process dissolves the minimum amount of bulk steel necessary to give the desired whitening effect (Covino *et al.*, 1984).

Stainless-steel and high-nickel alloy scales adhere tightly and are difficult to remove with the acids used for plain steel, although hot 10% sulfuric acid containing 1–2% sodium thiosulfate or hydrosulfite, or 2% hydrofluoric acid with 6–8% ferric chloride, is often effective. Moderate or light scale is removed with 20% nitric acid containing 2–4% hydrofluoric acid. Nitric acid is a widely used pickling agent and does not affect the stainless character of the steel; in fact, these steels are passivated in nitric acid at greater than 20% concentration. Hydrochloric acid may be used as an activator or as a first treatment to remove scale (Schneberger, 1981).

(c) Other processes

Other processes involving acid treatment of metals, for which some occupational exposure data were available, include electroplating and electrowinning. Electroplating is the application of a metal coating through the action of an electric current. Types of plating include chromium (see IARC, 1990a), nickel (see IARC, 1990a), copper, brass, silver, gold, cadmium (see IARC, 1987), zinc, lead (see IARC, 1987) and tin. Some strong inorganic acids used are chromic, sulfuric, hydrochloric and nitric acids; different solutions are used depending on the metal to be electrodeposited (Soule, 1982). Galvanizing refers specifically to the plating of zinc onto a ferrous metal. Electrowinning, or electrolytic refining, is the process of extracting a metal from its soluble salt using an electrolytic cell (Sax & Lewis, 1987).

1.2.4 *Sulfuric acid manufacture*

In ancient times, sulfuric acid was probably made by distilling nitre (potassium nitrate) and green vitriol (ferrous sulfate heptahydrate). Weathered iron pyrites were usually the source of the green vitriol. Around 1740, the acid was made in England by burning sulfur in the presence of potassium nitrate in a gas balloon flask. The vapours united with water to form acid, which condensed on the walls of the flask. In 1746, the glass balloon flask was replaced by a large lead-lined box or chamber, giving rise to the name 'chamber process'. In 1827, Gay-Lussac, and in 1859, Glover, changed the circulation of gases in the plant by adding towers, which are now known as Gay-Lussac and Glover towers. These permit the recovery from the exit gases of the nitrogen oxides that are essential to the economic production of 'chamber acid'. The acid produced by this method has a maximum acid strength of 75–85% H_2SO_4 (West & Duecker, 1974; West & Smith, 1983). Once of great importance in western Europe and North America, chamber process plants have become almost extinct. Whereas the chamber process accounted for about 80% of sulfuric acid production in these regions in 1910, the figure had decreased to about 15% in 1960; and, by 1980, virtually no sulfuric acid was being produced by this process. Today, most sulfuric acid is produced by the contact process, based on technology developed around 1900 and thereafter (West & Duecker, 1974; West & Smith, 1983; Sander *et al.*, 1984).

In the chamber process, chemical reactions involve sulfur dioxide, oxygen, nitrogen oxides and water vapour. A series of intermediate compounds are formed which decompose to yield sulfuric acid and nitrogen oxides. The overall effect is that the sulfur dioxide is oxidized to sulfur trioxide, which combines with water vapour to form sulfuric acid ($2SO_2 + O_2 + 2H_2O \rightarrow 2H_2SO_4$). Nitrogen dioxide acts as the oxidant and is reduced to nitric oxide, which must be reoxidized continually by oxygen in the air. When all the sulfur dioxide has been consumed, the nitrogen oxides are absorbed in sulfuric acid in the Gay-Lussac tower as nitrosylsulfuric acid. The solution of nitrosylsulfuric acid (nitrose) from the Gay-Lussac tower is pumped to the denitration (Glover) tower, where heat releases the nitrogen oxides for re-use in the cycle. In the Glover tower, the denitrated sulfuric acid is concentrated to approximately 78%. Part of this acid is returned to the Gay-Lussac tower for recovery of the nitrogen oxides from the exit gases. The balance is available for use or sale (West & Duecker, 1974).

The basic features of the contact process for making sulfuric acid, as practised today, were described in a British patent in 1831. It disclosed that if sulfur dioxide, mixed with oxygen or air, is passed over heated platinum, the sulfur dioxide is rapidly converted to sulfur trioxide, which can be dissolved in water to make sulfuric acid. A demand for acid stronger than that which could be produced readily by the chamber process stimulated this development. The heart of the contact sulfuric acid plant is the converter in which sulfur dioxide is converted catalytically to sulfur trioxide. Over the course of time, a variety of catalysts have been used, including platinum and the oxides of iron, chromium, copper, manganese, titanium, vanadium and other metals. Platinum and iron catalysts were the main catalysts used prior to the First World War. At present, vanadium catalysts in various forms are generally used. The principal steps in a contact plant burning sulfur are: (1) oxidation of sulfur to sulfur dioxide with dry air; (2) cooling of the gas; (3) conversion or oxidation of the sulfur dioxide to sulfur trioxide; (4) cooling of the sulfur trioxide gas; and (5) absorption of the sulfur trioxide in water to produce sulfuric acid (West & Duecker, 1974; West & Smith, 1983; Mannsville Chemical Products, 1987).

Various attempts have been made to increase the conversion of sulfur dioxide to sulfur trioxide. In one of these, the double catalyst–double absorption system, the process flow is modified so that after the second or third pass in the converter the gases are withdrawn and passed through the absorber to remove the sulfur trioxide. The remaining gases are reheated and sent through the last pass over the catalyst; further absorption follows. Increased conversion, up to 99.5–99.7%, is obtained. This process has been used in new sulfuric acid plants in many industrialized countries to meet strict regulatory restrictions on emissions (United Nations Industrial Development Organization, 1978; West & Smith, 1983; Sander et al., 1984).

Sulfur dioxide for sulfuric acid production is obtained from pyrite and pyrrhotite. It can be obtained from calcium sulfate (as natural gypsum or natural anhydrous calcium sulfate) by calcining with coke (Müller-Kühne method) (United Nations Industrial Development Organization, 1978).

Oleum (fuming sulfuric acid), which consists of solutions of sulfur trioxide in 100% sulfuric acid, is produced in contact process plants by adding sulfur trioxide to sulfuric acid in a special oleum tower (Sander et al., 1984).

Users of sulfuric acid confronted with the task of disposing of waste or spent acid find it advantageous to arrange with an independent producer to exchange the waste acid for fresh acid. Methods have been developed which permit such producers to reprocess the waste acid and obtain a product of virgin quality. In addition, they can operate large, centrally located plants which can produce acid at a much lower cost than can small plants. The end-use of sulfuric acid, more than any other factor, determines the location of sulfuric acid plants; however, sulfuric acid plants in which metallurgical gas is used as the source of sulfur are usually located near smelters producing the gas (West & Smith, 1983).

Enormous amounts of spent sulfuric acid are reprocessed, since most of the sulfuric acid used for industrial processes, other than in the fertilizer industry, acts only as a reaction medium and does not form part of the final product. The largest quantities of spent sulfuric acid come from the organic chemical and petrochemical industries. The range of grades of spent sulfuric acid produced in these industries is very wide, from extremely dilute to comparatively concentrated forms, which may at the same time be lightly or heavily contaminated with organic and inorganic compounds. Another important source of spent sulfuric acid is inorganic chemical factories, particularly those for processing titanium dioxide pigment (see IARC, 1989). The spent acid produced is relatively uniform, with about 20–23% sulfuric acid and 7–15% metal sulfates. Spent acids of similar composition are produced in the metallurgical industry from pickling processes. Wash acids from gas cleaning plants (especially in sulfide ore roasting plants) may have widely varying contents of impurities (Sander *et al.*, 1984).

Sulfuric acid is made in numerous grades and strengths. A discussion of the different grades and purities of sulfuric acid is given in the Annex to this monograph.

Production levels of sulfuric acid in a number of countries and regions are presented in Table 3. A more detailed analysis of the worldwide production and movement of sulfuric acid stocks in 1982 is presented in Table 4.

China is the third largest producer of sulfuric acid, after the USA and the USSR. Since 1876, the Chinese sulfuric acid industry has been based on pyrite as the main raw material. With the national emphasis on agricultural production and the consequent demand for phosphate fertilizers, a large number of small-scale sulfuric acid plants utilizing local resources have been constructed throughout China since the 1960s. In 1984, there were more than 400 sulfuric acid plants in China, with the largest plants producing over 550 000 tonnes per year and the smaller plants producing 9 000–36 000 tonnes. About 60% of the sulfuric acid produced in China in the early 1980s was used in the production of phosphate fertilizers (Zengtai, 1984).

1.2.5 *Soap and detergent manufacture*

Soaps are metallic salts of fatty acids. Detergents are substances that reduce the surface tension of water and include soaps and synthetic detergents, such as the linear alkyl sulfonates and alkyl benzene sulfonates (Sax & Lewis, 1987).

Soap is believed to be one of the oldest materials obtained by purposely reacting two chemical substances to get a useful product. The word 'soap' is derived from the latin *sapo*, first used by Pliny the Elder around 75 AD. Although Pliny is credited with the first written reference to soap, its use is believed to have begun long before recorded history. Soap *per se* was probably never actually discovered but evolved from various crude mixtures of alkali and fatty materials (Feierstein & Morgenthaler, 1983).

With time, it was learnt that soap is not a mixture of alkali and fat but results from a chemical reaction, later called saponification; thus, soap-making changed from an art to an industry. Indeed, soap remained the principal cleaning product, or surface active agent, well into the twentieth century. The development of synthetic detergents in the 1930s dramatically reduced world dependence on soap. Nonetheless, a significant market remains for

Table 3. Production of sulfuric acid in a number of countries and regions (thousand tonnes)

Country or region	1980	1981	1982	1983	1984	1985	1986	1987	1988	1989	1990
Australia	2 175	1 963	2 027	1 782	1 726	1 773	1 788	1 678	1 818	1 904	1 464
Bulgaria	852	920	916	861	908	810	807	689	840	846	NA
Canada	4 295	4 117	3 131	3 686	4 043	3 890	3 536	3 437	3 805	3 560	3 311
China	7 640	7 810	8 175	8 696	8 172	6 764	7 510	9 620	10 981	11 408	11 689
Czechoslovakia	1 284	1 315	1 252	1 244	1 240	1 297	1 292	1 264	1 249	1 142	1 033
France	4 941	4 498	4 018	4 093	4 490	4 279	4 005	3 909	4 012	4 146	3 768
Germany[a]	5 065	5 038	4 700	4 559	4 515	4 317	4 214	4 159	4 059	3 250	3 352
Hungary	608	573	571	606	549	541	540	573	512	482	244
India	2 320	2 780	2 270	2 270	NA	NA	NA	NA	NA	NA	NA
Italy	2 821	2 539	4 000	4 115	4 250	4 349	4 159	4 350	4 299	3 213	3 303
Japan	6 777	6 572	6 530	6 662	6 458	6 580	6 561	6 541	6 766	6 885	6 887
Korea (Republic of)	1 702	1 304	1 596	1 610	1 975	2 028	1 898	2 039	NA	NA	NA
Poland	3 019	2 776	2 682	2 786	2 770	2 863	2 966	3 149	3 154	3 114	1 850
Romania	1 756	1 814	1 600	1 941	1 915	1 835	1 971	1 693	1 825	1 687	1 112
Taiwan	769	819	685	678	762	733	727	742	664	768	658
United Kingdom	3 375	2 885	2 582	2 582	2 644	2 550	2 325	2 176	2 253	2 152	1 997
USA	40 059	36 961	30 148	33 188	37 922	36 188	32 653	35 612	38 630	39 283	40 171
USSR	23 033	24 095	23 801	24 714	25 338	26 037	27 847	28 531	29 372	28 276	27 300

From Anon. (1984a,b, 1986, 1988, 1991); NA, not available
[a]Figures for 1989 and 1990 are for western Germany only.

Table 4. Worldwide sulfuric acid production and trade in 1982 (thousand tonnes 100% H_2SO_4)

Geographical area	Production	Imports	Exports
World total	130 263	3 185	3 247
Western Europe	24 094	1 143	1 595
Belgium	1 798	492	64
France	3 927	134	154
Germany (western)	3 750	34	766
Italy	2 360	2	39
Netherlands	1 692	179	195
Spain	2 690	48	75
United Kingdom	2 587	115	67
Africa	10 141	124	NA
Morocco	3 072	NA	NA
South Africa	3 382	105	NA
Tunisia	2 525	1	NA
North America	32 490	582	496
Canada	3 131	203	260
USA	29 359	379	237
Central America	2 979	477	2
Mexico	2 920	453	2
South America	3 329	175	6
Argentina	260	NA	NA
Brazil	2 229	91	NA
Chile	460	1	NA
Asia	20 872	329	785
China	8 174	103	0
India	2 232	NA	0
Japan	6 531	NA	0
Republic of Korea	1 596	141	785
Taiwan	680	22	0
Oceania	2 491	1	NA
Australia	1 971	1	NA
New Zealand	520	NA	NA
Eastern Europe	9 136	355	166
Czechoslovakia	1 252	164	2
Germany (eastern)	920	NA	6
Poland	2 682	NA	94
Romania	1 669	NA	NA
Yugoslavia	1 120	93	NA
USSR	23 801	90	197

From Sander *et al.* (1984); NA, not available

soap-based products, for personal use, primarily as bars, and for industrial use (Feierstein & Morgenthaler, 1983).

Free fatty acids are a raw material not only for soap but increasingly for other chemical products. Although fatty acids are sometimes synthesized, most of those used commercially are produced by the hydrolysis of naturally occurring fats and oils. Fatty acids have been produced by four basic processes: saponification of fats followed by acidulation; the Twitchell process; batch autoclave splitting; and continuous high-pressure, high-temperature hydrolysis. The Twitchell process is described in detail as it is the only process in which a strong acid is used (Feierstein & Morgenthaler, 1983).

The Twitchell process is batch acid hydrolysis of fats at atmospheric pressure in the presence of a catalyst called Twitchell's reagent. The original Twitchell's reagent was benzenestearosulfonic acid, but sulfonated petroleum products were commonly used later. After impurities have been removed, the fats are mixed with water, the catalyst (0.75–1.25%) and a small amount of sulfuric acid (0.5–1.0%) and are boiled with steam for one to two days. Spent water is removed and replaced with fresh water and sulfuric acid, and then another boiling cycle is conducted. After two to four boiling cycles, the hydrolysis reaction approaches completion, and the crude fatty acids are drawn off for purification. While the Twitchell process is the simplest to run, it has several drawbacks compared to more modern techniques, one of which is the emission of noxious, acidic fumes (Feierstein & Morgenthaler, 1983).

Alkylbenzene sulfonates account for approximately 50% of the total volume of synthetic anionic detergents used in liquid and spray-dried formulations. Two chemicals are routinely used for sulfonation: oleum (fuming sulfuric acid) and sulfur trioxide; the latter has gained increased popularity in recent years. The oleum process normally yields sulfonic acid of 88–91% purity; the remainder, after neutralization, consists of sulfuric acid and a small amount of unsulfonated oils. The air–sulfur trioxide process normally produces a 95–98% pure sulfonic acid, the remainder consisting of sodium sulfate after neutralization. Another process for making anionic surfactants is sulfation of fatty alcohols or ethoxylated fatty alcohols and alpha olefins. Sulfamic acid and chlorosulfonic acid have also been used in commercial sulfation (Feierstein & Morgenthaler, 1983).

1.2.6 *Nitric acid manufacture*

Nitric acid has been known since the thirteenth century. Glauber synthesized it from strong sulfuric acid and sodium nitrate; however, it was Lavoisier who showed that nitric acid contained oxygen and Cavendish who showed that it could be made from moist air with an electric spark. In the oldest methods used, Chile saltpetre (sodium nitrate) was reacted with concentrated sulfuric acid in heated cast iron retorts; the evolved nitric acid vapours were condensed and collected in stoneware vessels (Green & Li, 1983).

Nitric acid is currently made by oxidation of ammonia with air over a precious-metal catalyst at atmospheric or higher pressures and at 800–950 °C. The overall reaction is: $NH_3 + 2O_2 \rightarrow HNO_3 + H_2O + 98.7$ kcal [413.2 kJ] evolved. The concentration of nitric acid produced with conventional equipment is usually about 60%; if higher concentrations are desired, special equipment or processes are required. Typical processes used for nitric acid manufacture have included low-pressure (800 °C; atmospheric pressure; 50–52% acid strength); medium-pressure (Montecatini process: 850 °C; 40 psi [276 kPa]; 60% acid strength); medium-pressure (Kuhlman process: 850 °C; 40 psi; 70% acid strength); high-pressure (DuPont process: 950 °C; 120 psi [827 kPa]; 60% acid strength); and Pintsch Bamag's 'Hoko Process' (850 °C; atmospheric pressure; 98-99% acid strength) (Green, 1974; Green & Li, 1983).

The first processes for oxidation of ammonia operated at atmospheric pressure. Both high-pressure and dual-pressure processes have been used, but the latter is widely used today. In this process, ammonia is oxidized at 72.5 psi [500 kPa], and the oxidation products are absorbed at 160 psi [1 MPa]. The low pressure used for oxidation promotes high conversion efficiency and minimizes losses of the precious-metal catalyst (Green & Li, 1983).

Nitric acid is produced by the standard ammonia-oxidation processes as an aqueous solution at a concentration of 50-70 wt%. Such concentrations are suitable for the production of ammonium nitrate, but anhydrous nitric acid is required for use in organic nitrations. Since nitric acid forms an azeotrope with water at 68.8 wt%, water cannot be separated from the acid by simple distillation. Two industrial methods for concentrating nitric acid are extractive distillation and reactions with additional nitrogen oxides; these latter reactions are the direct, strong nitric processes (Newman, 1981).

Extractive distillation is the most widely used method for concentrating nitric acid. It consists of mixing 60% nitric acid with strong (93%) sulfuric acid and passing the mixture through a distillation system from which concentrated (95-98%) nitric acid and denitrated, residual sulfuric acid containing approximately 70% H_2SO_4 are obtained. The dilute, residual sulfuric acid may be reconcentrated for further use. In the Pintsch Bamag process, nitric acid is concentrated on the basis of the difference in the composition of the nitric acid-water constant boiling mixtures at different pressures in a two-column distillation system (Green & Li, 1983).

Modifications of a concentration process that was described in 1932, direct, strong nitric processes, have been widely used in Europe. Nitrogen tetroxide is separated from the process gases that leave the ammonia converter by refrigeration or by absorption in concentrated nitric acid. The tetroxide then reacts with weak nitric acid and air or oxygen to yield a 98 wt% product (Newman, 1981).

Worldwide production of nitric acid is presented in Table 5. White fuming nitric acid usually contains 90-99 wt% nitric acid, 0-2 wt% nitrogen dioxide and up to 10 wt% water. Red fuming nitric acid usually contains about 70-90 wt% nitric acid, 2-25 wt% nitrogen dioxide and up to 10 wt% water. Over time, concentrated nitric acids tend to decompose to nitrogen dioxide, water and oxygen; as a result, pressure builds up in storage vessels. Decomposition of concentrated acid is reduced by adding such substances as quaternary ammonium compounds, organic sulfones, inorganic persulfates and organic sulfonium compounds. Nitric acid is also very corrosive, and stabilizers and corrosion inhibitors are sometimes used; for instance, corrosion of aluminium by red fuming nitric acid is reduced by adding 4 wt% of hydrogen fluoride (52% HF) (Green, 1974; Green & Li, 1983).

1.2.7 *Phosphate fertilizer manufacture*

The phosphate minerals fluorapatite [$3Ca_3(PO_4)_2 \cdot CaF_2$] and hydroxyapatite [$3Ca_3(PO_4)_2 \cdot Ca(OH)_2$] (Hudson & Dolan, 1982) supply the bulk of the phosphorus in

Table 5. Trends in production of nitric acid in some countries (thousand tonnes)

Country	1980	1981	1982	1983	1984	1985	1986	1987	1988	1989	1990
Brazil	381.0	349.0	308.0	321.1	355.6	364.8	389.8	407.6	387.5	NR	NR
Canada	712.6	1157.7	976.8	1060.8	1100.5	1128.3	1023.9	899.9	919.3	1026.6	965.0
China	227.6	184.4	246.1	255.9	257.7	273.9	275.3	290.2	302.1	NR	NR
Germany[a]	3172.4	2883.0	2286.1	2620.9	2850.4	2885.3	2816.8	2639.0	2312.4	2180.4	1879.7
India	454.0	561.0	487.0	551.0	529.0	NR	NR	NR	NR	NR	NR
Italy	1011.5	1005.5	1029.7	1027.8	1099.9	1181.5	1091.6	1195.2	1193.3	1108.1	1040.1
Japan	NR	470.7	531.1	540.0	581.0	578.4	563.4	573.0	618.0	NR	NR
Mexico	170.0	161.0	167.0	167.0	171.0	173.0	154.0	NR	NR	NR	NR
Spain	1266.4	1225.9	1199.5	1054.7	1285.0	1245.8	1292.9	1211.0	1247.8	1266.9	NR
United Kingdom	NR	2973.2	3083.8	3144.8	NR	NR	NR	NR	2364.9	NR	NR
USA	8374.2	8249.0	6704.1	6139.8	7008.9	6922.7	6109.0	6554.4	7249.3	7574.1	7029.8

From Anon. (1983, 1987, 1991); Dialog Information Services (1991); NR, not reported
[a]Data are for western Germany only.

fertilizers manufactured all over the world. The powdered rock itself is useless as a fertilizer, however, because the phosphorus it contains is not water-soluble and thus not readily available to plants. Reacting the rock with sulfuric, nitric or hydrochloric acid produces phosphoric acid (H_3PO_4) and superphosphoric acid—important intermediates in the production of phosphate fertilizers (United Nations Industrial Development Organization, 1978; Fertilizer Institute, 1982).

The oldest commercial fertilizer is normal superphosphate (containing 19–20% phosphorus as P_2O_5), first made in about 1840. This was the leading phosphate fertilizer for many years, but by the 1970s it had been supplanted to a large extent by ammonium phosphates and triple superphosphate. One reason for its long tenure is the ease with which it can be manufactured: All that is necessary is to mix pulverized phosphate rock with sulfuric acid, wait until the mixture sets into a solid and cures (completes the reaction), and then break up the mass. About half of the normal weight of superphosphates is gypsum (calcium sulfate) (Fertilizer Institute, 1982).

By using a higher ratio of sulfuric acid to phosphate rock, phosphoric acid (52–54% phosphorus as P_2O_5) rather than normal superphosphate can be produced. The crude product contains phosphoric acid with solid calcium sulfate in suspension. The calcium sulfate is separated by filtration, giving a large quantity of waste by-product (nearly 5 tonnes per tonne of P_2O_5 in phosphoric acid). Phosphoric acid (H_3PO_4) made in this way is called 'wet-process' acid. The acid is concentrated by evaporation to the usual commercial grade of 52–54% P_2O_5. It is used in making triple superphosphate, ammonium phosphate and liquid mixed fertilizers. 'Furnace'-grade phosphoric acid is made by smelting phosphate rock with coke and silica in an electric furnace. The elemental phosphorus produced is burned and converted to phosphoric acid. This relatively pure acid is now used almost entirely in the detergent and food industries, as the high production cost essentially eliminated use of 'furnace' acid in the production of commercial fertilizers by the early 1970s (Fertilizer Institute, 1982).

Superphosphoric acid (68–72% phosphorus as P_2O_5) (Herrick, 1982) is made by concentrating wet-process acid past the point needed for the usual 52–54% P_2O_5 grade. The composition of superphosphoric acid differs radically from that of ordinary phosphoric acid: It contains mainly polyphosphates rather than orthophosphate. It is a fluid at ordinary temperature, even though there is little or no water present, and this property confers certain advantages—higher solubility and readier solubilization of impurities when it is used to make fluid fertilizers. Polyphosphates in superphosphoric acid became the backbone of high-quality liquid fertilizers in the 1960s and 1970s (Fertilizer Institute, 1982).

When phosphate rock is treated with phosphoric acid, triple superphosphate (44–51% phosphorus as P_2O_5) results (Herrick, 1982). The operation is similar to that for making normal superphosphate, but the product has more than twice the P_2O_5 content because phosphoric acid is used rather than sulfuric acid. It is produced in granular and nongranular forms. Triple superphosphate is second to ammonium phosphates in use among phosphate fertilizers worldwide (Fertilizer Institute, 1982).

Phosphoric acid treated with ammonia produces ammonium phosphates. The high nitrogen and phosphorus content, high water solubility, good physical characteristics and low production costs of granular ammonium phosphates have made these compounds the leading fertilizers in the world. The most popular type is diammonium phosphate (18% nitrogen and 46% phosphorus as P_2O_5), which is made in very large plants and used widely in bulk blending. Other types are monoammonium phosphate, produced with various ratios of nitrogen and phosphorus, and ammonium phosphate plus ammonium sulfate, typically containing 16% nitrogen and 20% phosphorus as P_2O_5. Monoammonium phosphate is also produced in nongranular form and used in the production of granular nitrogen–phosphorus–potassium and suspension fertilizers (Fertilizer Institute, 1982).

Worldwide production of phosphate fertilizers is presented in Table 6.

Table 6. Regional phosphate fertilizer production (thousand tonnes)

Region	1960	1965	1970	1975	1980	1985	1987
North America	2736	3991	5451	7229	9786	10321	8613
Western Europe	3839	4825	5579	6275	5574	4812	4133
Eastern Europe	553	1209	1909	2641	3207	3165	3096
USSR	879	1407	2072	3504	5083	6330	7687
Oceania	728	1140	1134	1029	1330	870	830
Africa	244	377	742	956	1103	1573	1771
Latin America	91	183	328	769	1510	1714	1921
Asia	705	1466	2237	3432	4634	6832	7503

From Bumb (1989)

1.2.8 *Lead battery (accumulator) manufacture*

In 1860, Gaston Planté presented the first working model of the lead–acid secondary battery to the French Academy of Science. Lead–acid batteries, or accumulators, are used to store electrical energy. The basic components of a lead–acid battery are the container (case, cover and vent plugs) and the cell; the cell contains the plates (positive, lead dioxide on lead grid; negative, lead on lead grid), separators and electrolyte solution (approx. 33 wt% aqueous H_2SO_4). There are three principal categories of lead–acid battery: *automotive* (for cranking internal combustion engines); *industrial or stationary* (heavy-duty applications, such as motive power, and stand-by power for vital facilities, such as power stations, telephone exchanges and hospitals); and *consumer* (emergency lighting and security systems, cordless appliances and tools and small engine starting) (Doe, 1978; Sander *et al.*, 1984; Berndt, 1985).

A lead–acid battery may contain any number of cells, depending on the voltage: Stationary batteries contain up to 120 cells (240 volts), whereas automobile batteries generally contain three or six cells (6 or 12 volts). Lead–acid storage batteries vary in size and weight (100 g to several tonnes), depending on the capacity required (US Environmental Protection Agency, 1989a).

The manufacture of lead–acid batteries has been described in detail by Hehner (1986). Battery manufacture begins with grid casting and paste mixing. Two grids are generally cast at the same time from molten lead, to which calcium (0.1%), antimony (2.5–6.0%), arsenic (see IARC, 1987) (0.3–0.6%) or tin (0.1–0.6%) is added as an alloy component. These grids are coated with either positive or negative paste, formed, cured, cut into two (a process called slitting) and then sent to be assembled (Hehner, 1986; US Environmental Protection Agency, 1989a).

The paste mixing operation is a batch-type process in which lead oxide is added to the mixer, water and sulfuric acid are added, and the mixture is blended to form a stiff paste. Approximately 1 wt% of expander (generally a mixture of barium sulfate, carbon black (see IARC, 1987) and organic compounds) is added to batches of paste to make negative plates. The paste is then applied to the grids, which are flash dried and then stacked and sent to curing ovens. After the plates have been cured, they are sent to the three-process operation, which includes plate stacking, welding and assembly of elements into the battery case (US Environmental Protection Agency, 1989a).

During formation, the inactive lead oxide–sulfate paste is converted chemically into an active electrode. Formation is essentially an oxidation–reduction reaction, in which the lead oxide in the positive plates is oxidized to lead dioxide (PbO_2) and that in the negative plates is reduced to metallic lead. This is accomplished by placing the unformed plates in a dilute (10–25%) sulfuric acid solution and connecting the positive plates to the positive pole and the negative plates to the negative pole of the direct current source. During the formation process, hydrogen is released in the form of small bubbles, which carry sulfuric acid with them as they break through the surface of the solution and enter the atmosphere above the container. The emissions of sulfuric acid mist generally increase with increasing temperature and rate of charge; and, as the formation cycle nears the end, the release of hydrogen bubbles increases, augmenting emissions of sulfuric acid (US Environmental Protection Agency, 1989a).

In the manufacture of lead–acid batteries using the wet ('jar') formation process, the elements are assembled in the case before forming. It is common practice to place the cells in the battery case, put the lid on the battery and add sulfuric acid. After formation, additional acid is added to fill the battery completely or the spent acid is dumped from the battery and new acid is added. Wet formation generally takes one to four days. In most plants, a 36- to 48-h forming cycle is used; the charging rate is high during the first 24–36 h and lower during the remaining 12 h (US Environmental Protection Agency, 1989a).

The dry ('tank') formation process can be performed in several ways. In some cases, the plates are formed individually in tanks of sulfuric acid and then assembled. Most often, however, the plates are assembled into elements before formation, and these elements are placed in large tanks of sulfuric acid and connected electrically. Dry formation typically lasts 16 h, plates or elements being loaded into tanks during the day shift and formed during the evening and night shifts (US Environmental Protection Agency, 1989a).

Global shipments of automotive batteries in 1990 amounted to 233.8 million units: 84.9 million units for North America; 67.3 million units for Europe; 53.7 million units for Asia and the Pacific; 17.9 million units for Latin America; and 10.0 million units for Africa and the Middle East (Ficker, 1991).

1.3 Analysis

Methods for the measurement and analysis of strong acids in atmospheric samples have been reviewed. These include thermal volatilization, extraction with pH measurement or proton titration, specific extraction of atmospheric acids, specific extraction with derivatization and continuous and/or real-time analysis using flame photometric detection (Tanner, 1987).

1.4 Exposures in the workplace

In this section, occupational exposures to mists, vapours and gases of sulfuric acid, hydrochloric acid, nitric acid and phosphoric acid in various industries and occupations are summarized. Table 7 lists industries in which exposures to these acids may occur. Most of the sulfuric acid consumed in the USA is in phosphate fertilizer production, where it is used to convert phosphate rock to phosphoric acid. Other industrial uses include production of pigments, textiles (see IARC, 1990b), explosives, alcohols and detergents, petrochemical refining and chemical manufacturing, plating and pickling of metals and lead–acid battery production. Nitric acid is used primarily in making synthetic fertilizers and in explosives, plastics, fibres, dyestuffs and other chemical manufacturing industries. Most of the hydrochloric acid produced in the USA is used within the chemical industry in oxyhydrochlorination processes, e.g., making vinyl chloride and chlorinated solvents. Hydrochloric acid is also produced as a by-product in the manufacture of vinyl chloride (see IARC, 1987), chlorinated ethanes and ethylenes, fluorocarbons and other chlorinated organics, and isocyanates. Phosphoric acid is used primarily in phosphate fertilizer production, with additional consumption for the production of detergents, animal feed supplements, metal treatment agents, water softeners and fire retardants.

A list of occupations in which workers may be exposed to strong inorganic acids is presented in Table 8. Very few data exist on the numbers of workers exposed. In the USA, the National Occupational Exposure Survey conducted by the National Institute for Occupational Safety and Health between 1981 and 1983 provided estimates of the numbers of US workers with potential exposure to sulfuric (776 000), hydrochloric (1 239 000), nitric (298 000) and phosphoric (1 257 000) acids (US National Institute for Occupational Safety and Health, 1990). The occupations listed and the estimates of numbers of workers were based on a survey of US companies and did not involve measurements of actual exposures.

The following sections address eight industries in which exposures to acid mists, vapours and gases occur. Exposures in each of these industries are described, and mechanisms by which acid mists, vapours and gases may be generated are given when that information was available for specific processes. In general, the factors that affect generation of gases and vapours include temperature and pressure; additional factors that influence the generation of vapours from solutions are solution strength and evaporative surface area. Mists may be formed by either condensation of vapour or disturbance of liquid solutions, such as release of dissolved gases or mechanical agitation. Occupational exposures also depend on the proximity of a worker to sources of mists and vapours and on process control measures such as ventilation and containment.

1.4.1 *Isopropanol manufacture*

No measurement has been published of exposure to sulfuric acid in isopropanol plants. Potential exposures include propylene and sulfuric acid (raw materials), diisopropyl and isopropyl hydrogen sulfates (intermediates), isopropanol (product), isopropyl ether and

Table 7. Industries in which there is potential exposure to strong inorganic acids

Industry	Sulfuric acid	Hydrochloric acid	Nitric acid	Phosphoric acid
Aerospace		+	+	
Building and construction	+	+	+	+
Chemical manufacture	+	+	+	+
– isopropanol	+			
– sulfuric acid	+			
– synthetic ethanol	+			
– vinyl chloride		+		
Detergents	+			
Electric and electronic equipment	+	+	+	+
Fertilizers	+		+	+
Food products	+	+	+	+
Health services	+	+	+	+
Instruments	+	+	+	+
Lead–acid batteries	+			
Leather	+	+	+	+
Metal plating	+	+	+	+
Metal cleaning and pickling	+	+	+	+
Metal extraction and ore processing	+	+	+	+
Oil and gas extraction	+	+		+
Petroleum and coal products	+	+	+	+
Photography shops	+	+	+	+
Printing and publishing	+	+	+	+
Paper and allied products	+	+	+	+
Rubber and plastic products	+	+		+
Semiconductors		+	+	
Soap	+			
Steel	+	+	+	
Textile products	+	+	+	+
Zinc galvanizing		+		

From US National Institute for Occupational Safety and Health (1974, 1976); Burgess (1981); Soule (1982); US National Institute for Occupational Safety and Health (1990)

isopropyl oil (by-products), and benzene (process chemical) (see section 1.2.1). According to veteran employees of a plant in the USA where synthetic ethanol was produced from 1930 to 1968 and isopropanol from 1928 to 1949 by the strong-acid method, the process was initially poorly controlled, and misting of sulfuric acid and other agents took place during the opening of reaction vessels; later, the process was operated from a well-ventilated remote-control office (Teta *et al.*, 1992). Maximal air concentrations of diisopropyl sulfate over a spill in the USA have been calculated (Lynch *et al.*, 1979; see the monograph on diisopropyl sulfate, section 1.3.2).

Table 8. Occupations in which there is potential exposure to strong inorganic acids

Occupation	Sulfuric acid	Hydrochloric acid	Nitric acid	Phosphoric acid
Alloy workers	+	+	+	
Anodizers	+	+	+	+
Artists	+	+	+	
Battery workers	+			
Cement workers		+		
Chemical workers	+	+	+	+
Chemists	+	+	+	+
Coke production	+	+	+	+
Corn millers	+			+
Crane operators	+	+	+	+
Detergent manufacturers	+			
Dyers		+	+	
Electroplaters	+	+	+	+
Electrowinners		+	+	
Explosives manufacturers			+	
Firefighters		+		
Fertilizer processors	+		+	+
Jewellers		+	+	
Laboratory workers	+	+	+	+
Leather manufacturers	+	+	+	+
Maintenance workers	+	+	+	+
Metal cleaners, picklers, cranemen	+	+	+	+
Metal workers	+	+	+	+
Oil workers	+	+		
Paper mill workers	+	+	+	+
Petrochemical workers	+	+	+	+
Photography lab workers	+	+	+	+
Platers	+	+	+	+
Printing machine operators	+	+	+	+
Refinery operators	+	+	+	
Soap manufacturers	+			
Sheet metal workers	+	+	+	
Steel workers	+	+	+	
Textile workers	+	+	+	+
Toll-booth workers	+		+	
Wire millers		+	+	
Zinc die casters	+	+	+	+

From Burgess (1981); Soule (1982); US National Institute for Occupational Safety and Health (1990)

1.4.2 *Synthetic ethanol manufacture*

No measurements of exposure to sulfuric acid in synthetic ethanol plants have been published. Potential exposures include ethylene and sulfuric acid (raw materials), diethyl and ethyl hydrogen sulfates (intermediates), ethanol (product), diethyl ether (by-product), phosphoric acid (catalyst) and benzene, cyclohexane or ethylene glycol (process chemicals) (see section 1.2.1). According to interviews with supervisors at a synthetic ethanol plant in the USA, there is opportunity for exposure to acid mist in the general plant area and particularly in operations involving vat-type acid coolers operated in an open mode. Exposure to diethyl sulfate is also possible, e.g., during pump seal leakages and maintenance and cleaning of absorbers and extract soakers. Maximal air concentrations of diethyl sulfate over a spill have been calculated (Lynch *et al.*, 1979; see the monograph on diethyl sulfate, section 1.3.2).

1.4.3 *Pickling and other acid treatment of metals*

Most of the data on occupational exposures to acid aerosols have been obtained in the plating and pickling industries; in general, these data represent the highest measured exposures. These data are summarized in Table 9. Sulfuric, hydrochloric, nitric and phosphoric acids are all used in pickling processes. Phosphoric acid use is generally limited to pickling, chemical polishing and phosphate conversion coatings. Sulfuric, hydrochloric and nitric acids are also used for electroplating. Plating processes that involve one of these acids include decorative (bright) and hard chromium, nickel, copper, tin and platinum plating.

(a) Pickling, cleaning, etching

Arithmetic means of the concentrations of sulfuric acid in the air during pickling and acid cleaning ranged from < 0.01 to 5.6 mg/m^3.

Arithmetic mean concentrations of hydrochloric acid in the air of Finnish and US plants ranged from < 0.2 to 13.6 mg/m^3; in a study in China, a mean value of 59 mg/m^3 was observed (Xu & Zhang, 1985). Individual measurements of hydrochloric acid in air ranged from 0.2 to 49.8 in French (Lamant *et al.*, 1989), German (Mappes, 1980) and Russian (Muravyeva *et al.*, 1987) studies. Geometric mean air concentrations of hydrochloric acid at six sites in a Dutch zinc galvanizing plant were 1.8–12.4 mg/m^3; the estimated arithmetic means (assuming a lognormal distribution) were approximately 2.3–15 mg/m^3 (Remijn *et al.*, 1982).

Few measurements are available of exposure to nitric acid; individual concentrations in air are 0.01–0.4 mg/m^3. The concentrations of phosphoric acid in air were measured in three studies: ≤ 0.04 mg/m^3 (Ruhe & Donohue, 1980), < 0.67 mg/m^3 (Daniels & Orris, 1981) and 0.03 mg/m^3 (Geissert, 1977).

Other exposures that may occur during acid cleaning of metals are to chromic acid, chromates, hydrogen fluoride, sodium fluoride, sodium hydroxide and alkaline salts. In an evaluation by the US National Institute for Occupational Safety and Health of health hazards in one steel manufacturing facility in the USA, detectable quantities of iron oxide (average, 0.8 mg/m^3; range, 0.34–2.7 mg/m^3) and lead (average, 0.04 mg/m^3; range, none detected to 0.27 mg/m^3) were measured in 14 full-shift personal samples (Price, 1977). Copper, manganese, chromium, zirconium, hafnium, respirable free silica, phenol and formaldehyde were not detected.

Table 9. Occupational exposures to strong inorganic acid mists and vapours during acid treatment of metals

Operation	Acid	Industry	Sample type	No. of samples	Air concentration (mg/m³) Mean	Air concentration (mg/m³) Range	Year of measurement	Country	Reference
Pickling									
Batch	H$_2$SO$_4$	Surface treatment	NR	2	5.6	0.7–10.5	1957, 1966	Finland	FIOH (1990)
Pickle hooker		Steel	Personal	7	0.15	0.07–0.25	1975	USA	Beaumont et al. (1987)
Ass't pickle hooker			Personal	4	0.20	<0.03–0.48			
Crane operator			Personal	4	0.22	0.15–0.29			
		Wire manufacture (cleaning department)	Personal	20	0.22	<0.01–0.64	1976–77	USA	Haas & Geissert (1977)
Pickle tanks		Steel	Area	2	0.15	0.12–0.27	1977	USA	Beaumont et al. (1987)
Crane operator			Area	10	0.25	0.01–0.50			
		Steel	Personal	6	0.15	0.09–0.19	1977	USA	Price (1977)
			Area	2	0.20	0.12–0.27			
Crane operator		Steel and alloy wire mill	Area	8	0.29	0.13–0.50	1977	USA	Geissert (1977)
Crane cab and catwalk			Area	13	0.68	0.11–2.94			
Cold finishing		Steel rod and wire mill	Area	3	0.032	0.016–0.05	1979	USA	Young (1979a)
		Seamless steel tubing manufacture	Personal full shift	13	0.17	0.08–0.47	1980	USA	Daniels & Orris (1981)
			Personal short term	6	NR	<0.67–0.97			
		Radio tower manufacture	Personal	13	0.11	0.05–0.18	1981	USA	Kominsky (1981a)
			Area	5	2.97	1.05–5.66			
Milling area near pickling area		Steel	Personal	4	<0.1		1986	USA	Ahrenholz (1987)
			Area	4	<0.1				
Continuous		Steel	Personal	8	0.1	<0.01–0.16	1977	USA	Anania et al. (1978)
			Area	2	0.05	<0.01–0.09			
Crane operator			Area	2	0.1	0.09–0.14			
			Personal	2	0.16	NR			
Cold strip mill		Nonfabricated steel	Area	3	0.92	0.35–1.20	1979	USA	Young (1979b)
Finishing			Area	2	0.09	0.039–0.14			

Table 9 (contd)

Operation	Acid	Industry	Sample type	No. of samples	Air concentration (mg/m³) Mean	Air concentration (mg/m³) Range	Year of measurement	Country	Reference
Pickling (contd)									
Batch	HCl	Zinc galvanizing	Personal	51	5.3[a]	2.09[b]	1978-82	Netherlands	Remijn et al. (1982)
				50	4.1[a]	2.00[b]			
				51	2.3[a]	1.82[b]			
				52	1.8[a]	2.00[b]			
				47	3.4[a]	2.29[b]			
				52	12.4[a]	1.82[b]			
Crane cab		Steel and alloy wire mill	Area	12	0.4	<0.004–2.72	1977	USA	Geissert (1977)
Crane cab detector tubes			Personal	4	1.0	0.5–1.5			
Continuous		Welding wire	Area	2	0.15	0.1–0.2	1979	USA	Lee (1980)
		Steel	NR	10	59	5–175	NR	China	Xu & Zhang (1985)
'Acid pickling'		Surface treatment	NR	2	5.66	4.47–6.7	1952–67	Finland	FIOH (1990)
'Pickling'		Steel	NR	3	29.2	26.5–33.5	1980	Germany	Mappes (1980)
				4	3.73	1.7–5.2			
				8	5.74	3.8–8.4			
				6	2.05	0.8–4.5			
'Pickling'		Galvanization	NR	NR		1.36–6.88	NR	France	Lamant et al. (1989)
Milling area near pickling area		Steel	Personal	4	<0.2		1986	USA	Ahrenholz (1987)
			Area	4	<0.2				
Batch Short term	H₃PO₄	Steel	Personal	NR	<0.67		1981	USA	Daniels & Orris (1981)
Cab and catwalk		Steel and alloy wire mill	Area	3	0.03	0.02–0.05	1977	USA	Geissert (1977)

Table 9 (contd)

Operation	Acid	Industry	Sample type	No. of samples	Air concentration (mg/m³) Mean	Air concentration (mg/m³) Range	Year of measurement	Country	Reference
Cleaning									
	H_2SO_4	Coin manufacture	NR	2	0.8	0.3–1.2	1952	Finland	FIOH (1990)
		Metal processing	NR	3	1.7	0.6–3.2	1960	Finland	FIOH (1990)
		Metalware manufacture	NR	2	0.2	ND–0.3	1974, 1975	Finland	Skyttä (1978)
		Aircraft manufacture	Area	3	<0.01		1977	USA	Hervin et al. (1977)
		Small electronic parts	Area	1	0.01		1980	USA	Sheehy et al. (1982a)
		Semiconductors	Area	1	<0.01		1981	USA	Gunter (1982)
Strip acid, enclosed process, ventilation		Steel	Area	48	0.333	<0.248–>1.205	NR	Wales (UK)	Anfield & Warner (1968)
Small steel components		Automobile manufacture	Area	85	2.96	<0.360–>14.43	NR		
	HCl	Surface treatment	NR	2	1.79	1.34–2.1	1952–67	Finland	FIOH (1990)
		Small electronic parts	Area	2	0.25	0.22–0.28	1980	USA	Sheehy et al. (1982a)
Continuous	HCl	Continuous coiled steel galvanizing	Personal	9	0.23	0.16–0.29	1981	USA	Kominsky (1981b)
Attendant's desk			Area	1	0.27				
Crane cab			Area	7	0.87	0.48–2.20			
	HNO_3	Semiconductors	Area	2	<0.25		1981	USA	Gunter (1982)
		Small metal components	Area	2	0.021	0.014–0.027	1975–76	USA	Geissert (1976)
		Small electronic parts	Area	NR	0.03		1980	USA	Sheehy et al. (1982a)
	H_3PO_4	Semiconductors	Personal	4	0.12	ND–0.4	1983	USA	Moseley (1983)
Chromic acid stripping		Automobile trim	Personal	2	<0.01		1976	USA	Ruhe & Andersen (1977)

Table 9 (contd)

Operation	Acid	Industry	Sample type	No. of samples	Air concentration (mg/m^3) Mean	Air concentration (mg/m^3) Range	Year of measurement	Country	Reference
Etching	H_2SO_4	Aircraft maintenance	Personal	3	0.067	<0.047–0.106	1981	USA	Godbey (1982)
			Area	4	0.062	0.053–0.083			
	HCl	Galvanizing	NR	NR	4.14	0.2–49.8	NR	USSR	Muravyeva et al. (1987)
	HNO_3	Aircraft manufacture	Area	4	0.1	NR	1977	USA	Hervin et al. (1977)
Titanium			Area	8	0.10	0.01–0.30			
Titanium			Area	6	0.027	0.01–0.05			
Aluminium		Semiconductors	Personal	7	0.03	ND–0.2	1983	USA	Moseley (1983)
Electrolytic refining									
Tank house	H_2SO_4	Secondary copper smelting and refining	Personal	4	0.072	0.056–0.097	1982–83	USA	Kominsky & Cherniack (1984)
			Area	2	0.043	0.031–0.055			
Millwright			Personal	3	0.114	0.065–0.191			
Tank house			Personal	4	0.13	0.083–0.265	1978	USA	Kominsky & Kreiss (1981)
			Area	1	0.042				
Electrowinning		Copper cathode	Personal	12	0.27	0.02–0.79	1978	USA	Ruhe & Donohue (1980)
			Area	4	0.21	0.08–0.35			
Electrowinning cell house		Zinc plant	NR	NR	NR	0.5–1.0	1977	Finland	Roto (1980)
Sulfatizing, roasting		Cobalt plant	NR	4	5.6	3.3–8.2	1968	Finland	FIOH (1990)
Dissolving			NR	4	0.93	0.5–1.6			
Electrolysis	H_2SO_4	Metal processing	NR	8	0.3	0.2–0.4	1960	Finland	FIOH (1990)
		Nickel manufacture	NR	11	0.6	0.2–1.2	1966	Finland	FIOH (1990)
		Metal manufacture	NR	2	1.3	1.2–1.4	1972–73	Finland	Skyttä (1978)
Incineration		Secondary silver smelting and refining	Area	2	0.01	NR	1981	USA	Apol (1981a)
Slag removal	HCl	Cable manufacture	NR	1	3		1972	Finland	Skyttä (1978)
Refining	HNO_3	Secondary silver smelting and refining	Personal	2	0.41	NR	1981	USA	Apol (1981a)
			Area	2	0.39	0.36–0.41			

Table 9 (contd)

Operation	Acid	Industry	Sample type	No. of samples	Air concentration (mg/m³) Mean	Air concentration (mg/m³) Range	Year of measurement	Country	Reference
Plating	H_2SO_4								
		Electronic instrument	Personal	2	0.14	0.02–0.26	1975–76	USA	Ruhe (1976)
		Aerospace component	Personal	3	<0.09		1978	USA	Evans (1978)
		Small electronic parts	Area	4	0.12	0.04–0.23	1980	USA	Sheehy et al. (1982a)
		Chrome plating	Personal	6	<0.04	<0.04–<0.05	1980	USA	Sheehy et al. (1982b)
			Area	1	0.06				
Over liquid			Area	3	<0.05	SD, 0.01			
On tank perimeter			Area	6	1.7	SD, 1.87			
Before ventilation			Area	2	7.3	NR			
After ventilation			Area	2	4.4	NR			
Mixed acid bath			Area	6	5.15	0.74–11.84			
		Hard chrome plating	Personal	8	0.2	<0.2–0.4	1981	USA	Sheehy et al. (1982c)
			Area	12	0.4	0.2–0.7			
			Area	6	0.4	0.3–0.5			
			Area	15	0.4	0.2–0.8			
			Personal	5	0.11	0.10–0.12	1981	USA	Mortimer et al. (1982)
			Area	15	<0.11	<0.11–0.15			
			Area	3	0.013	0.010–0.015	1981	USA	Ahrenholz & Anderson (1981)
		Electroplating	NR	NR	1.8	NR	NR	USSR	Kuprin et al. (1986)
Cadmium covering			NR	NR	0.58	0.08–1.33	NR	USSR	Muravyeva et al. (1987)
Copper covering			NR	NR	0.47	0.05–0.7	NR		
Tin-bismuth covering			NR	NR	0.74	0.01–2.33	NR		
Copper coating		Welding wire	Area	2	0.05	ND–0.1	1979	USA	Lee (1980)
Plating tank		Hard chrome plating	Area	10	0.48	0.17–1.4	1981	USA	Spottswood et al. (1983)
				8	0.30	0.13–0.36			
				15	0.38	0.21–0.60			
				23	0.82	0.53–1.28			
				12	0.12	NR			

Table 9 (contd)

Operation	Acid	Industry	Sample type	No. of samples	Air concentration (mg/m³) Mean	Air concentration (mg/m³) Range	Year of measurement	Country	Reference
Plating (contd)									
General area			Area	4	0.18	0.15–0.27			
				2	0.10	NR			
			Personal	4	0.433	0.109–0.903			
				4	0.421	0.107–0.967			
				2	0.128	0.110–0.145			
		Fishing rod component	Personal	1	<0.06		1986	USA	Daniels & Gunter (1987)
			Area	3	<0.19				
	HCl	Electronic instrument	Personal	4	0.30	0.001–0.48	1975–76	USA	Ruhe (1976)
			Area	1	0.15				
		Small electronic parts	Area	6	0.14	<0.006–0.54	1980	USA	Sheehy et al. (1982a)
Bright dip tank		Fishing rod component	Personal	1	<0.06		1986	USA	Daniels & Gunter (1987)
Zinc coating	HCl	Surface treatment	NR	3	7.45	3.58–14.5	1952–67	Finland	FIOH (1990)
Tin coating			NR	1	0.75				
Cadmium coating			NR	1	0.75				
Before ventilation	HNO₃	Aerospace component	Personal	9	0.034	0.01–0.13	1978	USA	Evans (1978)
After ventilation		Chrome plating	Area	2	0.76		1980	USA	Sheehy et al. (1982b)
Nitric acid bath			Area	2	0.48				
Mixed acid bath			Area	6	1.3	0.05–2.8			
			Area	17	0.97	0.05–2.76			
			Personal	5	0.26	<0.04–0.64			
Bright dip tank		Small electronic parts	Area	6	0.05	0.03–0.10	1980	USA	Sheehy et al. (1982a)
Anodizing	H₂SO₄	Aluminium galvanizing	NR	NR	0.65	0.05–2.1	NR	USSR	Muravyeva et al. (1987)
		Automobile trim	Personal	2	<0.01		1976	USA	Ruhe & Andersen (1977)
	HCl	Aircraft component	Personal	3	0.09	0.03–0.2	1976	USA	Gunter (1976)
	HNO₃	Aircraft component	Personal	3	0.03	0.01–0.04			
	HNO₃	Automobile trim	Personal	3	0.05	0.02–0.10	1976	USA	Ruhe & Andersen (1977)

Table 9 (contd)

Operation	Acid	Industry	Sample type	No. of samples	Air concentration (mg/m^3) Mean	Air concentration (mg/m^3) Range	Year of measurement	Country	Reference
Miscellaneous									
Acid recovery	H$_2$SO$_4$	Steel	Area	42	0.795	<0.227-2.626	NR	Wales (UK)	Anfield & Warner (1968)
Dip		Copper pipe	Personal	5	0.06	<0.05-0.17	1974	USA	Gunter & Bodner (1974)
Hydrolysis		Ferrovanadium	Area	NR	4.7	2.0-7.5	NR	USSR	Kazimov (1977)
Electrochemical drilling		Jet engine components	Personal	17	0.09	<0.1-1.27	1975	USA	Kominsky (1975)
			Area	4	<0.1				
Photo-resist		Semiconductors	Area	4	0.03	<0.01-0.11	1981	USA	Gunter (1981)
Aluminium finishing		Custom finishing	Personal	7	0.10	0.04-0.19	1979	USA	Ruhe & Donohue (1980)
			Area	1	0.11				
Acid testing office		Steel sheet and tin plate	Area	1	0.026		1979	USA	Young et al. (1979)
Surface treatment		Metalware	NR	11	0.3	0.01-0.7	1971-76	Finland	Skyttä (1978)
Electrochemical drilling	HCl	Jet engine component	Area	1	0.83	0.03-0.09	1975	USA	Kominsky (1981a)
			Personal	2	0.06				
Leaching		Titanium sponge model	Area	2	0.31	0.15-0.47	1978	USA	Moseley et al. (1980)
Lighting		Galvanization	NR	NR	1.03	0.66-2.3	NR	USSR	Muravyeva et al. (1987)
Sintering		Steel	NR	8	ND		1955	Finland	FIOH (1990)
Opening of oven		Metalware	NR	2	13.6	9.4-17.9	1975	Finland	Skyttä (1978)
Surface treatment			NR	4	1.55	0.5-3.4	1971, 1975		
Diffusion	HNO$_3$	Semiconductors	Personal	8	0.01	ND-0.03	1983	USA	Moseley (1983)
Aluminium finishing		Custom finishing	Personal	7	0.046	0.02-0.15	1979	USA	Ruhe & Donohue (1980)
			Area	1	0.06				
Surface treatment		Metalware	NR	1	0.3		1971	Finland	Skyttä (1978)
Aluminium finishing	H$_3$PO$_4$	Custom finishing	Personal	7	0.01	<0.003-0.04	1979	USA	Ruhe & Donohue (1980)
			Area	1	0.04				

ND, not detected; NR, not reported
[a] Geometric mean
[b] Geometric standard deviation

(b) Electrolytic refining

Mean exposures to sulfuric acid during electrolytic refining were 0.01–5.6 mg/m^3. Other exposures in smelters and in the secondary metals industry are to arsenic, sulfur dioxide, cadmium and other metal dusts (Kaminsky & Cherniack, 1984).

(c) Plating and anodizing

During chromium plating in US facilities, the mean concentrations of sulfuric acid in air ranged from 0.01 to 7.3 mg/m^3. Information on exposure during anodizing is limited; however, the air concentrations of nitric, hydrochloric and sulfuric acids appear to be lower than during plating. Other exposures in plating and anodizing processes may be to hydrogen fluoride, ammonium chloride, zinc chloride, zinc oxide, sulfurous anhydride, nitrogen oxides, chromic acid, hydrogen cyanide, alkaline salts, alkaline mists, metal salts and metal dusts, depending on the process (Soule, 1982; Lamant et al., 1989).

1.4.4 *Sulfuric acid manufacture*

In a sulfuric acid plant in Sweden, area samples taken in 1979–80 contained sulfuric acid at 0.1–3.1 mg/m^3; breathing zone samples contained < 0.1–2.9 mg/m^3. Sulfur dioxide concentrations measured in 1969–84 ranged from 2.4 to 124 mg/m^3 in area samples (mean, 9.1 mg/m^3) and 1.1–23 mg/m^3 in breathing zone samples (mean, 3.6 mg/m^3). Other potential exposures in sulfuric acid plants include iron disulfide (starting material for sulfur dioxide), ferric oxide (end-product of roasting of iron disulfide), sulfur trioxide (intermediate), vanadium pentoxide (catalyst) and sulfuric acid (end-product). If iron disulfide includes arsenic as an impurity, small amounts of arsenic oxides may also be present in the air of the roasting departments of the plants. Concentrations of total dust, arsenic and quartz were reported (Englander et al., 1988).

In a Finnish sulfuric acid plant, the concentration of sulfuric acid in seven air samples ranged from none detected to 1.7 mg/m^3, with a mean concentration of 0.9 mg/m^3 (Skyttä, 1978). Air concentrations of sulfuric acid in three area samples taken in a sulfuric acid plant at a US copper smelter in 1984 were 0.15–0.24 mg/m^3 (mean, 0.21 mg/m^3) (Gunter & Seligman, 1984). The concentration of sulfuric acid in working area samples in a Russian sulfuric acid plant ranged from 1.8 to 4.6 mg/m^3 (Petrov, 1987); that in general area samples was 0.5–2.4 mg/m^3.

1.4.5 *Soap and detergent manufacture*

Sulfuric acid concentrations measured in 1974 in the air in a soap production plant in Italy were 0.64–1.12 mg/m^3 in the hydrolysis and saponification areas. Other exposures were to soap powder, glycerol, fatty acids, nickel and its compounds (up to 0.07 mg/m^3) and mineral oils (see IARC, 1987) (1.2 mg/m^3) (Forastiere et al., 1987).

1.4.6 *Nitric acid manufacture*

Most nitric acid is manufactured by the catalytic oxidation of ammonia in air in the presence of a platinum catalyst. No data on occupational exposures have been published.

1.4.7 *Phosphate fertilizer manufacture*

Table 10 summarizes occupational exposures to acid mists and vapours in the phosphate fertilizer manufacturing industry. Workers in the phosphate fertilizer industry are potentially exposed to calcium phosphate minerals (including calcium fluoride), sulfuric acid, phosphoric acid (partly as phosphorus pentoxide), calcium sulfate, ammonia and ammonium phosphate (see section 1.2.7). Other potential exposures during mining and chemical processing of phosphate rocks include silica, chromium, arsenic, vanadium and alpha and gamma radiation from uranium-238 and radium-226 impurities of phosphate minerals. In two studies, exposure to ionizing radiation was reported to be low in comparison with recommended standards (Herrick, 1982; Checkoway *et al.*, 1985a).

1.4.8 *Lead battery (accumulator) manufacture*

Sulfuric acid is used in the manufacture of lead–acid batteries. The highest exposures have been found in plate forming, where lead plates are immersed in tanks of dilute sulfuric acid through which a current is passed. Gas bubbles generate an acid mist above the tanks. In the forming process, the lead plates are fused and then encased in a shell to prepare them for charging; or the battery is filled with acid and charged with direct current. Table 11 presents the available data on occupational exposures to sulfuric acid in this industry, the highest value found being 11.6 mg/m^3.

In a study of five battery manufacturing plants in the USA, the highest levels of sulfuric acid mist were usually measured in forming, and sometimes in charging, assembly and battery repair. The concentrations of lead, arsine and stibine in air during forming also tend to be higher than in most other operations (Jones & Gamble, 1984).

Only one study was available to the Working Group on the particle size distribution of acid mists in the work environment. In a study of five US battery manufacturing plants, the average mass median aerodynamic diameter of H_2SO_4 mist was 5–6 μm, with an average geometric standard deviation of 4–5 μm, depending on the impactor used (Jones & Gamble, 1984).

1.4.9 *Other industries*

Table 12 summarizes the available data on occupational exposures in other industries in which acid mists or vapours may be generated. Although the numbers of measurements were often limited, the highest exposures were to hydrochloric acid during titanium dioxide production in the USSR (Feigin, 1986), in the sand chlorination area of a zirconium and hafnium plant in the USA (Apol & Tanaka, 1978), during short-term exposure of fire fighters during a training exercise in the USA (Zey & Richardson, 1989) and during painting in Finland (FIOH, 1990) and to phosphoric acid during fertilizer production in Finland (FIOH, 1990).

1.5 Regulations and guidelines

Occupational exposure limits for sulfuric acid in some countries or regions are presented in Table 13; those for nitric acid and for phosphoric acid are presented in Tables 14 and 15, respectively. Those for hydrochloric acid are given in the monograph on p. 196.

Table 10. Occupational exposures to strong inorganic acid mists and vapours during phosphate fertilizer manufacture

Operation/process	Acid	Sample	No. of samples	Air concentration (mg/m^3) Mean	Air concentration (mg/m^3) Range	Year of measurement	Country	Reference
Acid tanks, compressors, precipitation	HNO$_3$	NR	5	38.7	1.8–14.5	1965	Finland	FIOH (1990)
Process operator	HNO$_3$	NR	1	1.3		1975	USA	Cassady et al. (1975)
Cleaning phosphoric acid reactor vessel in phosphate fertilizer/-phosphoric acid production	H$_2$SO$_4$ H$_3$PO$_4$	Area Area	8 9	<0.07 0.25	<0.005–2.12			
Cleaning H$_3$PO$_4$ reactor vessel	H$_3$PO$_4$ H$_2$SO$_4$	NR NR	NR NR	NR NR	0.02–0.08 0.08–0.13	1975	USA	Wolf & Cassady (1976)
Cleaning H$_3$PO$_4$ reactor vessel	H$_3$PO$_4$ H$_2$SO$_4$	Personal Personal	9 11	0.075 0.571	0.03–0.129 0.16–3.31	1976	USA	Stephenson et al. (1977a)
Cleaning H$_3$PO$_4$ reactor vessel	H$_3$PO$_4$ H$_2$SO$_4$	Personal Personal	4 3	0.183 0.068	0.03–0.25 0.013–0.16	1976	USA	Stephenson et al. (1977b)
General area	H$_3$PO$_4$ H$_2$SO$_4$	Area Area	4 5	0.31 0.136	0.17–0.52 0.03–0.22			
Phosphoric acid evaporation and agitation in ammonium phosphate fertilizer production	H$_3$PO$_4$ H$_2$SO$_4$	Personal Personal	11 11	0.34 0.13	<0.05–3.43 <0.05–1.26	1985	USA	Apol & Singal (1987)
Drilling level in superphosphate fertilizer manufacture	H$_2$SO$_4$ H$_2$SO$_4$[a]	NR NR	1 1	0.3 8.3		1957 1951	Finland	FIOH (1990)
Superphosphate plant, work area	H$_2$SO$_4$ H$_2$SO$_4$	NR NR	NR NR	NR NR	5.2–9.2 2.7–4.4	NR	USSR	Tadzhibaeva & Gol'eva (1976)

NR, not reported
[a] Concentration of sulfur trioxide calculated as sulfuric acid

Table 11. Occupational exposures to sulfuric acid mists during lead battery (accumulator) manufacture

Operation/process	Sample	No. of samples	Air concentration (mg/m^3)		Year of measurement	Country	Reference
			Mean	Range			
Accumulator room in electricity plant, worst case		1	11.6		1955	Finland	FIOH (1990)
Plate forming		NR	>16 (humid day)	3.0–16.6 (dry day)	NR	USA	Malcolm & Paul (1961)
Charging		NR		<0.8–2.5			
Plate forming	Area	38	1.38	<0.183–>5.618	NR	Wales (UK)	Anfield & Warner (1968)
	Area	12	0.971	<0.221–3.517			
Battery manufacture	Area	>12		26.1–35.0	NR	Egypt	El-Sadik et al. (1972)
		>12		12.6–13.5			
Forming		3	0.16	0.07–0.25	1971, 1973, 1975	Finland	Skyttä (1978)
Charging in brewery battery shop		33	<0.1		1976	USA	Rivera (1976)
Acid room	Area	1	0.03		1978	USA	Young (1979c)
Charging	Area	1	0.04				
Assembly	Area	1	0.03				
Charging	Area	1	0.107		1978	USA	Young (1979d)
Wetdown area	Area	1	0.064				
Acid room	Area	1	0.141				
Forming	NR	1	1.03		1978	USA	Young (1979e)
Acid room	NR	1	0.09				
Charging	NR	1	0.03				
Various	Personal	2		0.1–>0.1	1979	USA	Costello & Landrigan (1980)
	Personal	4		0.08–0.1			
	Personal	14		0.06–0.08			
	Personal	15		0.04–0.06			
	Personal	9		0.02–0.04			
	Personal	3		<0.02			

Table 11 (contd)

Operation/process	Sample	No. of samples	Air concentration (mg/m³) Mean	Air concentration (mg/m³) Range	Year of measurement	Country	Reference
Charging in municipal transit battery shop	Personal Area	1 1	0.029 0.068		1980	USA	Hartle (1980)
Charging in diesel engine and locomotive manufacture	Personal Area	12 12	0.015 0.024	0.01–0.027 0.008–0.040	1980	USA	Lucas & Cone (1982)
Various Forming	Personal Area	9 1	<0.18 <0.19		1984	USA	Singal et al. (1985)
Various	Personal	18 55 37 57 58	0.08 0.14 0.08 0.35 0.16	SD, 0.07 SD, 0.14 SD, 0.08 SD, 0.35 SD, 0.21	NR	USA	Jones & Gamble (1984)
Lead-acid battery recharge Short term Full shift	Area Personal Personal	4 4 1	0.01 0.09 0.015	0.009–0.011 0.05–0.12	1988	USA	Daniels (1988)

NR, not reported

Table 12. Occupational exposures to strong inorganic acid mists and vapours in various industries

Acid	Operation	Sample type	No. of samples	Air concentration (mg/m^3) Mean	Air concentration (mg/m^3) Range	Year of measurement	Country	Reference
H$_2$SO$_4$	Acid preparation in paper mill	NR	3	4.5	0.3–11.5	1951	Finland	FIOH (1990)
	Paper machine	NR	4	6.3	2.7–8.9	1951–59		
	Hall near acid tanks and storage	NR	3	0.6	0.5–0.8	1959		
	Copper smelter[a]	NR	17	1.0	<0.1–3.7	1952–57		
	Nitrocellulose manufacture: oleum storage, denitration, acid centrifuge, mixing of acid	NR	4	0.7	0.2–1.2	1952		
	Sulfite pulp production: acid plant[a]	NR	3	<0.2		1954–55		
	leakage	NR	1	18				
	Reaction, filtering, evaporation in titanium dioxide manufacture							Skyttä (1978)
	Reaction	NR	5	0.4	0.3–0.8	1961		
	Dissolving	NR	1	2.3		1971–74		
	Filtering	NR	1	1.0				
	control	NR	2	0.4	0.2–0.5			
	Waste treatment plant in aircraft maintenance facility	NR	2	<0.015		1972	USA	Hervin & Reifschneider (1973)
	Heating, slag removal, water treatment at power plant	NR	1	0.6		1972	Finland	Skyttä (1978)
	Electrolytic treatment in offset printing	NR	3	0.2	ND–0.5	1974–76		
	Extraction in ammonium phosphate production	NR	NR	NR	2.5–14	NR	USSR	Danielyants (1976)
	Tollbooth in national park	Personal and area	11	0.52	0.18–1.14	1976	USA	Haas & Geissert (1976)
	Guard booth at border crossing	NR	4	ND		1979	USA	Markel & Ruhe (1981)
	Desulfurization control room in coke plant	Area	1	0.014		1979	USA	Lewis (1980)
	Volcano observation	NR	1	1.0		1979	USA	Belanger (1980)
	Cement company	Area	10	0.05	ND–0.2	1980	USA	Jankovic (1980)
		Personal	4	0.15	0.1–0.22			

Table 12 (contd)

Acid	Operation	Sample type	No. of samples	Air concentration (mg/m^3) Mean	Air concentration (mg/m^3) Range	Year of measurement	Country	Reference
H_2SO_4 (contd)	Paper machine tending	Personal and area	27	0.01	<0.01–0.06	1981	USA	Apol (1981b)
	Alum batch processing	Personal	3	0.5	0.09–0.38	1981	USA	McGlothlin et al. (1982)
		Area	4	0.08	0.03–0.2			
	Deliming and bating in chrome leather tannery	NR	6	0.48	0–0.96	1981	USA	Stern et al. (1987)
	Belly pickling in leather manufacture	Personal	2	0.18	0.16–0.20	1982	USA	Fajen (1982)
	Tanning	Area	3	0.16	0.12–0.20			
	Wet milling in corn starch production	Area	NR	NR	<0.04–0.05	1985	USA	Almaguer & London (1986)
	Photography lab	Personal	1	0.02		1985	USA	Hunninen (1986)
		Area	1	<0.003				
	Pigmentary titanium dioxide production area	Area	NR	NR	2.03–3.66	NR	USSR	Feigin (1986)
	Mixing of odourizing chemicals	Area	4	<0.02		1987	USA	Pryor (1987)
		Personal	2	<0.02				
	Wet milling of corn products	Area	3	1.7	0.7–2.5	1988	USA	Gunter (1988)
HCl	Agricultural research	Personal	2	11.8	8.5–15	1951	Finland	FIOH (1990)
	Cooling department in HCl plant	NR	1	4		1954		
	Reaction department in TiO$_2$ plant	NR	4	2	0.08–0.5	1961		
	Furnaces, HCl absorption plant, charging in NaSO$_2$ plant	NR	28	6.4	1.3–23.8	1963–67		
	Reactor, evaporators, driers in CaCl$_2$ plant	NR	13	1.3	ND–6.9	1963–67		
	Etching of offset printing plates	NR	1	15		1966		
	Pressing of records	NR	4	ND		1966		
	Acid room in electric bulb plant	NR	1	3.1		1966		
	Tin soldering with HCl	NR	4	8.2	6.0–10.4	1967–68		
	Welding in metalware plant	NR	2	ND		1967–68		
	Etching of offset printing plates	NR	9	3.7	0.15–18	1971–76		
	Drying of offset printing plates	NR	1	3.9		1974		Skyttä (1978)
	Burning resin in offset printing plant	NR	1	0.45		1976		

Table 12 (contd)

Acid	Operation	Sample type	No. of samples	Air concentration (mg/m³) Mean	Air concentration (mg/m³) Range	Year of measurement	Country	Reference
HCl (contd)	Chemical storage	NR	1	60		1972	Finland	Skyttä (1978)
	Mixing of lime, drying of sewage sludge	NR	2	0.75				
	Sand chlorination in zirconium and hafnium extraction	Area	9	3.6	0.08–7.3	1975–77	USA	Apol & Tanaka (1978)
	Heating slag removal, water treatment in power plant	NR	2	0.6	0.5–0.7	1976	Finland	Skyttä (1978)
	Zinc die casting in automobile parts plant	Area	2	0.05	ND–0.1	1977	USA	Gilles et al. (1977)
	Superwash treatment, seaming	NR	2	2.16	0.75–3.58	1975, 1976	Finland	Skyttä (1978)
	Organic flocculant batch mixing	Area	3	0.08	ND–0.14	1981	USA	McGlothlin et al. (1982)
		Personal	1	ND				
	Extrusion in polyvinyl chloride container plant	Area	3	0.25	0.19–0.28	1982	USA	Lucas & Schloemer (1982)
		Area	6	<0.005				
		Personal	2	<0.005				
	Wet milling in corn starch plant	Area	NR	NR	<0.02–0.93	NR	USA	Almaguer & London (1986)
	Working area in TiO₂ production	NR	NR	9.67	4.46–13.39	NR	USSR	Feigin (1986)
	Smoke bomb during firefighting training	NR	8	18.2	1.9–44	1987	USA	Zey & Richardson (1989)
HNO₃	Wet milling in corn products plant	Area	3	0.04	0.03–0.06	1988	USA	Gunter (1988)
	Pumps, presses in lanthanide plant	NR	2	1.6	1.0–1.8	1965	Finland	FIOH (1990)
	Printing machines (relief)	NR	1	1.03		1971	Finland	Skyttä (1978)
	Cleaning relief printing plates	NR	1	1.3		1971		
	Print-making in art college	Personal	2	0.83	0.50–1.15	1976	USA	Levy (1976)
		Area	1	0.06				
	Wet milling in corn products plant	Area	3	ND		1988	USA	Gunter (1988)
H₃PO₄	Phosphoric acid production	NR	NR	0.31	0.07–0.62	1974	Italy	Fabbri et al. (1977)
	Wet milling in corn products plant	Area	3	0.40	0.23–0.68	1988	USA	Gunter (1988)

NR, not reported; ND, not detected or below detection limit
[a]Concentration of sulfur trioxide calculated as sulfuric acid

Table 13. Occupational exposure limits and guidelines for sulfuric acid

Country or region	Year	Concentration (mg/m^3)	Interpretation[a]
Australia	1990	1	TWA
Austria	1982	1	TWA
Belgium	1990	1	TWA
		3	STEL
Bulgaria	1984	1	TWA
Chile	1983	0.8	TWA
China	1979	2	TWA
Czechoslovakia	1990	1	TWA
		2	STEL
Denmark	1990	1	TWA
Finland	1990	1[b]	TWA
		3[b]	STEL (15 min)
France	1990	1	TWA
		3	STEL
Germany	1990	1[b]	TWA
Hungary	1990	1	STEL
India	1983	1	TWA
Indonesia	1978	1	TWA
Italy	1978	1	TWA
Japan	1990	1	TWA
Mexico	1983	1	TWA
Netherlands	1985	1	TWA
Norway	1990	1	TWA
Poland	1990	1	TWA
Romania	1975	0.5	TWA
		1.5	Ceiling
Sweden	1990	1	TWA
		3	STEL (15 min)
Switzerland	1990	1	TWA
		2	STEL
Taiwan	1981	1	TWA
United Kingdom	1990	1	TWA
USA			
ACGIH	1990	1	TWA
		3	STEL
OSHA	1989	1	TWA
USSR	1990	1[b]	STEL

Table 13 (contd)

Country or region	Year	Concentration (mg/m^3)	Interpretation[a]
Venezuela	1978	1	TWA
		1	Ceiling
Yugoslavia	1971	1	TWA

From Cook (1987); US Occupational Safety and Health Administration (OSHA) (1989); American Conference of Governmental Industrial Hygienists (ACGIH) (1990); Direktoratet for Arbeidstilsynet (1990); International Labour Office (1991)
[a]TWA, full-shift time-weighted average; STEL, short-term exposure limit
[b]Skin irritant notation

Table 14. Occupational exposure limits and guidelines for nitric acid (CAS No. 7697-37-2)

Country or region	Year	Concentration (mg/m^3)	Interpretation[a]
Australia	1990	5	TWA
		10	STEL
Austria	1990	5.2	TWA
		10	STEL
Belgium	1990	5.2	TWA
		10	STEL
Chile	1983	4	TWA
Czechoslovakia	1990	2.5	TWA
		5	STEL
Denmark	1990	5	TWA
Germany	1990	25[b]	TWA
Finland	1990	5	TWA
		13	STEL (15 min)
France	1990	5	TWA
		10	STEL
Hungary	1990	5	STEL
India	1983	5	TWA
		10	STEL
Indonesia	1978	5	TWA
Italy	1978	5	TWA
Japan	1990	5.2	TWA
Mexico	1983	5	TWA
Netherlands	1986	5	TWA
Norway	1990	5	TWA
Poland	1990	10	TWA
Romania	1975	4	TWA
		10	Ceiling
Sweden	1990	5	TWA
		13	STEL (15 min)

Table 14 (contd)

Country or region	Year	Concentration (mg/m^3)	Interpretation[a]
Switzerland	1990	5	TWA
		10	STEL
Taiwan	1981	25	TWA
United Kingdom	1990	5	TWA
		10	STEL (10 min)
USA			
ACGIH	1990	5.2	TWA
		10	STEL
OSHA	1989	5	TWA
Venezuela	1978	5	TWA
		10	Ceiling
Yugoslavia	1971	25	TWA
USSR	1990	2	STEL

From Cook (1987); US Occupational Safety and Health Administration (OSHA) (1989); American Conference of Governmental Industrial Hygienists (ACGIH) (1990); Direktoratet for Arbeidstilsynet (1990); International Labour Office (1991)
[a]TWA, full-shift time-weighted average; STEL, short-term exposure limit
[b]Skin irritant notation

Table 15. Occupational exposure limits and guidelines for phosphoric acid (CAS No. 7664-38-2)

Country or region	Year	Concentration (mg/m^3)	Interpretation[a]
Australia	1990	1	TWA
		3	STEL
Belgium	1990	1	TWA
		3	STEL
Denmark	1990	1	TWA
Finland	1990	1[b]	TWA
		3[b]	STEL (15-min)
France	1990	1	TWA
		3	STEL
Indonesia	1978	1	TWA
Italy	1978	1	TWA
Japan	1990	1	TWA
Netherlands	1986	1	TWA
Norway	1990	1	TWA
Sweden	1990	1	TWA
		3	STEL (15-min)
Switzerland	1990	1	TWA

Table 15 (contd)

Country or region	Year	Concentration (mg/m^3)	Interpretation[a]
United Kingdom	1990	1	TWA
		3	STEL (10-min)
USA			
ACGIH	1990	1	TWA
		3	STEL
Venezuela	1978	1	TWA
		3	Ceiling
Yugoslavia	1971	1	TWA

From Cook (1987); American Conference of Governmental Industrial Hygienists (ACGIH) (1990); Direktoratet for Arbeidstilsynet (1990); International Labour Office (1991)
[a]TWA, full-shift time-weighted average; STEL, short-term exposure limit
[b]Skin irritant notation

2. Studies of Cancer in Humans

2.1 Case reports

Fifteen of the 30 cases of primary bronchial cancer seen in a hospital ward in Frankfurt, Germany, were from a plant which produced, up to 1931, sulfuric acid, hydrochloric acid and sulfates, secondary to the production of chromate (Alwens *et al.*, 1936). Four cases occurred among workers exposed only to acids for 24, 28, 31 and 42 years. Six of the 15 workers had worked exclusively in the chromate workshop, with employment periods ranging from 22 to 40 years.

2.2 Cohort studies

The cohort studies described below are summarized in Table 16 (p. 90).

2.2.1 *Isopropanol manufacture*

A cohort study of US chemical workers (Weil *et al.*, 1952) based on death claims for employees active in 1928–50 revealed 258 deaths from all causes; 34 (13.2%) were deaths due to cancer. This did not represent an excess when compared to US proportional mortality rates. A total of 182 workers had been employed in the isopropanol unit of the South Charleston plant studied by Teta *et al.*, 1992 (see p. 82) between 1928 and 1950; 71 had worked for more than five years, and 37 had worked for more than 10 years. Four of the six respiratory tract cancers observed were in the sinuses (in two workers who died and in two who survived), one was of the lung (in one dead worker) and one was of the larynx (in one surviving worker). The three who died were aged 30 to early 40s, but the age at diagnosis of the remaining three cases was not given. All six workers with cancer had worked for more than five years in the unit, and their exposure had started in the early 1930s, before any change was made in the unit. A highly significant excess risk for cancer of the paranasal sinuses was seen on comparison with the expected number, based on the US rate of 0.2%. [The Working Group noted that it was not clear what methods were used to enumerate the cohort; however, the excess was so large as to render this concern inconsequential.]

Hueper (1966) reviewed the data described by Weil *et al.* (1952) and a report by Eckardt (1959) of three cases of sinus cancer and two of cancer of the intrinsic larynx among workers at another isopropanol manufacturing plant. Hueper calculated a highly significant, age-specific excess incidence in men aged 45–54 years with at least nine years in isopropanol production; the relative risk is 21 for cancers of the nasal sinuses and larynx combined based on four cases [95% confidence interval (CI), 5.7–53.9]. [The Working Group noted that the basis for the comparison is not clear.]

A cohort study was carried out among 262 men who had been employed for at least one year during 1949–75 at an isopropanol plant in the United Kingdom and followed up to 1975 (Alderson & Rattan, 1980). There were 26 deaths (standardized mortality ratio [SMR], 1.10 [95% CI, 0.72–1.61]), including nine from cancer (SMR, 1.45 [95% CI, 0.67–2.76]). One man died from nasal cancer (0.02 expected), and two each from lung cancer (SMR, 0.78 [95% CI, 0.09–2.8]), kidney cancer (SMR, 6.45 [95% CI, 0.8–23.3]) and brain tumour (SMR, 16.67 [95% CI, 2.0–60.2]).

Enterline (1982) briefly reported results for 54 deaths among 433 workers employed for more than three months in an isopropanol unit in Texas (USA) between 1941 and 1965, with follow-up through 1978. Compared to rates in Texas, mortality from all causes was significantly low (54 deaths; SMR, 0.65 [95% CI, 0.49–0.84]), while the SMR for cancers at all sites was 0.99 (16 deaths [95% CI, 0.57–1.61]); there were two deaths from cancer of the buccal cavity and pharynx (0.50 expected) and seven deaths from lung cancer (SMR, 1.18 [95% CI, 0.47–2.43]). Four of the seven subjects who died from lung cancer had also worked in an epichlorohydrin unit (SMR, 2.48 [95% CI, 0.67–6.36]); the other three had a low risk of lung cancer (SMR, 0.69 [95% CI, 0.14–2.02]). Neither of the subjects with cancer of the buccal cavity and pharynx had worked with epichlorohydrin, and their high risk was attributed to employment in the isopropanol unit.

2.2.2 *Manufacture of synthetic ethanol and isopropanol by the strong acid process*

A historical cohort study was conducted of 335 process workers (Lynch *et al.*, 1979) who had had one month or more employment in an isopropanol plant and an ethanol plant in a petrochemical complex in Baton Rouge, LA (USA), between 1950 and 1976. A total of 255 were still alive, 48 dead and 32 lost to follow-up; two women were excluded from the analyses. Comparison rates were based on US white male rates from the Third National Cancer Survey for 1969–71. The standardized incidence ratio (SIR) for laryngeal cancer in this cohort was 5.04 [95% CI, 1.36–12.90], based on four cases. In an expanded cohort of 740 men, including both process workers and mechanical craftsmen and supervisors, the SIR was 3.2 [1.3–6.6], based on seven cases. Presumed exposure to diethyl sulfate was tentatively implicated. (See also the study by Soskolne *et al.*, 1984, p. 89.)

The mortality experience of 538 men employed as ethanol and isopropanol process workers in a Union Carbide chemical plant in South Charleston (SC) and 493 at a plant in Texas City (TC), all of whom had been employed for one month or more from 1941 through 1978, was followed from the early 1940s to 1983 (Teta et al., 1992). The SC plant produced ethanol from 1930 to 1968 and isopropanol from 1928 to 1949, using strong sulfuric acid in each process. The TC plant used strong sulfuric acid in the production of ethanol from 1941 to 1968 but switched in 1969 to a process employing the hydration of ethylene; this plant also used strong sulfuric acid for the production of isopropanol from 1941 to 1949, when they changed to a weak-acid process. External comparisons were made to national US and regional rates. For the two plants combined, there were 300 deaths (29% of the cohort), and nine subjects were lost to follow-up. All subjects who died in the SC plant had had an exposure assignment to the strong sulfuric acid units. Mortality from all causes and from malignant neoplasms at all sites for the combined cohort of strong-acid workers in the two plants was approximately as expected. The mortality rate for lung cancer was not elevated (22 deaths [SMR, 0.94; 95% CI, 0.59–1.43]); there were two deaths from laryngeal cancer [SMR, 2.00; 95% CI, 0.22–7.22] and three from cancer of the buccal cavity and pharynx [SMR, 1.36; 95% CI, 0.27–3.98]). A significant excess of deaths from lymphoma and reticulosarcoma was restricted to workers at the SC plant who had had fewer than five years of employment. One sinus cancer was reported among workers at the SC plant prior to 1950, but no reference rates were available. No cancer death was seen among weak-acid workers (1.9 expected). The one death due to laryngeal cancer and the two deaths due to cancer of the buccal cavity and pharynx in the SC plant (strong-acid process) were seen in men with fewer than five years of employment in the plant.

2.2.3 Pickling and other acid treatment of metals

Mazumdar et al. (1975) reported on a cohort study of mortality among white sheet and tin mill workers, including pickling workers, in an updating of their longitudinal study of Allegheny County (USA) steelworkers, 1953–66. Men involved in batch pickling and sheet drying (n = 55), coating (n = 328), continuous pickling and electric cleaning (n = 205), sheet finishing and shipping (n = 1733), stainless annealing, pickling and processing (n = 46) and tin finishing and shipping (n = 396) were included. Cancer of the respiratory organs occurred in 27 of 2763 men employed in these areas [SMR, 1.10; 95% CI, 0.73–1.60]. [The Working Group combined results for the work areas where there was assumed to be opportunity for exposure to acid aerosols and mists.]

Ahlborg et al. (1981) reported three incident cases of 'medium, differentiated' squamous laryngeal cancers diagnosed between 1971 and 1978 among 110 men employed for at least one year between 1951 and 1979 in a small Swedish factory unit for the pickling and processing of stainless-steel pipes, whereas 0.06 were expected on the basis of reference rates from the Swedish Cancer Registry. All three men had smoked 10–15 cigarettes per day for many years. All three had first been employed ≥ 10 years before the cancer was diagnosed. Exposure during the 1950s was to pickling baths containing sulfuric and nitric acids and that during the 1960s and 1970s to oxalic acid, ammonium bifluoride and soap. There was also one case of bronchial carcinoma.

In a cohort study undertaken by the US National Institute for Occupational Safety and Health (NIOSH) (Beaumont et al., 1987), the mortality patterns of 1165 male workers employed from 1940 to 1964 and exposed to sulfuric and other acid mists (primarily hydrochloric acid mist) in three steel-pickling operations for at least six months were examined through October 1981. Of the full cohort, 722 had been exposed only to sulfuric acid (595 probably had daily exposure) and 254 to sulfuric acid and other acid mists; 189 had been exposed to acids other than sulfuric. The exposure of all workers averaged 8.8 years (Steenland & Beaumont, 1989). Pickling workers who had ever been employed in coke ovens were excluded. In a health hazard evaluation conducted by NIOSH in 1977 in the largest facility, exposures to a number of agents were measured, including iron oxide, lead, nickel, chromium and respirable silica; detectable levels were found only of iron oxide and lead. There were 326 deaths in the cohort; death certificates were not obtained for 22, and vital status was not ascertained for 15 (1.3%) individuals. Mortality from causes of death other than lung cancer was unremarkable. Analysis of the full cohort for exposure to any acid, using US death rates as the standard, showed mortality from lung cancer to be significantly elevated (SMR, 1.64; 95% CI, 1.14–2.28), based on 35 observed deaths. The SMR was 1.85 (95% CI, 1.25–2.64) for men with more than 20 years since first exposure to any acid, but was not related to duration of exposure. For those with probable daily exposure to sulfuric acid, all of the excess risk occurred 20 years or more after first employment (SMR, 1.93; 95% CI, 1.10–3.13). For men exposed to sulfuric acid only, the SMR for lung cancer was 1.39 ([95% CI, 0.84–2.17], 19 deaths); for those with probable daily exposure to sulfuric acid only, it was 1.58 ([95% CI, 0.94–2.50], 18 deaths); for those exposed to sulfuric and other acids, it was 1.92 ([95% CI, 0.77–3.95], seven deaths); for those exposed to acids other than sulfuric acid, it was 2.24 [95% CI, 1.02–4.25]; 9 deaths). No dose–response relationship was evident for men who had held jobs with probable daily exposure to sulfuric acid, using length of employment as the measure of exposure. Using another steelworker group for comparison and adjusting for the probable distribution of smoking habits, it was shown that smoking was unlikely to explain the increased lung cancer risk entirely.

Steenland and Beaumont (1989) extended the period of follow-up of the cohort of Beaumont et al. (1987) from November 1981 through early 1986 and obtained additional information: 73% of the men themselves or their next-of-kin were contacted to determine vital status and smoking habits. Indirect adjustment was made for smoking using the technique of Axelson (1978), taking into account observed differences in smoking habits between the cohort and the US referent population. The SMR for lung cancer was 1.55 (95% CI, 1.12–2.11), based on 41 deaths and unadjusted for smoking; the adjusted SMR was 1.36 (95% CI, 0.97–1.84). For men with 20 or more years since first exposure, the unadjusted SMR was 1.72 (95% CI, 1.21–2.39); that adjusted for smoking was 1.50 (95% CI, 1.05–2.27). Using duration as a measure of exposure did not result in a dose–response trend, although the authors state that duration may be a poor surrogate of exposure.

Steenland et al. (1988) conducted an interview-based study of laryngeal cancer incidence, using a subset (77%) of the population studied by Beaumont et al. (1987) comprising all men for whom adequate information could be obtained to determine the incidence of laryngeal cancer. Follow-up through 1985 rendered 47 additional deaths, for a total of 373 deaths, or 32% of the entire cohort. The smoking habits of 795 and the drinking habits of 593 male steelworkers exposed to acid mists during pickling operations were determined. The average duration of exposure was 9.5 years. Nine laryngeal cancer cases were confirmed. Using data from national surveys of cancer incidence as referent rates, 3.44 laryngeal cancers would have been expected [relative risk, 2.6; 95% CI, 1.2–5.0]. As the exposed cohort smoked more than the US population, the expected number of cases was raised to 3.92, giving an SIR of 2.30 [95% CI, 1.05–4.36].

2.2.4 *Sulfuric acid manufacture*

Seven lung cancer cases were diagnosed during an 11-year period (1957–67) in a group of 259 blue-collar workers at a sulfuric acid plant in Germany (Thiess *et al.*, 1969). The patients had been employed at the plant for periods of six months to 32 years. Six were smokers (the smoking habits of the other case were unknown). The authors calculated an incidence of 268 per 10 000 employees at the sulfuric acid plant and 39.8 per 10 000 among other workers in the factory. A further lung cancer case occurred in an office worker at the same plant, who was a smoker. [The Working Group noted the incomplete reporting of methodology; e.g., the extent of follow-up of the employees.]

Mortality and cancer incidence were evaluated among workers employed at a sulfuric acid plant that has been operating since 1932 in Sweden (Englander *et al*, 1988). Industrial hygiene data, available between 1969 and 1984, indicated possible exposure of the respiratory zone to the following substances: sulfur dioxide (median of yearly time-weighted averages, 3.6 mg/m^3), arsenic (11 µg/m^3), total dust (2.2 mg/m^3), respirable dust (0.6 mg/m^3) and sulfuric acid (occasional measurements; range, < 0.1–2.9 mg/m^3). A total of 400 workers who had been employed for at least six months during the period 1 July 1960 to 31 December 1981 were identified from company records and followed up through 1985; two subjects were lost to follow-up. The vast majority of the workers had been employed for fewer than 25 years. Information about tumours diagnosed between 1961 and 1985 among cohort members and reference rates for cancer incidence in the county were obtained from the Southern Swedish Regional Tumour Register. Mortality from all causes was higher than expected (53 deaths (all with death certificates available); SMR, 1.48 [95% CI, 1.11–1.94]), whereas the number of cancer deaths was about that expected (eight deaths; SMR, 0.88 [95% CI, 0.38–1.73]; 23 cancers diagnosed; SIR, 1.34 [95% CI, 0.85–2.02]). There were excess numbers of respiratory cancers (five cases; SIR, 2.00 [95% CI, 0.50–4.67]) and bladder cancers (five cases; SIR, 3.77 [95% CI, 1.25–8.98]). The risk for bladder cancer was higher among workers with five or more years since first employment (five cases; SIR, 4.36 [95% CI, 1.35–9.72]), but the risk for respiratory cancer was not higher in this subgroup (four cases; SIR, 1.83 [95% CI, 0.50–4.69]).

Sulfuric acid was manufactured at some of the smelters on which studies are reported in the monograph on sulfur dioxide. The predominant exposure at the smelters, however, was to sulfur dioxide, and results on exposure to acid mists were not reported.

2.2.5 *Soap and detergent manufacture*

Workers at a factory in central Italy which produced solid soap were studied for mortality and incidence of laryngeal cancer (Forastiere *et al.*, 1987). According to measurements taken in 1974, workers were exposed to sulfuric acid mists (0.64–1.12 mg/m^3), nickel and its compounds (up to 0.07 mg/m^3) and mineral oils (1.2 mg/m^3); soap powder, glycerol and fatty acids were also present. From company records, 361 men active on 1 January 1964 or hired thereafter until 1972 and employed for at least one year were enrolled. Follow-up for vital status lasted from 1 January 1969 to 30 June 1983 and was completed for 347 (96%) cohort members. Cause of death was obtained for all deceased individuals. Laryngeal cancer incidence was ascertained (from 1 January 1972 to 30 June 1983) by reviewing the discharge files of the ear, nose and throat departments of local hospitals. SMRs were calculated using the mortality figures of the province as reference; expected numbers of laryngeal cancer cases were estimated according to both incidence rates from four European cancer registers and data derived from the local search. Fewer than the expected number of deaths occurred from all causes (30 deaths; SMR, 0.70; 95% CI, 0.47–1.00) as well as from all cancers (eight deaths; SMR, 0.71; 95% CI, 0.31–1.39). One subject died of laryngeal cancer (0.6 expected), and five lung cancer deaths were recorded (SMR, 1.69; 95% CI, 0.55–3.86). Five laryngeal cancer cases were detected (including the death), yielding an SIR of [6.94 (95% CI, 2.25–16.2)] or [3.47 (95% CI, 1.13–8.10)], depending on the reference population chosen. All of the cancers occurred among subjects with more than 10 years since first employment and with 4–27 years' duration of exposure.

2.2.6 *Nitric acid manufacture*

Cancer incidence was investigated among production and maintenance workers at a nitric acid production plant within an electrochemical industrial complex in southern Norway (Hilt *et al.*, 1985). A group of 287 men who had been exposed to asbestos between 1928 and 1980 was divided according to degree of exposure to asbestos. The 190 workers who were only indirectly exposed to asbestos (mechanics, plumbers, welders and production workers) but were also exposed to nitrous gases, nitric acid vapours and ammonia and who had had at least one year of exposure at the plant are considered here. Mortality from all causes in this group in 1953–80 was about as expected (75 deaths; SMR, 1.07 [95% CI, 0.84–1.34]), and the incidence of cancers at all sites in the same period was not increased (19 cases; SIR, 0.95; 95% CI, 0.6–1.5). Five cases of cancer of the lung and one of the pleura were detected, while a total of 2.5 cases was expected (SIR, 2.4; 95% CI, 0.92–5.4); there were also five cancers of unknown origin (SIR, 5.4; 95% CI, 1.8–13.0). These excesses were present mainly in maintenance workers, both with regard to respiratory cancer (three cases; SIR, 5.0; 95% CI, 1.03–14.61) and to cancers of unknown origin (four cases; SIR, 21.0; 95% CI, 5.5–51.2); in production workers, three lung cancers and one cancer of unknown origin were observed, while the expected numbers were 1.9 and 0.7, respectively. [The Working Group noted that the possiblity of concomitant exposure to asbestos limits the interpretability of this study with respect to exposure to nitric acid.]

2.2.7 *Phosphate fertilizer manufacture*

Mining and chemical processing of phosphate rocks to obtain phosphate fertilizer involves exposures to several toxic substances (see also section 1.2.7), including ionizing radiation from decay products of uranium (Checkoway *et al.*, 1985a). Concern about possible adverse health effects, especially lung cancer, of exposure to low levels of ionizing radiation during work in phosphate mining and phosphate fertilizer production motivated three independent historical cohort studies among workers in the Florida (USA) phosphate industry (Checkoway et al., 1985a; Stayner et al., 1985; Block et al., 1988).

Men employed for a minimum of three months' continuous service with one of 16 member companies of the Florida Phosphate Council during the years 1949-78 and with at least 12 months' cumulative service were enrolled in a cohort (Checkoway et al., 1985a). Vital status was ascertained for 17 601 white and 4722 non-white men from 1 January 1949 to 31 January 1978: 1620 white and 650 non-white men had died (no death certificate for 56 and 20, respectively); 191 white and 81 non-white subjects were lost to follow up. Race-specific SMRs were calculated, taking both the US and Florida (the latter only for cancer) male populations as comparisons. Among white men, the SMR for all causes was 1.00 and that for overall cancer was 0.95 (289 deaths [95% CI, 0.84-1.07]). Fewer deaths from laryngeal cancer were seen than expected both on the basis of US (three deaths; SMR, 0.66 [95% CI, 0.14-1.93]) and Florida (SMR, 0.59 [95% CI, 0.12-1.72]) standards. Lung cancer mortality was higher than expected on the basis of rates for the US population (117 deaths; SMR, 1.22 [95% CI, 1.01-1.46]); the excess, however, was non-significant when Florida rates were used for comparison (SMR, 1.03 [95% CI, 0.85-1.23]). No clear trend in lung cancer mortality was evident from an analysis of duration of employment, but consistently elevated SMRs were found for men with 30-39 years since first employment (21 deaths; SMR (USA), 1.71; SMR (Florida), 1.52) and for men with 40 or more years since first employment (10 deaths; SMR (USA), 2.08; SMR (Florida), 2.04). Among non-white subjects, the SMR for overall deaths was low (0.80 [95% CI, 0.74-0.86]), whereas it was close to 1.0 for all malignant neoplasms (131 deaths; SMR, 1.02 [95% CI, 0.85-1.21]). Again, lung cancer mortality was increased on the basis of US standards (46 deaths; SMR, 1.24; [95% CI, 0.91-1.65]); this effect was not seen when Florida rates were taken as the comparison (SMR, 1.02 [95% CI, 0.75-1.36]). There was no consistent trend in the SMR for lung cancer with length of employment or with latency since first employment among non-whites. [The Working Group noted that no information was given on the smoking habits of cohort members, which would have been important in view of the possible interaction between smoking and radiation.]

The same data were used for an internal comparison of rates of mortality from lung cancer within the Florida phosphate industry (Checkoway et al., 1985b). Job histories were obtained from the companies, and workers were classified into 16 work areas (one of which included sulfuric and phosphoric acid manufacture) and into several kinds of potential exposure (including phosphoric acid and soluble phosphate, sulfuric acid, sulfur oxides, hydrofluoric acid and soluble fluorides). The analysis was conducted by computing standardized rate ratios (SRRs), adjusted for age and calendar period, within each exposure group across three strata of employment duration (less than one year, the referent category; 1-9 years; 10 years or more). Only subjects employed in skilled crafts and in plant-wide services had a trend for increased risk of lung cancer with duration of employment. No consistent increase in relative risk for lung cancer was found for workers in sulfuric and phosphoric acid production (1-9 years: eight deaths; SRR, 1.34 [95% CI, 0.58-2.64]; > 10 years: three deaths; SRR, 0.87 [95% CI, 0.81-2.54]) or among subjects with potential exposure to acids. Subjects exposed to α radiation or mineral (rock) dust had an excess relative risk, but this did not increase consistently with duration of exposure. [The Working Group noted that the job and exposure categories overlapped.]

A report of three lung cancer cases among workers involved in the cleaning of a phosphoric acid reaction vessel at a phosphate fertilizer production facility in Polk County, Florida, prompted an investigation by researchers at NIOSH (Stayner et al., 1985). In an industrial hygiene survey of the plant, personal and air samples were collected; fluorides (average, 3.39 mg/m^3), sulfuric acid (average, 0.11 mg/m^3) and phosphoric acid (0.25 mg/m^3) were the main contaminants. A total of 3199 subjects, including 212 women, who had worked at the plant from 1953–76 were enrolled and followed-up through December 1977; 113 subjects (3.5%) were lost to follow-up. There were 176 deaths, but death certificates were available for only 163 individuals (calculations were done using only 155 cases). US sex-, age-, time- and race-specific death rates were used to calculate expected number of deaths. Both overall mortality (155 deaths; SMR, 0.82 [95% CI, 0.69–0.96]) and mortality from all cancers (22 deaths; SMR, 0.76 [95% CI, 0.48–1.15]) were lower than expected. The risk for lung cancers among all study subjects was increased only slightly (10 deaths; SMR, 1.13 [95% CI, 0.54–2.08]), but five deaths occurred among black subjects, to yield an SMR of 1.82 [95% CI, 0.59–4.26]. Among black men with ≥ 20 years of duration of exposure and latency, two cases of lung cancer were seen, whereas 0.16 were expected. The initial three cases of lung cancer, which also occurred among black men, gave an SMR of [1.27; 95% CI, 0.26–3.71].

Male workers employed for six months or more between 1950 and 1979 at a Florida phosphate company were included in a cohort followed up through 1981 (Block et al., 1988). Individuals were categorized according to the job area in which they had worked the longest. Workers in chemical/fertilizer had potential exposure to chemical fumes (sulfuric acid, sulfur dioxide and fluorides), silica dust and radiation from radon decay products. Of the 3451 subjects in the study, 486 (for 18 of whom there was no information about cause of death) were found to be deceased, while vital status was unknown for 226 (6.5%). The expected number of deaths was calculated on the basis of race-, age- and time-specific US rates; Florida rates were also considered. A questionnaire including questions on smoking habits was sent to 2155 subjects with one year or more of employment; 992 (46%) replied. Information on cancer occurrence was confirmed from medical records, and SIRs were computed using incidence rates for Connecticut. Mortality from all causes of death was similar to that expected among whites (346 deaths; SMR, 1.00) but was significantly lower among blacks (127 deaths; SMR, 0.74 [95% CI, 0.62–0.88]). Overall cancer rates were increased among whites (86 deaths; SMR, 1.26 [95% CI, 1.01–1.56]) but not among blacks (26 deaths; SMR, 0.93 [95% CI, 0.61–1.36]). Two deaths from laryngeal cancer were reported among whites (SMR, 1.91 [95% CI, 0.23–6.90]) but none among blacks. There was a significant excess of lung cancer deaths (37) among white workers, in comparison to both US rates (SMR, 1.62 [95% CI, 1.14–2.23]) and Florida rates (SMR, 1.50 [95% CI, 1.06–2.07]); no excess of lung cancer was observed among blacks (nine deaths; SMR, 1.04 [95% CI, 0.48–1.97]). Among workers with one year or more of employment, there was an increasing trend in numbers of deaths from lung cancer according to duration of employment, which was especially evident when 20 years or more of latency had elapsed. In the group with 20 years or more of both duration and latency, an SMR of 2.48 [95% CI, 1.19–4.56] (10 deaths) was recorded. The results for respiratory cancer were confirmed by using incidence data (SIR, 1.55). [The Working Group noted that the number of incident cases was not reported.] An indirect adjustment for smoking was made using the data from the questionnaire: The authors reported that smoking could not completely explain the excess of lung cancer. When an internal comparison of job categories was made with regard to lung cancer, an SMR of 2.83 [95% CI, 0.58–8.27] (three deaths) was found for drying/shipping, whereas no increase was found for workers exposed to chemical/fertilizer.

Hagmar et al. (1991) conducted a historical cohort study on workers employed in a Swedish fertilizer factory. The factory produced superphosphate (raw phosphate treated with a mixture of sulfuric acid and phosphoric acid) from its foundation in 1882 until 1937; from 1907, sulfuric acid was also produced. Production of PK fertilizers (mainly superphosphate and potash) began in 1937, and that of phosphoric acid in 1940; production of nitrogen-containing fertilizers began in 1963. Two cohorts were assembled: 'nitrate fertilizer workers', 2131 men who had been employed in the factory for three months or longer during 1963–85 (these were omitted from consideration here); and 'other fertilizer workers', 1236 men who had been employed for three months or longer during 1906–62 but not after 1962. Follow-up for cancer incidence was carried out for the period 1958–86 through the national Swedish and southern Swedish regional tumour registries. Expected numbers of tumours were calculated from county rates, taking into consideration calendar year and age. A total of 128 cancer cases was observed in the 'other fertilizer workers' cohort (SIR, 0.97; 95% CI, 0.81–1.16). Significant excesses were seen of cancer of the respiratory tract (29 cases; SIR, 1.52; 95% CI, 1.03–2.20) and of cancer of the lung and pleura (25 cases; SIR, 1.51; 95% CI, 0.99–2.25); the remaining four cases were nasal and laryngeal cancers (RR, 1.6; 95% CI, 0.4–4.1). The elevated risks remained when analyses were restricted to 10 or more years of latency. Nine cancers of the oral cavity and pharynx were seen (SIR, 1.76; 95% CI, 0.81–3.35).

2.2.8 Lead battery (accumulator) manufacture

Cohort studies of workers employed in lead–acid battery manufacture have been reviewed previously (IARC, 1980, 1987). The results of a cohort study of 7032 US workers in six lead production facilities and 10 battery plants, first reported by Cooper and Gaffey (1975), were reported by Cooper et al. (1985) for 34 years of follow-up (1947–80). Of 4519 workers who had been exposed in the battery plants for at least one year, 1718 had died (82 without a death certificate). Total mortality was greater than in the US white male population (SMR, 1.07; 95% CI, 1.02–1.12), and there was a significant excess of deaths due to all malignant neoplasms (344 deaths; SMR, 1.13; 95% CI, 1.02–1.26). The excess was due mainly to more deaths than expected from stomach cancer (34 deaths; SMR, 1.68; 95% CI, 1.16–2.35) and from lung cancer (109 deaths; SMR, 1.24; 95% CI, 1.02–1.50). An examination of cancer mortality in terms of cumulative years of employment in the battery plants showed no evident trend for either stomach or lung cancer.

Long-term employees who received a pension from four lead–acid battery companies in the United Kingdom were studied by Malcolm and Barnett (1982). A total of 1898 subjects (1644 men) were followed up from 1925 through 1976. In addition, a list of all 553 employees who had died while still employed in the largest of the four factories was available. Death certificates were obtained mostly from the company pension scheme. National statistics provided reference numbers. Workers were classified into three groups of potential occupational exposure to lead on the basis of their jobs. SMRs were calculated for the cohort of pensioners and proportionate mortality rates (PMRs) for the workers who had died while still employed. There were 754 deaths from all causes in male pensioners (SMR, 0.99 [95% CI, 0.92–1.06]). Mortality during service from all malignant neoplasms was slightly elevated (136 observed; PMR, 1.15 [95% CI, 0.96–1.06]), particularly among people in the highest category of lead exposure. [The Working Group noted that exposure to lead may not be correlated with exposure to acid and that incomplete reporting of the follow-up of the total cohort and emphasis on retirees limit the usefulness of the study.]

2.2.9 *Other industries*

Cumulative exposure to sulfuric acid was calculated in a study of deceased workers from a US copper smelter (Rencher *et al.*, 1977), described in detail in the monograph on sulfur dioxide (p. 159). Workers who died of lung cancer had higher indices of exposure to arsenic, lead, sulfur dioxide and sulfuric acid than workers who died of non-respiratory cancer.

In a follow-up study of workers with potential exposure to acrylamide in four chemical plants in USA and the Netherlands, Collins *et al.* (1989) reported an excess of lung cancer at one of the facilities studied. The excess was due partly to an increased number of lung cancer deaths (11 deaths) observed among men who had worked in a muriatic acid [hydrochloric acid] department. [The Working Group noted that the expected numbers were not reported.]

2.3 Case–control studies

Results of case–control studies are summarized in Table 17 (p. 97).

2.3.1 *Laryngeal cancer*

A case–control study of workers at the refinery and chemical plant in Baton Rouge, LA (USA), previously studied by Lynch *et al.* (1979), was designed to examine the association between upper respiratory cancers (including the oropharynx) and exposure to sulfuric acid (Soskolne *et al.*, 1984). Fifty incident cases, diagnosed between 1944 and 1980, were ascertained from company medical records, social security administration records and the county cancer registry and matched to 175 controls for sex, age, race, duration of employment and year of first employment. Only workers who had been employed for one or more years were included. Occupational exposures to sulfuric acid and several other substances were estimated for the job of each subject by the plant industrial hygienist. The odds ratios for cancer were increased for workers with exposure to sulfuric acid at moderate (2.2; 95% CI, 0.78–6.36) and high levels (4.0; 95% CI, 1.26–12.7) compared with the no/low category, using the mean grade exposure measure and adjusting for the effects of tobacco, previous history of ear, nose and throat diseases and alcoholism. The odds ratios were higher when laryngeal cancer cases were considered (4.6; 0.83–25.35; and 13.4; 2.08–85.99, respectively). Asbestos, nickel and wood dust were not related to the risk for laryngeal cancer. Industrial hygiene information was not available about the presence of dialkyl sulfates in all units and processes, so this exposure could not be included in the analysis; however, an analysis excluding workers in both the ethanol and isopropanol units and an analysis of workers exposed only in the weak-acid process gave odds ratios and exposure–response relationships of the same order of magnitude.

Table 16. Cohort studies of workers in industries which involve potential exposure to inorganic acid aerosols

Reference (country)	Number of workers	Larynx			Lung			Comments
		N^a	RR^b	95% CI	N^a	RR^b	95% CI	
Isopropanol manufacture								
Weil et al., 1952 (USA)	182 (71 exposed for >5 years)	1^c	–	–	1	–	–	Method of enumeration of cohort unclear. Four sinonasal cases represent an apparent, large excess (2 dead, 2 surviving). Cases of cancer found in workers exposed >5 years
Alderson & Rattan, 1980 (UK)	262				2	0.78	[0.09–2.8]	Increased risks for cancers of kidney (6.5 [0.8–23.3]) and brain (16.7 [2.0–60.2]) based on 2 cases each and sinonasal cancer (50.0 [0.65–278.2]) based on 1 case
Enterline, 1982 (USA)	433 (125 also exposed to epichlorohydrin)				4	2.48	[0.67–6.36]	Workers also exposed to epichlorohydrin
					3	0.69	[0.14–2.02]	Workers not exposed to epichlorohydrin
Synthetic ethanol and isopropanol manufacture by the strong-acid process								
Lynch et al., 1979 (USA)	335	4^c	5.04	[1.36–12.90]				Isopropanol + ethanol manufacture. Assumed to be due to diethyl sulfate
Teta et al., 1992 (USA)	1031	2	[2.0]	[0.22–7.22]	22	[0.94]	[0.59–1.43]	Ethanol, 1930–68, isopropanol, 1928–49, both by strong-acid process
Pickling and other acid treatment of metals								
Mazumdar et al., 1975 (USA)								
Batch pickling and sheet dryers					0^d	–	–	
Coating					4^d	[1.43]	[0.4–3.66]	
Continuous pickling and electric cleaning					0^d	–	–	
Sheet finishing and shipping					19^d	1.22	[0.7–1.9]	

Table 16 (contd)

Reference (country)	Number of workers	Larynx			Lung			Comments
		N^a	RR^b	95% CI	N^a	RR^b	95% CI	

Pickling and other acid treatment of metals (contd)

Reference (country)	Number of workers	N^a	RR^b	95% CI	N^a	RR^b	95% CI	Comments
Mazumdar et al., 1975 (USA) (contd)								
Stainless annealing, pickling and processing					2^d	[3.3]	[0.4-12.0]	
Tin finishing and shipping					2	[0.56]	[0.1-2.01]	
Ahlborg et al., 1981 (Sweden)	110							
> 10 years' induction time		3^c		(Exp: 0.06)	1		(Exp: 0.60)	
		3^c		(Exp: 0.05)	1		(Exp: 0.50)	
Beaumont et al., 1987 (USA)	1165							SMR = 1.85 (1.25-2.64) for any acid and SMR = 1.93 (1.10-3.13) for sulfuric acid daily with ≥ 20 year latency. Adjustment for smoking in some analyses. Associations lower when comparisons made to a steelworker population
Any acid		2	1.93	0.23-6.99	35	1.64	1.14-2.28	
Sulfuric acid only					19	1.39	[0.84-2.17]	
Sulfuric acid, daily								
Mixed sulfuric and other acids					18	1.58	[0.94-2.50]	
Other acid only (primarily hydrochloric)					7	1.92	[0.77-3.95]	
Steenland & Beaumont, 1989 (USA)	1165				9	2.24	[1.02-4.25]	Extension of cohort of Beaumont et al. (1987). RRs indirectly adjusted for smoking. No increase in risk with duration of employment
20 years since first exposure					41	1.36	0.97-1.84	
					NR	1.50	1.05-2.27	
Steenland et al., 1988 (USA)	879	9^c (5 dead, 4 alive)	2.3	[1.05-4.36]				RRs adjusted for smoking and alcohol. Four cases exposed to sulfuric acid only, three to mixed acids, and two only to acids other than sulfuric (primarily hydrochloric)

Table 16 (contd)

Reference (country)	Number of workers		Larynx			Lung			Comments
			N[a]	RR[b]	95% CI	N[a]	RR[b]	95% CI	
Sulfuric acid manufacture									
Thiess et al., 1969 (Germany)	259					8	[6.7]	–	Crude ratio, not age-adjusted. One case was an office worker.
Englander et al., 1988 (Sweden)	400					5[c]	2.00	[0.50–4.67]	SMR = 1.83 [95% CI, 0.50–4.69] for ≥5-year latency. Excess of bladder cancer
Soap and detergent manufacture									
Forastiere et al., 1987 (Italy)	361		1	2.30	0.09–11.43	5	1.69	0.55–3.86	Nickel potential confounder
			5[c]	[6.94] [3.47]	[2.25–16.2] [1.13–8.10]				Two SIRs according to reference population
Nitric acid manufacture									
Hilt et al., 1985 (Norway)	190	All				6[c]	2.4	0.92–5.4	Exposure to nitric acid not qualified
		Maintenance				3[c]	5.0	1.03–4.61	One pleural mesothelioma included; asbestos a potential confounder
		Production				3[d]	[1.6]	[0.31–4.61]	
Phosphate fertilizer manufacture									
Checkoway et al., 1985a,b (USA)	17 601 white men		3	0.66	[0.14–1.93]	117	1.22	[1.01–1.46]	RR based on US male rates. Trend of lung cancer risk with latency. No excess of lung cancer among non-whites using local reference rates. No trend with duration of employment in departments with exposure to sulfuric or phosphoric acids. Radon decay products a potential confounder.
	4 722 non-white men		1	0.42	[0.006–2.34]	46	1.24	[0.91–1.65]	

Table 16 (contd)

Reference (country)	Number of workers		Larynx			Lung			Comments
			N^a	RR^b	95% CI	N^a	RR^b	95% CI	
Phosphate fertilizer manufacture (contd)									
Stayner et al., 1985 (USA)	3199	All Blacks	0		(Exp: 0.43)	10 5	1.13 1.82	[0.54–2.08] [0.59–4.26]	Trend with duration of employment and length of follow-up among blacks, not among whites. Radon decay products a potential confounder.
Block et al., 1988 (USA)	2607 white men 840 black men		2 0	1.91	[0.23–6.90]	37 9	1.62 1.04	[1.14–2.23] [0.48–1.97]	Trend in risk of lung cancer death or incidence with duration of employment among long-term workers. No major confounding by smoking; radon decay products a potential confounder.
Hagmar et al., 1991 (Sweden)	1236		[4]^e	[1.6]	[0.4–4.1]	25^f	1.51	0.99–2.25	SMR = 1.50 (0.98–2.26) with 10-year latency
Lead battery (accumulator) manufacture									
Cooper et al., 1985 (USA)	4519*		6	1.28	0.47–2.80	109	1.24	1.02–1.50	No trend in lung cancer risk with duration of employment. Stomach cancer: SMR = 1.68 (1.16–2.35)
Other industries									
Collins et al., 1989 (USA)	8854					161	1.32	[1.1–1.5]	Excess lung cancer in two groups in one facility, including muriatic acid department (11 cases). No expected number of deaths given

RR, relative risk; CI, confidence interval; NR, not reported
^{a}Number of events; deaths from specified cancer except where noted otherwise
^{b}Estimate
^{c}Incident case
^{d}Respiratory tract
^{e}Sinonasal and larynx combined
^{f}Lung and pleura combined

A case–control study of laryngeal cancer was conducted at the Institute of Oncology in Gliwice, Poland (Zemla et al., 1987), comprising 328 histologically confirmed laryngeal cancer cases among men referred for the first time to the hospital for treatment during 1980–84. Controls were 656 individuals with no neoplastic disease. Information about occupational and life-style factors was derived from questionnaires. The authors reported increased odds ratios for manual workers 'constantly' exposed to vapours of sulfuric acid, hydrochloric acid and nitric acid (relative risk [RR], 4.27; $p < 0.001$, based on 11 exposed cases). A nonsignificantly increased risk (RR, 1.66) was observed for manual workers 'constantly' exposed to dust and vapours, based on 20 exposed cases. [The Working Group noted that the methods were inadequately described.]

A population-based case–control study was conducted on the Texas Gulf Coast, USA (Brown et al., 1988). Cases were 183 incident cases (136 living, 47 dead) of squamous-cell carcinoma of the larynx diagnosed during 1975–80 among white men aged 30–79 years; 250 controls (179 living, 71 dead) were frequency matched. Interviews were completed for 69.5% of living and 67.5% of dead cases and for 62.8% of dead controls, 60.9% of controls less than 65 years old and 85.7% of controls over 65 years of age. Exposure assessment was based on an industrial hygienists's evaluation of complete job histories. A significantly increased risk was found (odds ratio, 2.11; 95% CI, 1.17–3.78) for any exposure in metal fabricating. For all workers with potential exposure to sulfuric acid, the odds ratio was 0.76 (95% CI, 0.42–1.35). Both odds ratios were controlled for tobacco and alcohol intake. [The Working Group noted the relatively low participation rates.]

In a population-based case–control study, 183 incident male cases of histologically confirmed carcinoma of the larynx diagnosed between 1977 and 1979 in southern Ontario, Canada, and 183 controls matched for sex, age and neighbourhood were compared for exposure to sulfuric acid (Soskolne et al., 1992). (The response rate was 79% for cases; 77.5% of controls agreed to participate at initial approach [Burch et al., 1981]). Detailed work histories and information on tobacco and alcohol use were obtained by personal interview. Concentration and frequency of exposure to sulfuric acid for each job were estimated by the same method described by Siemiatycki (1991) (see below) and were assessed independently using three four-point scales; the degree of confidence of the industrial hygienist in the reliability of these assessments was included in the exposure scheme. The product of these measures for each job was squared and then multiplied by the time spent in that job, and this value was summed over all jobs. This total was then divided by the total time of exposure to the concentration and/or frequency scores of 1 or more to calculate 'average exposure level'. Conditional logistic regression analysis using two categories of exposure and controlling for tobacco and alcohol use resulted in an odds ratio of 3.04 (95% CI, 1.67–5.53). Omitting exposures in the five years prior to diagnosis and including only the most specific exposure scale resulted in a significant dose–response effect, with an odds ratio of 2.52 (95% CI, 0.80–7.91) at the lowest level and 6.87 (95% CI, 1.00–47.06) at the highest. Asbestos was not a significant confounder.

2.3.2 *Multiple myeloma*

A population-based case–control study of multiple myeloma addressed the potential carcinogenicity of several toxic substances, including acids and fertilizers (Morris et al.,

1986). Cases were identified through cancer registries serving four areas in the USA. For 698 cases (89% of those recruited initially) diagnosed between 1977 and 1981, either a direct (68%) or a next-of-kin interview was available. Controls were chosen randomly from among residents of the areas inhabited by the cases under study; 1683 controls (83%) were interviewed (99% in person). After excluding interviews with next-of-kin of cases, the odds ratio (adjusted for several potential confounders) was somewhat increased for exposures to acids (1.5; 95% CI, 0.8–2.8); when all subjects were considered, the ratio was 1.0 (95% CI, 0.6–1.9).

2.3.3 Cancers at multiple sites

A population-based case–control study of cancer included histologically confirmed cases of cancer at 11 major sites (not including larynx), newly diagnosed between 1979 and 1985 among male residents of Montréal, Canada, aged 35–70, ascertained in 19 major hospitals (Siemiatycki, 1991). With a response rate of 82%, 3730 cancer patients were successfully interviewed. For each site of cancer analysed, two control groups were used, giving rise to two separate sets of analyses and results: one control group selected from among cases of cancer at the other sites studied (cancer controls) and the other consisting of 533 population controls representing those successfully interviewed from an age-stratified sample of the general population (response rate, 72%). The interview was designed to obtain detailed lifetime job histories and information on potential confounders. Each job was reviewed by a trained team of chemists and hygienists who translated jobs into occupational exposures. Of these, 293 of the most common occupational substances were then analysed as potential risk factors in relation to each site of cancer included. Cumulative exposure indices were created for each substance, on the basis of duration, concentration, frequency and the degree of certainty in the exposure assessment itself, and these were analysed at two levels: 'any' and 'substantial' exposure; the latter is a subset of 'any'. Analyses were repeated for a French-Canadian subset, comprising about 60% of the total sample and providing a population that is relatively homogeneous from both a genetic and social perspective, in order to eliminate important sources of confounding and effect modification. Among the substances on the checklist was the general category 'inorganic acid solutions', described as mainly solutions of hydrochloric, sulfuric and nitric acids, to which 13% of the entire study population had been exposed at some time (i.e., lifetime exposure prevalence). Unless otherwise stated, the results quoted are based on cancer controls and the 'any' exposure level. For inorganic acid solutions, there were two significant associations: a RR of 2.0 for oat-cell carcinoma of the lung (33 cases; 90% CI, 1.3–2.9) and a RR of 1.7 for cancer of the kidney (32 cases; 90% CI, 1.2–2.4). The RRs at the 'substantial' levels of exposure were about the same but were based on fewer cases and thus had wider CIs. No excess risk for other histological types of lung cancer was seen, and the RR for all lung cancers combined was 1.2 for any exposure to inorganic acid solutions (129 cases; 90% CI, 1.0–1.6) and 1.1 (0.7–1.6) for substantial exposure. When the category of sulfuric acid alone was analysed, 9% of the entire study population had been exposed at some time. Some evidence of an association with exposure to sulfuric acid was found for all lung cancers and for oat-cell carcinoma of the lung in the French-Canadian subset of the population and for squamous-cell carcinoma of the lung in the whole population. An elevated RR of 2.2 was found for oesophageal cancer (15 cases; 90% CI, 1.3–3.6) in the whole population, again with no indication of higher risk at the substantial exposure level. There was weak evidence of an excess risk for kidney cancer, restricted to the French-Canadian subset of the study population with substantial exposure (four cases; RR, 2.5; 90% CI, 1.0–6.1).

3. Studies of Cancer in Experimental Animals

No data were available to the Working Group.

4. Other Relevant Data

4.1 Absorption, distribution, metabolism and excretion

4.1.1 *Humans*

The impact of an inhaled acidic agent on the respiratory tract depends on a number of interrelated factors which include whether it is a gas or an aerosol; particle size, small particles being more able to penetrate deeply into the lung (Martonen *et al.*, 1985; Jarabek *et al.*, 1989; US Environmental Protection Agency, 1989b); water solubility, agents of higher solubility being more likely to be deposited in the nose and mouth; free hydrogen ion concentration; rate and breathing pattern; and the buffering capacity of the airways and of the local deposition site (Utell *et al.*, 1989). The specific anion may modulate acute effects directly or indirectly. The impact also depends upon the presence of any other chemicals that are carried along with the aerosol particle.

Given the general lack of information on the particle size of aerosols of acids during occupational exposures, it is difficult to clarify the principal deposition site within the respiratory tract. For example, 90% of an aerosol of sulfuric acid (mass median aerodynamic diameter of particles, 5 µm) to which lead–acid battery workers are exposed would be deposited in the extrathoracic portion of the respiratory tract, whereas only 50% of an aerosol with a 2-µm particle size would be deposited in that portion of the respiratory tract. This relationship of size to deposition makes estimation of the changes in pH of the mucus problematic, as diffuse deposition challenges the buffering capacity much less than does deposition of large particles at local sites (Gamble *et al.*, 1984a; Jarabek *et al.*, 1989).

Using an average particle size of 1 µm and exposure concentrations of 0.4–1.0 mg/m^3, Amdur *et al.* (1952) showed that 77% of inhaled sulfuric acid was retained in the airways of exposed human subjects. Martonen *et al.* (1985) calculated the growth of ≤ 1-µm particles of several inorganic acids within the respiratory tract and found that it depended on humidity, particle size, respiratory characteristics and the hygroscopic nature of the particle.

In the moist environment of the respiratory tract, sulfur trioxide reacts instantaneously with water to form sulfuric acid (see Annex, section 3.2, p. 123); therefore, the toxicology of sulfur trioxide would be expected to be the same as that of sulfuric acid. Ammonia produced by the respiratory tract can partially neutralize the acidity of acid aerosols (Larson *et al.*, 1977; Utell *et al.*, 1989) in the mucous lining of the respiratory tract. Inhalation studies of

Table 17. Case–control studies of risks associated with exposure to inorganic acid aerosols

Reference (country)	Study population	Definition of exposure (source of data)		Exposed cases	OR	95% CI	Comments
Laryngeal cancer							
Soskolne et al., 1984 (USA)	Nested in cohort of workers in refinery and chemical plant (50 upper respiratory cancers of which 30 laryngeal; 175 controls)	Average sulfuric acid (industrial hygienist's evaluation based on work history from personnel records)	'Moderate' 'High'	– –	4.6 13.4	0.83–25.4 2.08–86.0	Adjusted for tobacco smoking and history of alcoholism and ear, nose and throat diseases. Matched analysis; number of discordant sets not available
Zemla et al., 1987 (Poland)	(328 cases; 656 controls)	Sulfuric, hydrochloric, nitric acids (interview included 'occupational factors')		11	4.27	Not reported	Lack of details on methods; insufficient data to calculate CIs; $p \leq 0.001$
Brown et al., 1988 (USA)	Population-based (183 cases; 250 controls)	Sulfuric acid (industrial hygienist's evaluation based on complete work history from interview)		22	0.76	0.42–1.35	Adjusted for smoking and alcohol consumption; low response rate
Soskolne et al., 1992 (Canada)	Population-based (183 cases; 183 controls)	Sulfuric acid mists (job exposure matrix; full occupational history from interview)		134	3.04	1.67–5.53	Trend with level of exposure. Similar results with more specific definition of exposure.
Multiple myeloma							
Morris et al., 1986 (USA)	Population-based (698 cases; 1683 controls)	Acids (self-reported by interview)	Direct interviews Both direct and next-of-kin interviews	– –	1.5 1.0	0.8–2.8 0.6–1.9	Adjusted for age, sex and race
Multiple sites							
Siemiatycki, 1991 (Canada)	Population-based (lung cancer: 857 cases, 1360 controls; kidney cancer: 177 cases, 2481 controls; oesophageal cancer: 99 cases, 2546 controls)	Inorganic acid solutions	Lung Any exposure Substantial exposure	129 32	1.2 1.1	1.0–1.6[a] 0.7–1.6[a]	No excess cancers of oesophagus, stomach, colon, rectum, pancreas, prostate or bladder, skin melanoma or non-Hodgkin's lymphoma

Table 17 (contd)

Reference (country)	Study population	Definition of exposure (source of data)		Exposed cases	OR	95% CI	Comments
Multiple sites (contd)							
		Inorganic acid solutions (contd)	Kidney				No excess cancers of stomach, colon, rectum, pancreas, kidney, prostate or bladder, skin melanoma or non-Hodgkin's lymphoma
			Any exposure	32	1.7	1.2–2.4[a]	
			Substantial exposure	11	1.8	1.0–3.1[a]	
		Sulfuric acid	Lung				
			Any exposure	60[b]	1.2	0.8–1.9[a]	
			Substantial exposure	8[b]	2.9	0.8–10.4[a]	
			Oat-cell (any exposure)	16[b]	1.7	1.0–2.9[a]	
			Squamous-cell (any exposure)	38	1.5	1.0–2.4[a]	
			Oesophagus				
			Any exposure	15	2.2	1.3–3.6[a]	
			Substantial exposure	3	2.1	0.8–5.8[a]	

OR, odds ratio; CI, confidence interval
[a]90% CI
[b]French Canadians only

ammonium sulfate may therefore be relevant to an assessment of the carcinogenicity of inhaled sulfuric acid.

The breathing pattern (e.g., mouth *versus* nose breathing with normal augmentation through the mouth) also influences deposition. The dose deposited regionally below the nasopharynx is higher for mouth breathers for all particle sizes. The effect of mouth breathing is most pronounced in increasing deposition in the oropharynx, larynx and upper trachea (Jarabek *et al.*, 1989).

4.1.2 *Experimental systems*

Generally, similar information is available for animals and humans. Regional deposition of sulfuric acid aerosols in experimental animals is thus also dependent on particle size (e.g., Dahl *et al.*, 1983). Animal species differ from humans with regard to the dimensions and architecture of the respiratory tract, and deposition patterns of aerosols vary accordingly (Jarabek *et al.*, 1989). Ammonia production by the respiratory tract is important in partial neutralization of acid aerosols, but larger particles are neutralized less efficiently than smaller particles (e.g., Larson *et al.*, 1982).

4.2 Toxic effects

4.2.1 *Humans*

The toxic effects of acid aerosols, including those containing sulfuric acid, have been reviewed (Fouts & Lippmann, 1989; US Environmental Protection Agency, 1989b). Of the acidic mists, sulfuric acid has been studied most extensively. As for deposition, the toxicity of acid mists to the lung depends in part on aerosol size, smaller particles penetrating more deeply into the lung (Lippmann *et al.*, 1987).

Acids are highly corrosive and irritating and give rise to local effects on the skin, eye and other mucous epithelia when there is direct exposure to sufficient concentrations (see also monograph on hydrochloric acid).

Sulfur dioxide and related acid mists of sulfuric acid have caused respiratory irritation, bronchitis and death (WHO Working Group, 1986; WHO, 1987; American Thoracic Society, 1991) (see also the monographs on sulfur dioxide and hydrochloric acid).

Concern about the health effects of acidic aerosols, and particularly sulfuric acid and acid sulfates, was accentuated by the episodes of smog in London in the 1950s and 1960s, during which thousands more deaths than expected were recorded. People at particular risk were those with pre-existing cardiovascular and pulmonary disease. Similar gas–aerosol complexes have been responsible for acute and chronic lung disease, including potentiation of respiratory tract infections and chronic bronchitis in geographical areas where there is significant air pollution from stationary sources of fossil fuel combustion (Thurston *et al.*, 1989). Although sulfuric acid is only one component of these complexes, it has been suggested that hydrogen ion concentration, presumably primarily reflecting sulfuric and nitric acids, is correlated with bronchitic symptoms in children (Speizer, 1989; US Environmental Protection Agency, 1989b). Levels of sulfate and fine particles may also be better predictors of mortality than are concentrations of total suspended particles or inhalable particles (Özkaynak & Thurston, 1987).

The historical cohort study of mortality among 22 323 workers in the Florida phosphate industry, described on pp. 85–86 (Checkoway *et al.*, 1985a), showed increased mortality from emphysema (31 cases; SMR = 1.48; $p < 0.05$). No clear trend with length of employment or years since first employment was seen, but the excess mortality was more pronounced among workers first hired before 1940 (9 cases) than among those hired after 1940 (22 cases). [The Working Group noted, as did the authors, that this finding is difficult to interpret in the light of the many exposures of these workers, the absence of information on tobacco smoking and variation in the diagnoses of chronic respiratory diseases.]

Airway mucus has a high buffering capacity and protects the epithelial cells of the respiratory mucous membranes. Its viscosity depends on pH, and acidified mucus of increased viscosity diminishes lung function. People who have acidic mucus with a low protein concentration (e.g., people with infections or inflammations and some asthmatics) may be at high risk when exposed to acids (Holma, 1989).

Estimates of the pH of mucus range from 6.5 to 7.5, with a mean of approximately 6.9. [The Working Group noted that chemical composition, and therefore the pH of mucus, vary within the respiratory tract and can be changed by sampling techniques.] The US Environmental Protection Agency (1989b) has estimated that exposure to sulfuric acid at 390–780 μg [1300 μg/m^3] for 30 min at a ventilation rate of 20 litres/min and 50% deposition (for a particle size of 2 μm) would lower the pH of the mucus in the tracheo-bronchial region by approximately 1 unit. This calculation assumes that the distribution of sulfuric acid is uniform; non-uniform distribution would alter the change in pH in specific regions. The calculation does not take into consideration neutralization of acid in the airways by ammonia.

Dental erosion has been observed as a result of industrial exposure to acid mists. Bruggen Cate (1968) studied dental erosion in 555 workers from several industries in the United Kingdom where acid processes (pickling, galvanizing and battery manufacture) were used. Control subjects were selected from among workers in other departments in the same firms where acid was not used. Exposure to acids was not measured. The prevalence of dental erosion was highest among battery formation workers and lower among picklers. A similar association was seen in a sample of 186 workers from battery factories in Finland (Tuominen *et al.*, 1989). Various degrees of dental erosion were seen in 90% of picklers in a zinc galvanizing plant in the Netherlands; the threshold limit value for hydrochloric acid (7 mg/m^3) was exceeded for 27% of the working time (Remijn *et al.*, 1982).

Controlled human exposures to relatively high levels of sulfuric acid resulted in acute symptoms and other findings suggestive of bronchoconstriction (Balmes *et al.*, 1989). Effects have generally not been observed in healthy adults exposed acutely to levels of less than 500 μg/m^3 over a broad range of particle sizes, although delayed symptomatology (mild throat irritation and increased carbachol bronchorestrictor response) was noted after exposure to 450 μg/m^3 for 4 h while exercising moderately (Utell, 1985). Concentration (0, 500, 1000 and 2000 μg/m^3)-related increases in upper respiratory symptoms (cough) without change in pulmonary function have also been noted (Avol *et al.*, 1988). Exercising asthmatics were reported to be highly responsive (in terms of decreased forced expiratory volume in 1 sec) to a low level of sulfuric acid (100 μg/m^3) (Koenig *et al.*, 1989).

Acute exposure of human volunteers to 100 μg/m³ of sulfuric acid resulted in increased mucociliary clearance of particles from the large proximal airways; at higher levels (1000 μg/m³), the opposite occurred. Clearance from the distal airways was reduced at both levels (Leikauf et al., 1984).

The acute and chronic effects of sulfuric acid were studied in five lead–acid battery plants. Personal monitoring of 225 workers revealed mean exposures to sulfuric acid of 0.18 mg/m³ (range, 0.08–0.35 mg/m³) at an average mass median aerodynamic diameter of close to 5 μm. No difference was noted in acute symptoms between groups exposed to high (> 0.3 mg/m³) and low (< 0.07 mg/m³) levels of sulfuric acid, although eye irritation and cough were more prevalent in the groups with higher exposure. The possibility that workers became acclimatized to the acute effects of sulfuric acid was considered: neither short-term nor long-term changes in pulmonary function (as measured by spirometry) were observed, and the prevalence of respiratory symptoms was not related to cumulative acid exposure. Dental etching and erosion occurred about four times more frequently in the group exposed to high levels of acid (Gamble et al., 1984a,b).

Other health effects have been reported in industries in which acidic mists occur, which have been attributed to other pollutants. For instance, haematological effects seen in the lead battery industry have been presumed to be due to lead (IARC, 1980).

4.2.2 Experimental systems

In donkeys (Lippmann et al., 1982) and in rabbits (Schlesinger, 1990), repeated exposures to sulfuric acid at levels that initially increased mucociliary clearance of particles led over time to decreased clearance, indicating chronic effects. Sulfuric acid significantly reduced the phagocytic capacity of alveolar macrophages in rabbits exposed by inhalation to ≥ 1000 μg/m³ for 1 h per day for five days (Schlesinger et al., 1990).

The alveolar phagocytotic response *in vitro* was related linearly to exposure *in vitro* to H^+, whereas the response *in vivo* was not (Schlesinger et al., 1990).

Changes in particle bronchial clearance and an increased number of mucus secretory cells were observed in rabbits exposed to sulfuric acid at 250 μg/m³ for 1 h per day on five days per week for up to 12 months; no change in the pulmonary tissues was observed by routine histological procedures (Gearhart & Schlesinger, 1986; Schlesinger & Gearhart, 1986; Gearhart & Schlesinger, 1989). Sulfuric acid may induce hyperresponsiveness of the airways in exposed rabbits (Gearhart & Schlesinger, 1986).

Long-term, continuous exposure to sulfuric acid mist had no effect in three groups of 100 guinea-pigs exposed for 52 weeks to filtered air (control), to 0.10 mg/m³ sulfuric acid with a particle size of 2.78 μm mass median aerodynamic diameter or to 0.08 mg/m³ sulfuric acid with a particle size of 0.84 μm. In a similar study, five groups of nine cynomolgus monkeys were exposed continuously for 78 weeks to sulfuric acid. Deleterious effects were seen on pulmonary function and respiratory histology, depending on the concentration and particle size of the sulfuric acid. Effects were particularly prominent in monkeys exposed to 4.79 mg/m³ with a particle size of 0.73 μm mass median aerodynamic diameter. At 0.48 mg/m³ (0.54 μm) and 0.38 mg/m³ (2.15 μm), only minimal effects were noted (Alarie et al., 1973).

4.3 Reproduction and developmental effects

4.3.1 *Humans*

No data were available to the Working Group.

4.3.2 *Experimental systems*

Groups of 35–40 CF-1 mice and 20 New Zealand rabbits were exposed *via* inhalation to aerosols containing sulfuric acid (purity, 95.7%) at 0, 5 or 20 mg/m^3 for 7 h per day on days 6–15 or 6–18 of gestation, respectively. The count medium diameters of particles in the chambers were 0.4, 1.6 and 2.4 μm in the control, low-dose and high-dose groups. Animals were deprived of food and water during exposure. Mouse fetuses were examined on day 18 and rabbit fetuses on day 29 of gestation. In dam mice, body weight was not significantly lower than that of controls; food consumption was reported to be decreased during the first few days of exposure at 20 mg/m^3 but not at 5 mg/m^3; no alteration was noted in respiratory tract histology. In dam rabbits given the high dose, body weight was significantly reduced in the early part of the exposure period, and histological examination of the respiratory tract showed a dose-related increase in the incidence of subacute rhinitis and tracheitis. No significant effect on embryonic viability or growth was noted in either species, and no dose-related morphological effect was seen in mouse fetuses. One case of a very rare defect (conjoined twinning) was seen in the litter of a mouse given the high dose. The only significant effect seen in rabbit fetuses was an increased incidence of 'small non-ossified areas in the skull bones' in the high-dose group (Murray *et al.*, 1979). [The Working Group noted that actual data were not given.]

4.4 Genetic and related effects (see also Table 18 and Appendices 1 and 2)

4.4.1 *Humans*

(a) Sulfuric acid manufacture

The frequencies of sister chromatid exchange, micronuclei and chromosomal aberrations in cultured lymphocytes from 40 workers exposed to sulfur dioxide in a sulfuric acid factory in Taiyuan City, northern China, were compared with those of 42 controls working and studying at a university situated in the same city as the factory, who were matched according to sex, age and smoking habits. The concentrations of sulfur dioxide in the factory varied irregularly from 0.34 to 11.97 mg/m^3 at the time of investigation. The mean number of sister chromatid exchanges/cell was 6.72 ± 0.22 for sulfur dioxide-exposed workers and 2.71 ± 0.31 for unexposed controls ($p < 0.01$); the mean frequency of micronuclei in cultivated lymphocytes was 0.168% in those from the workers and 0.071% for the control group ($p < 0.001$); and the mean frequency of severe types of chromosomal aberration (including rings, translocations and dicentrics) per 100 metaphases was 0.963% for the workers and 0.227% for controls ($p < 0.01$). No positive correlation was observed between the frequency of sister chromatid exchange, micronuclei or chromosomal aberrations and length of service of the workers. While there was no significant difference between smokers and nonsmokers with regard to the frequencies of sister chromatid exchange and chromosomal aberrations, smokers among both the workers and the control group had significantly more micronuclei than nonsmokers ($p < 0.001$) (Meng & Zhang,

1990a,b). [The Working Group noted that no information was provided on exposures other than to sulfur dioxide.]

(b) Lead battery (accumulator) manufacture

No data on exposure to acid mists were given in reports of studies of sister chromatid exchange or chromosomal aberrations in workers in lead battery manufacture (Grandjean *et al.*, 1983; Al-Hakkak *et al.*, 1986).

4.4.2 *Experimental systems*

Genotoxicity under extreme conditions of culture, including pH, has been reviewed (Scott *et al.*, 1991). No data were available on the genetic and related effects of exposures to acid mist in experimental systems; however, the effects of pH reduction have been investigated.

Low pH enhances the level of depurination of isolated DNA (Singer & Grunberger, 1983), and the fidelity of DNA replication and repair enzymes may be reduced by extremes of pH (Brusick, 1986). Low pH did not affect the frequency of point mutations in *Salmonella typhimurium* (with or without S9), *Escherichia coli*, *Neurospora crassa* or *Saccharomyces cerevisiae*, but it induced gene conversion in *S. cerevisiae*, chromosomal aberrations in *Vicia faba* root tips and a variety of mitotic abnormalities in sea urchin embryos and in offspring after treatment of sperm.

In mammalian systems, the genotoxic effects of low pH appear to be strongly enhanced by the presence of S9. Brusick (1986) reported that low pH induced chromosomal aberrations in Chinese hamster ovary cells only in the presence of S9. Morita *et al.* (1989), however, showed that in the same cells at low pH (5.5 or less) aberrations were also induced in the absence of S9, although S9 greatly enhanced the effect. No chromosomal effect was observed in rat lymphocytes incubated at pH 5.1, either with or without S9. Mutations have been reported in mouse lymphoma L5178Y cells exposed to low pH, both with and without S9, although the effect was only marginal (1.9 fold at pH 6.3) in the absence of S9. Reduction in pH from 7.35 to 6.70, achieved by lowering the concentrations of sodium bicarbonate in the medium, resulted in increased transformation frequency in Syrian hamster embryo cells.

5. Summary of Data Reported and Evaluation

5.1 Exposure data

Strong inorganic acids may be present in the work environment as mists, vapours or gases. The most prevalent acids are sulfuric, hydrochloric, nitric and phosphoric acids, which may be present in a wide variety of industries, including the extraction, fabrication and finishing of metal, fertilizer production, battery manufacture and various segments of the petroleum, chemical and petrochemical industries. Millions of workers worldwide are estimated to be potentially exposed to these acids.

Sulfuric acid is the most widely used of the strong inorganic acids. Average exposures to sulfuric acid mists in pickling, electroplating and other acid treatment of metals are frequently above 0.5 mg/m^3, while lower levels are usually found in the manufacture of

Table 18. Genetic and related effects of acidic pH

Test system	Result		Dose or pH	Reference
	Without exogenous metabolic system	With exogenous metabolic system		
SA0, *Salmonella typhimurium* TA100, reverse mutation	-	0	pH 3	Tomlinson (1980)
SA0, *Salmonella typhimurium* TA100, reverse mutation	-	-	pH 5.5	Cipollaro et al. (1986)
SA2, *Salmonella typhimurium* TA102, reverse mutation	-	-	pH 5.5	Cipollaro et al. (1986)
SA5, *Salmonella typhimurium* TA1535, reverse mutation	-	-	pH 3	Tomlinson (1980)
SA5, *Salmonella typhimurium* TA1535, reverse mutation	-	-	pH 5.5	Cipollaro et al. (1986)
SA9, *Salmonella typhimurium* TA98, reverse mutation	-	-	pH 5.5	Cipollaro et al. (1986)
SAS, *Salmonella typhimurium* TA97, reverse mutation	-	-	pH 5.5	Cipollaro et al. (1986)
ECR, *Escherichia coli*, (B/Sd-4/1,3,4,5) reverse mutation streptomycin[R]	-	0	0.002–0.005%	Demerec et al. (1951)
ECR, *Escherichia coli*, (B/Sd-4/3,4) reverse mutation streptomycin[R]	-	0	0.002–0.005%	Demerec et al. (1951)
SCG, *Saccharomyces cerevisiae*, gene conversion	+	0	pH 5.8	Nanni et al. (1984)
SCR, *Saccharomyces cerevisiae*, reverse mutation	-	0	pH 3.8	Nanni et al. (1984)
NCR, *Neurospora crassa*, reverse mutation	-	0	pH 3	Tomlinson (1980)
NCR, *Neurospora crassa*, reverse mutation	-	0	pH 3	Whong et al. (1985)
VFC, *Vicia faba*, chromosomal aberrations	+	0	pH 4.0	Bradley et al. (1968)
VFC, *Vicia faba*, chromosomal aberrations	+	0	pH 4.0	Zura & Grant (1981)
CIA, Chromosomal aberrations, *Sphaerechinus granularis* embryos, mitotic abnormalities	+	0	pH 6.0	Cipollaro et al. (1986)
CIA, Chromosomal aberrations, *S. lividus* embryos	+	0	pH 6.5	Pagano et al. (1985a)
CIA, Chromosomal aberrations, *Paracentrotus lividus* sperm, mitotic abnormalities	+	0	pH 6.5	Pagano et al. (1985b)
CIA, Chromosomal aberrations, *P. lividus* sperm, mitotic abnormalities	+	0	pH 5	Cipollaro et al. (1986)
CIA, Chromosomal aberrations, *S. granularis* sperm, mitotic abnormalities	+	0	pH 6.5	Cipollaro et al. (1986)
GST, Gene mutation, mouse lymphoma L5178Y cells, *tk*	(+)	+	pH 6.0	Cifone et al. (1987)
CIC, Chromosomal aberrations, Chinese hamster CHO cells *in vitro*	-	+	pH 5.5	Brusick (1986)
CIC, Chromosomal aberrations, Chinese hamster CHO cells *in vitro*	+	+	pH 5.5	Morita et al. (1989)
CIR, Chromosomal aberrations, rat lymphocytes *in vitro*	-	-	pH 5.1	Sinha et al. 1989)
TFS, Cell transformation, Syrian hamster embryo cells, focus assay	+	0	pH 6.7	Le Boeuf & Kerckaert (1986)

lead–acid batteries and in phosphate fertilizer production. Exposure to sulfuric acid also occurs during its manufacture and during the production of isopropanol, synthetic ethanol and detergents. Hydrochloric acid is used in industries that involve acid treatment of metals, where occupational exposure levels to hydrochloric acid mists and gas are frequently above 1 mg/m^3. Exposures to hydrochloric acid may also occur during its synthesis and use in various industrial processes. Pickling and other acid treatments of metal may entail occupational exposures to nitric and phosphoric acids, but these occur less frequently than exposures to sulfuric and hydrochloric acids. Exposure to nitric acid also occurs during its manufacture and exposure to phosphoric acid in phosphate fertilizer production.

5.2 Human carcinogenicity data

An early study of isopropanol manufacture in the USA using the strong-acid process demonstrated an excess of nasal sinus cancer. Studies of one US cohort of workers in pickling operations within the steel industry showed excesses of laryngeal and lung cancer after smoking and other potential confounding variables had been controlled for. A Swedish study of a cohort of workers in steel pickling also showed an excess risk for laryngeal cancer. A nested case–control study of workers in a US petrochemical plant showed an elevated risk for laryngeal cancer among workers exposed to sulfuric acid. Of two population-based case–control studies in Canada, one of laryngeal cancer showed an increased risk for exposure to sulfuric acid, and one of lung cancer suggested an excess risk; the latter also suggested a risk associated with exposure to mixed inorganic acids. In all these studies, sulfuric acid mists were the commonest exposure, and positive exposure–response relationships were seen in two of the studies.

Additional supporting evidence was provided by one cohort study in the soap manufacturing industry in Italy, which showed an increased risk for laryngeal cancer. Studies of three US cohorts and one Swedish cohort in the phosphate fertilizer manufacturing industry showed excess lung cancer, but there was potential confounding from exposure to radon decay products in some cohorts.

5.3 Animal carcinogenicity data

No data were available to the Working Group.

5.4 Other relevant data

Acid mists containing particles with a diameter of up to a few micrometers will be deposited in both the upper and lower airways. They are irritating to mucous epithelia, they cause dental erosion, and they produce acute effects in the lungs (symptoms and changes in pulmonary function). Asthmatics appear to be at particular risk for pulmonary effects.

Significant increases in the incidences of sister chromatid exchange, micronucleus formation and chromosomal aberrations in peripheral lymphocytes were observed in a single study of workers engaged in the manufacture of sulfuric acid.

The studies reviewed examined the effects of pH values < 7 specifically. In cultured mammalian cells at pH 6.7 or below, cell transformation, gene mutation and chromosomal aberrations were induced. Mitotic abnormalities were induced in sea urchins and clastogenic effects in plants. Gene conversion was induced in yeast cells. No point mutation was observed in fungi, yeast or bacteria. Acid pH caused depurination of isolated DNA.

5.5 Evaluation[1]

There is *sufficient evidence* that occupational exposure to strong-inorganic-acid mists containing sulfuric acid is carcinogenic.

Overall evaluation

Occupational exposure to strong-inorganic-acid mists containing sulfuric acid *is carcinogenic to humans (Group 1)*.

6. References

Ahlborg, G., Jr, Hogstedt, C., Sundell, L. & Åman, C.-G. (1981) Laryngeal cancer and pickling house vapors. *Scand. J. Work Environ. Health*, **7**, 239–240

Ahrenholz, S.H. (1987) *Health Hazard Evaluation, Empire-Detroit Steel Division, Mansfield, OH* (Report No. HETA 86-125-1853), Cincinnati, OH, National Institute for Occupational Safety and Health

Ahrenholz, S.H. & Anderson, K.E. (1981) *Health Hazard Evaluation, Valley Chrome Platers, Bay City, MI* (Report No. HETA 81-085-889), Cincinnati, OH, National Institute for Occupational Safety and Health

Alarie, Y., Busey, W.M., Krumm, A.A. & Ulrich, C.E. (1973) Long-term continuous exposure to sulfuric acid mists in cynomolgus monkeys and guinea pigs. *Arch. environ. Health*, **27**, 16–24

Alderson, M.R. & Rattan, N.S. (1980) Mortality of workers on an isopropyl alcohol plant and two MEK dewaxing plants. *Br. J. ind. Med.*, **37**, 85–89

Al-Hakkak, Z.S., Hamamy, H.A., Murad, A.M.B. & Hussain, A.F. (1986) Chromosomal aberrations in workers at a storage battery plant in Iraq. *Mutat. Res.*, **171**, 53–60

Almaguer, D. & London, M. (1986) *Health Hazard Evaluation, National Starch, Indianapolis, IN* (Report No. HETA 85-031-1706), Revised, Cincinnati, OH, National Institute for Occupational Safety and Health

Alwens, W., Bauke, E.E. & Jonas, W. (1936) Several bronchial cancers occurring in workers in the chemical industry (Ger.). *Arch. Gewerbepathol. Gewerbehyg.*, **7**, 69–84

Amdur, M.O., Silverman, L. & Drinker, P. (1952) Inhalation of sulfuric acid mist by human subjects. *Arch. ind. Hyg. occup. Med.*, **6**, 305–313

American Conference of Governmental Industrial Hygienists (1990) *1990–1991 Threshold Limit Values for Chemical Substances and Physical Agents and Biological Exposure Indices*, Cincinnati, OH, pp. 28, 30, 34

American Thoracic Society (1991) Health effects of atmospheric acids and their precursors. *Am. Rev. respir. Dis.*, **144**, 464–467

Anania, T.L., Price, J.H. & Evans, W.A. (1978) *Health Hazard Evaluation Determination, Midwest Steel Division, National Steel Corporation, Portage, IN* (Report No. HE 77-34-471), Cincinnati, OH, National Institute for Occupational Safety and Health

---

[1]For definition of the italicized terms, see Preamble, pp. 26–29.

Anfield, B.D. & Warner, C.G. (1968) A study of industrial mists containing sulphuric acid. *Ann. occup. Hyg.*, **11**, 185–194

Anon. (1983) Facts & figures for the chemical industry. *Chem. Eng. News*, **61**, 26–67

Anon. (1984a) Facts & figures for the chemical industry. *Chem. Eng. News*, **62**, 32–74

Anon. (1984b) II. Chemical industry statistics. 1. Statistical data of China chemical industry. In: Guangqi, Y., ed., *China Chemical Industry* (World Chemical Industry Yearbook), English ed., Beijing, Scientific & Technical Information, Research Institute of the Ministry of Chemical Industry of China, p. 530

Anon. (1986) Facts & figures for the chemical industry. *Chem. Eng. News*, **64**, 32–86

Anon. (1987) Facts & figures for the chemical industry. *Chem. Eng. News*, **65**, 24–76

Anon. (1988) Facts & figures for the chemical industry. *Chem. Eng. News*, **66**, 34–82

Anon. (1991) Facts & figures for the chemical industry. *Chem. Eng. News*, **69**, 28–81

Apol, A.G. (1981a) *Health Hazard Evaluation, Alaska Smelting and Refining Company, Wisilla, AK* (Report No. HETA 81-036-1023), Cincinnati, OH, National Institute for Occupational Safety and Health

Apol, A.G. (1981b) *Health Hazard Evaluation, Publishers Paper Company, Newberg, OR* (Report No. HETA 81-090-997), Cincinnati, OH, National Institute for Occupational Safety and Health

Apol, A.G. & Singal, M. (1987) *Health Hazard Evaluation, J.R. Simplot Company, Pocatello, ID* (Report No. HETA 84-488-1793), Cincinnati, OH, National Institute for Occupational Safety and Health

Apol, A.G. & Tanaka, S. (1978) *Health Hazard Evaluation Determination, Teledyne Wah Chang Albany, Albany, OR* (Report No. 75-161-454), Cincinnati, OH, National Institute for Occupational Safety and Health

Avol, E.L., Linn, W.S., Whynot, J.D., Anderson, K.R., Shamoo, D.A., Valencia, L.M., Little, D.E. & Hackney, J.D. (1988) Respiratory dose–response study of normal and asthmatic volunteers exposed to sulfuric acid aerosol in the sub-micrometer size range. *Toxicol. ind. Health*, **4**, 173–184

Axelson, O. (1978) Letter to the Editor. Aspects on confounding in occupational health epidemiology. *Scand. J. Work Environ. Health*, **4**, 98–102

Balmes, J.R., Fine, J.M., Gordon, T. & Sheppard, D. (1989) Potential bronchoconstrictor stimuli in acid fog. *Environ. Health Perspectives*, **79**, 163–166

Beaumont, J.J., Leveton, J., Knox, K., Bloom, T., McQuiston, T., Young, M., Goldsmith, R., Steenland, N.K., Brown, D.P. & Halperin, W.E. (1987) Lung cancer mortality in workers exposed to sulfuric acid mist and other acid mists. *J. natl Cancer Inst.*, **79**, 911–921

Belanger, P.L. (1980) *Health Hazard Evaluation Determination, University Corporation for Atmospheric Research, Mauna Loa Observatory, Hilo, HI* (Report No. HE 79-31-699), Cincinnati, OH, National Institute for Occupational Safety and Health

Berndt, D. (1985) Lead–acid batteries. In: Gerhartz, W., ed., *Ullmann's Encyclopedia of Industrial Chemistry*, 5th rev. ed., Vol. A3, New York, VCH Publishers, pp. 374–390

Block, G., Matanoski, G.M., Seltser, R. & Mitchell, T. (1988) Cancer morbidity and mortality in phosphate workers. *Cancer Res.*, **48**, 7298–7303

Bradley, M.V., Hall, L.L. & Trebilcock, S.J. (1968) Low pH of irradiated sucrose in induction of chromosome aberrations. *Nature*, **217**, 1182–1183

Brady, J.E. & Humiston, G.E. (1978) *General Chemistry: Principles and Structure*, 2nd ed., New York, John Wiley & Sons, pp. 375–428

Brown, L.M., Mason, T.J., Pickle, L.W., Stewart, P.A., Buffler, P.A., Burau, K., Ziegler, R.G. & Fraumeni, J.F., Jr (1988) Occupational risk factors for laryngeal cancer on the Texas Gulf coast. *Cancer Res.*, **48**, 1960–1964

Bruggen Cate, H.J.T. (1968) Dental erosion in industry. *Br. J. ind. Med.*, **25**, 249–266

Brusick, D. (1986) Genotoxic effects in cultured mammalian cells produced by low pH treatment conditions and increased ion concentrations. *Environ. Mutag.*, **8**, 879–886

Budavari, S., ed. (1989) *The Merck Index*, 11th ed., Rahway, NJ, Merck & Co., pp. 1417–1418

Bumb, B.L. (1989) *Global Fertilizer Perspective, 1960–95: The Dynamics of Growth and Structural Change* (Executive Summary), Muscle Shoals, AL, International Fertilizer Development Institute, pp. 10, 19

Burch, J.D., Howe, G.R., Miller, A.B. & Semenciw, R. (1981) Tobacco, alcohol, asbestos, and nickel in the etiology of cancer of the larynx. A case–control study. *J. natl Cancer Inst.*, **67**, 1219–1224

Burgess, W.A. (1981) *Recognition of Health Hazards in Industry*, New York, John Wiley & Sons

Cassady, M.E., Donaldson, H. & Gentry, S. (1975) *Industrial Hygiene Survey, Agrico Chemical Company, Pierce, Florida, June 22–26, 1975* (Report No. IWS 57-11), Cincinnati, OH, National Institute for Occupational Safety and Health

Checkoway, H., Mathew, R.M., Hickey, J.L.S., Shy, C.M., Harris, R.L., Jr, Hunt, E.W. & Waldman, G.T. (1985a) Mortality among workers in the Florida phosphate industry. I. Industry-wide cause-specific mortality patterns. *J. occup. Med.*, **27**, 885–892

Checkoway, H., Mathew, R.M., Hickey, J.L.S., Shy, C.M., Harris, R.L., Jr, Hunt, E.W. & Waldman, G.T. (1985b) Mortality among workers in the Florida phosphate industry. II. Cause-specific mortality relationships with work areas and exposures. *J. occup. Med.*, **27**, 893–896

Cifone, M.A., Myhr, B., Eiche, A. & Bolcsfoldi, G. (1987) Effect of pH shifts on the mutant frequency at the thymidine kinase locus in mouse lymphoma L5178Y TK$^{+/-}$ cells. *Mutat. Res.*, **189**, 39–46

Cipollaro, M., Corsale, G., Esposito, A., Ragucci, E., Staiano, N., Giordano, G.G. & Pagano, G. (1986) Sublethal pH decrease may cause genetic damage to eukaryotic cells: a study on sea urchins and *Salmonella typhimurium*. *Teratog. Carcinog. Mutag.*, **6**, 275–287

Collins, J.J., Swaen, G.M.H., Marsh, G.M., Utidjian, H.M.D., Caporossi, J.C. & Lucas, L.J. (1989) Mortality patterns among workers exposed to acrylamide. *J. occup. Med.*, **31**, 614–617

Cook, W.A. (1987) *Occupational Exposure Limits—Worldwide*, Akron, OH, American Industrial Hygiene Association, pp. 124, 125, 148, 150, 153, 204, 208, 216

Cooper, W.C. & Gaffey, W.R. (1975) Mortality of lead workers. *J. occup. Med.*, **17**, 100–107

Cooper, W.C., Wong, O. & Kheifets, L. (1985) Mortality among employees of lead battery plants and lead-producing plants, 1947–1980. *Scand. J. Work Environ. Health*, **11**, 331–345

Costello, R.J. & Landrigan, P.J. (1980) *Health Hazard Evaluation, Globe Union Battery Plant, Bennington, VT* (Project No. HE 78-98-710), Cincinnati, OH, National Institute for Occupational Safety and Health

Covino, B.S., Jr, Scalera, J.V. & Fabis, P.M. (1984) *Pickling of Stainless Steels—A Review* (Information Circular 8985; US NTIS PB85-111979), Washington DC, US Bureau of Mines

Dahl, A.R., Felicetti, S.A. & Muggenburg, B.A. (1983) Clearance of sulfuric acid-introduced ^{35}S from the respiratory tracts of rats, guinea pigs and dogs following inhalation or instillation. *Fundam. appl. Toxicol.*, **3**, 293–297

Daniels, W.J. (1988) *Health Hazard Evaluation, United States Air Force Reserve, Portland, Oregon* (Report No. HETA 88-255-0000), Cincinnati, OH, National Institute for Occupational Safety and Health

Daniels, W.J. & Gunter, B.J. (1987) *Health Hazard Evaluation, Olson Industries, Denver, CO* (Report No. HETA 86-063-1843), Cincinnati, OH, National Institute for Occupational Safety and Health

Daniels, W.J. & Orris, P. (1981) *Health Hazard Evaluation, US Steel, Tubing Specialties, Gary, IN* (Report No. HHE 80-025-989), Cincinnati, OH, National Institute for Occupational Safety and Health

Danielyants, L.A. (1976) Sanitation of working in the production of ammonium phosphate (Russ.). *Gig. Tr. Prof. Zabol.*, **11**, 48–50

Demerec, M., Bertani, G. & Flint, J. (1951) A survey of chemicals for mutagenic action on *E. coli*. *Am. Naturalist*, **85**, 119–136

Dialog Information Services (1991) *Chem-Intell Database* (File 318), Palo Alto, CA

Direktoratet for Arbeidstilsynet (Directorate of Labour Inspection) (1990) *Administrative Normer for Forurensning i Arbeidsatmosfaere 1990* [Administrative Norms for Pollution in Work Atmosphere 1990], Oslo, pp. 11, 18

Doe, J.B. (1978) Secondary cells, lead–acid. In: Mark, H.F., Othmer, D.F., Overberger, C.G., Seaborg, G.T. & Grayson, N., eds, *Kirk–Othmer Encyclopedia of Chemical Technology*, 3rd ed., Vol. 3, New York, John Wiley & Sons, pp. 640–663

Eckardt, R.E. (1959) *Industrial Carcinogens* (Modern Monographs in Industrial Medicine, No. 4), New York, Grune & Stratton, pp. 101–102

Eller, P.M., ed. (1984) *NIOSH Manual of Analytical Methods*, Method 7903, 3rd ed., Vol. 1 (DHHS (NIOSH) Publ. No. 84-100), Washington DC, US Government Printing Office, pp. 7903-1–7903-6

El-Sadik, Y.M., Osman, H.A. & El-Gazzar, R.M. (1972) Exposure to sulfuric acid in manufacture of storage batteries. *J. occup. Med.*, **14**, 224–226

Englander, V., Sjöberg, A., Hagmar, L., Attewell, R., Schütz, A., Möller, T. & Skerfving, S. (1988) Mortality and cancer morbidity in workers exposed to sulphur dioxide in a sulphuric acid plant. *Int. Arch. occup. environ. Health*, **61**, 157–162

Enterline, P.E. (1982) Importance of sequential exposure in the production of epichlorohydrin and isopropanol. *Ann. N.Y. Acad. Sci.*, **381**, 344–349

Evans, W. (1978) *Health Hazard Evaluation Determination, Western Gear Corporation, Flight Structures Division, North, Jamestown, ND* (Report No. HE 78-76-548), Cincinnati, OH, National Institute for Occupational Safety and Health

Fabbri, L., Mapp, C., Rossi, A., Cortese, S. & Saia, B. (1977) Chronic bronchopneumopathy and pneumoconiosis in workers employed in phosphoric acid production (It.). *Lav. Um.*, **29**, 50–57

Fajen, J. (1982) *In Depth Industrial Hygiene Survey Report of Howes Leather Company, Inc., Curwensville, PA* (Report No. IWS 132-13, US NTIS PB83-192989), Cincinnati, OH, National Institute for Occupational Safety and Health

Feierstein, G. & Morgenthaler, W. (1983) Soap and synthetic detergents. In: Kent, J.A., ed., *Riegel's Handbook of Industrial Chemistry*, 8th ed., New York, Van Nostrand Reinhold, pp. 450–487

Feigin, B.G. (1986) Occupational hygiene in the production of pigmentary titanium dioxide (Russ.). *Gig. Trud. Prof. Zab.*, **8**, 23–26

Fertilizer Institute (1982) *The Fertilizer Handbook*, Washington DC, pp. 47–49, 60–62

Ficker, J. (1991) 1990 Battery shipment review and five-year forecast report. In: *1991 Battery Council International 103rd Convention*, Chicago, IL, Delco Remy, General Motors

FIOH (Finnish Institute of Occupational Health) (1990) *Industrial Hygiene Measurements, 1950–69* (Data Base), Helsinki

Forastiere, F., Valesini, S., Salimei, E., Magliola, E. & Perucci, C.A. (1987) Respiratory cancer among soap production workers. *Scand. J. Work Environ. Health*, **13**, 258–260

Fouts, J.R. & Lippmann, M. (Organizers) (1989) Symposium on the health effects of acid aerosols. *Environ. Health Perspectives*, **79**, 1–205

Fowler, H.W. & Fowler, F.G., eds (1964) *The Concise Oxford Dictionary of Current English*, 5th ed., Oxford, Clarendon Press

Gamble, J., Jones, W. & Hancock, J. (1984a) Epidemiological–environmental study of lead acid battery workers. II. Acute effects of sulfuric acid on the respiratory system. *Environ. Res.*, **35**, 11–29

Gamble, J., Jones, W., Hancock, J. & Meckstroth, R.L. (1984b) Epidemiological–environmental study of lead acid battery workers. III. Chronic effects of sulfuric acid on the respiratory system and teeth. *Environ. Res.*, **35**, 30–52

Gearhart, J.M. & Schlesinger, R.B. (1986) Sulfuric acid-induced airway hyperresponsiveness. *Fundam. appl. Toxicol.*, **7**, 681–689

Gearhart, J.M. & Schlesinger, R.B. (1989) Sulfuric acid-induced changes in the physiology and structure of the tracheobronchial airways. *Environ. Health Perspectives*, **79**, 127–137

Geissert, J.O. (1976) *Health Hazard Evaluation Determination, Federal Products Corporation, Providence, RI* (Report No. 75-158-299), Cincinnati, OH, National Institute for Occupational Safety and Health

Geissert, J.O. (1977) *Health Hazard Evaluation Determination, Cleaning House at the Wire Mill, Bethlehem Steel Corporation, Johnstown, PA* (Report No. 77-42-452), Cincinnati, OH, National Institute for Occupational Safety and Health

Gilles, D., Anania, T.L. & Ilka, R. (1977) *Health Hazard Evaluation Determination, Airtex Products, Fairfield, IL* (Report No. 77-12-418), Cincinnati, OH, National Institute for Occupational Safety and Health

Godbey, F.W. (1982) *In Depth Survey Report: Control Technology For Trans World Airlines Maintenance Facility, Kansas City, MO* (Report No. CT-106-18b), Cincinnati, OH, National Institute for Occupational Safety and Health

Grandjean, P., Wulf, H.C. & Niebuhr, E. (1983) Sister chromatid exchange in response to variations in occupational lead exposure. *Environ. Res.*, **32**, 199–204

Green, R.V. (1974) Synthetic nitrogen products: nitric acid. In: Kent, J.A., ed., *Riegel's Handbook of Industrial Chemistry*, 7th ed., New York, Van Nostrand Reinhold, pp. 94–100

Green, R.V. & Li, H. (1983) Synthetic nitrogen products: nitric acid. In: Kent, J.A., ed., *Riegel's Handbook of Industrial Chemistry*, 8th ed., New York, Van Nostrand Reinhold, pp. 164–171

Gunter B.J. (1976) *Health Hazard Evaluation Determination, Western Gear Corporation, Jamestown, ND* (Report No. 76-23-319), Cincinnati, OH, National Institute for Occupational Safety and Health

Gunter, B.J. (1982) *Health Hazard Evaluation, Inmos Corporation, Colorado Springs, CO* (Report No. HETA 81-319-1114), Cincinnati, OH, National Institute for Occupational Safety and Health

Gunter, B.J. (1988) *Health Hazard Evaluation, Hubinger Company, Inc., Keokuk, IA* (Report No. HETA 86-159-1909), Cincinnati, OH, National Institute for Occupational Safety and Health

Gunter, B.J. & Bodner, A. (1974) *Health Hazard Evaluation Determination, EPC of Arkansas, Fayetteville, AR* (Report No. 73-177-147), Cincinnati, OH, National Institute for Occupational Safety and Health

Gunter, B.J. & Seligman, P.J. (1984) *Health Hazard Evaluation, Kennecott Smelter, Hurley, NM* (Report No. HETA 84-038-1513), Cincinnati, OH, National Institute for Occupational Safety and Health

Guthrie, J.P. (1978) Hydrolysis of esters of oxy acids: pKa values for strong acids: Brønsted relationship for attack of water at methyl; free energies of hydrolysis of esters of oxy acids; and a linear relationship between free energy of hydrolysis and pKa holding over a range of 20 pK units. *Can. J. Chem.*, **56**, 2342–2354

Haas, B.H. & Geissert, J.O. (1976) *Hazard Evaluation and Technical Assistance, Front Royal and Panorama Entrance Stations, Shenandoah National Park, Luray, VA* (Report No. TA 76-91), Cincinnati, OH, National Institute for Occupational Safety and Health

Haas, B.H. & Geissert, J.O. (1977) *Health Hazard Evaluation Determination, Rocky Mountain Manufacturing and Wire Company, Cleaning Department, Pueblo, CO* (Report No. 76-108-365), Cincinnati, OH, National Institute for Occupational Safety and Health

Haberstroh, W.H. & Collins, D.E. (1974) Synthetic organic chemicals: ethanol. In: Kent, J.A., ed., *Riegel's Handbook of Industrial Chemistry*, 7th ed., New York, Van Nostrand Reinhold, pp. 787–789

Haberstroh, W.H. & Collins, D.E. (1983a) Synthetic organic chemicals: isopropyl alcohol. In: Kent, J.A., ed., *Riegel's Handbook of Industrial Chemistry*, 8th ed., New York, Van Nostrand Reinhold, pp. 945–946

Haberstroh, W.H. & Collins, D.E. (1983b) Synthetic organic chemicals: ethanol. In: Kent, J.A., ed., *Riegel's Handbook of Industrial Chemistry*, 8th ed., New York, Van Nostrand Reinhold, pp. 935–936

Hagmar, L., Bellander, T., Andersson, C., Lindén, K., Attewell, R. & Möller, T. (1991) Cancer morbidity in nitrate fertilizer workers. *Int. Arch. occup. environ. Health*, **63**, 63–67

Hartle, R.W. (1980) *Health Hazard Evaluation, Long Island Rail Road, Richmond Hill, NY* (Report No. 80-057-781), Cincinnati, OH, National Institute for Occupational Safety and Health

Hehner, N.E. (1986) *Storage Battery Manufacturing Manual III*, 3rd ed., Largo, FL, Independent Battery Manufacturers Association

Herrick, R.F. (1982) *Industrial Hygiene Characterization of the Phosphate Fertilizer Industry* (US NTIS PB83-234963), Cincinnati, OH, National Institute for Occupational Safety and Health

Hervin, R.L. & Reifschneider, R. (1973) *Health Hazard Evaluation Determination, Trans World Airlines, Inc., Overhaul Base, Kansas City, MI* (Report No. 72-60), Cincinnati, OH, National Institute for Occupational Safety and Health

Hervin, R.L., Stroman, R., Belanger, P., Ruhe, R., Collins, C. & Dyches, T. (1977) *Health Hazard Evaluation Determination, McDonnell Aircraft Company, St Louis, MO* (Report No. 77-63-449), Cincinnati, OH, National Institute for Occupational Safety and Health

Hilt, B., Langård, S., Andersen, A. & Rosenberg, J. (1985) Asbestos exposure, smoking habits, and cancer incidence among production and maintenance workers in an electrochemical plant. *Am. J. ind. Med.*, **8**, 565–577

Hinds, W.C. (1985) *Aerosol Technology. Properties, Behavior and Measurement of Airborne Particles*, New York, John Wiley & Sons, p. 6

Holma, B. (1989) Effects of inhaled acids on airway mucus and its consequences for health. *Environ. Health Perspectives*, **79**, 109–113

Hudson, R.B. & Dolan, M.J. (1982) Phosphoric acids and phosphates. In: Mark, H.F., Othmer, D.F., Overberger, C.G., Seaborg, G.T. & Grayson, M., eds, *Kirk–Othmer Encyclopedia of Chemical Technology*, 3rd ed., Vol. 17, New York, John Wiley and Sons, pp. 426–472

Hueper, W.C. (1966) Occupational and environmental cancers of the respiratory system. *Recent Results Cancer Res.*, **3**, 105–107, 183

Hunninen, K. (1986) *Health Hazard Evaluation, Cuyahoga Community College, Cleveland, OH* (Report No. HETA 85-323-1677), Cincinnati, OH, National Institute for Occupational Safety and Health

IARC (1977) *IARC Monographs on the Evaluation of the Carcinogenic Risk of Chemicals to Man*, Vol. 15, *Some Fumigants, the Herbicides 2,4-D and 2,4,5-T, Chlorinated Dibenzodioxins and Miscellaneous Industrial Chemicals*, Lyon, pp. 223–243

IARC (1980) *IARC Monographs on the Evaluation of the Carcinogenic Risk of Chemicals to Humans*, Vol. 23, *Some Metals and Metallic Compounds*, Lyon, pp. 325–415

IARC (1987) *IARC Monographs on the Evaluation of Carcinogenic Risks to Humans*, Suppl. 7, *Overall Evaluations of Carcinogenicity: An Updating of* IARC Monographs *Volumes 1 to 42*, Lyon, pp. 100–106, 120–122, 139–142, 142–143, 198, 211–216, 229, 230–232, 252–254, 341–343, 373–376

IARC (1989) *IARC Monographs on the Evaluation of Carcinogenic Risks to Humans*, Vol. 47, *Some Organic Solvents, Resin Monomers and Related Compounds, Pigments and Occupational Exposures in Paint Manufacture and Painting*, Lyon, pp. 263–287, 307–326

IARC (1990a) *IARC Monographs on the Evaluation of Carcinogenic Risks to Humans*, Vol. 49, *Chromium, Nickel and Welding*, Lyon, pp. 49–256, 257–445

IARC (1990b) *IARC Monographs on the Evaluation of Carcinogenic Risks to Humans*, Vol. 48, *Some Flame Retardants and Textile Chemicals, and Exposures in the Textile Manufacturing Industry*, Lyon, pp. 215–278

International Labour Office (1991) *Occupational Exposure Limits for Airborne Toxic Substances*, 3rd ed. (Occupational Safety and Health Series 37), Geneva, pp. 290–291, 326–327, 372–373

Jankovic, J. (1980) *Health Hazard Evaluation Determination, Lehigh Portland Cement Company, Mason City, IA* (Report No. M-HHE 80-105-110), Cincinnati, OH, National Institute for Occupational Safety and Health

Japan Chemical Week (1990) *Japan Chemical Annual 1990—Japan's Chemical Industry*, Tokyo, The Chemical Daily Co., pp. 18–20

Jarabek, A.M., Menache, M.G., Overton, J.H., Jr, Dourson, M.L. & Miller, F.J. (1989) Inhalation reference dose (RfDi): an application of interspecies dosimetry modeling for risk assessment of insoluble particles. *Health Phys.*, **57** (Suppl. 1), 177–183

Jones, W. & Gamble, J. (1984) Epidemiological–environmental study of lead acid battery workers. I. Environmental study of five lead acid battery plants. *Environ. Res.*, **35**, 1–10

Kazimov, M.A. (1977) Occupational hygiene and new methods of ferrovanadium production (Russ.). *Gig. Tr. Prof. Zabol.*, **6**, 8–12

Koenig, J.Q., Covert, D.S. & Peirson, W.E. (1989) Effects of inhalation of acidic compounds on pulmonary function in allergic adolescent subjects. *Environ. Health Perspectives*, **79**, 173–178

Kominsky, J.R. (1975) *Health Hazard Evaluation Determination, General Electric Corporation, Evendale, OH* (Report No. 75-5-238), Cincinnati, OH, National Institute for Occupational Safety and Health

Kominsky J.R. (1981a) *Health Hazard Evaluation, American Bridge, Shiffler Plant, Pittsburgh, PA* (No. HETA-81-123-856), Cincinnati, OH, National Institute for Occupational Safety and Health

Kominsky, J.R. (1981b) *Health Hazard Evaluation, Wheeling Pittsburgh Steel Corporation, Martins Ferry, OH* (Report No. HETA 81-168-903), Cincinnati, OH, National Institute for Occupational Safety and Health

Kominsky, J.R. & Cherniack, M.G. (1984) *Health Hazard Evaluation, Chemetco, Incorporated, Alton, IL* (Report No. HETA 82-024-1428), Cincinnati, OH, National Institute for Occupational Safety and Health

Kominsky J.R. & Kreiss, K. (1981) *Health Hazard Evaluation, Copper Division, Southwire Company, Inc., Carrollton, GA* (Report No. HHE-78-132-818), Cincinnati, OH, National Institute for Occupational Safety and Health

Kosaric, N., Duvnjak, Z., Farkas, A., Sahm, H., Bringer-Meyer, S., Goebel, O. & Mayer, D. (1987) Ethanol. In: Gerhartz, W., ed., *Ullmann's Encyclopedia of Industrial Chemistry*, 5th rev. ed., Vol. A9, New York, VCH Publishers, pp. 587–653

Kuprin, A.I., Fedorenko, G.I., Voronin B.I., Fedko, S.A. & Budalovskaya, T.F. (1986) Abatement of air pollution in electroplating departments of industrial plants (Russ.). *Khim. Prom-st. (Moscow)*, **4**, 252

Lamant, V., Oury, B. & Peltier, A. (1989) A method for characterizing working environments in hot-dip galvanizing (Fr.). *Cah. Notes doc.*, **134**, 87–97

Larson, T.V., Covert, D.S., Frank, R. & Charlson, R.J. (1977) Ammonia in the human airways: neutralization of inspired acid sulfate aerosols. *Science*, **197**, 161–163

Larson, T.V., Frank, R., Covert, D.S., Holub, D. & Morgan, M.S. (1982) Measurements of respiratory ammonia and the chemical neutralization of inhaled sulfuric acid aerosol in anesthetized dogs. *Am. Rev. respir. Dis.*, **125**, 502–506

LeBoeuf, R.A. & Kerckaert, G.A. (1986) The induction of transformed-like morphology and enhanced growth in Syrian hamster embryo cells grown in acidic pH. *Carcinogenesis*, **7**, 1431–1440

LeBoeuf, R.A., Kerckaert, G.A., Poiley, J.A. & Raineri, R. (1989) An interlaboratory comparison of enhanced morphological transformation of Syrian hamster embryo cells cultured under conditions of reduced bicarbonate concentration and pH. *Mutat. Res.*, **222**, 205–218

Lee, S.A. (1980) *Health Hazard Evaluation Determination, Airco Welding Products, Chester, WV* (Report No. HE 80-27-704), Cincinnati, OH, National Institute for Occupational Safety and Health

Leikauf, G.D., Spektor, D.M., Albert, R.E. & Lippmann, M. (1984) Dose-dependent effects of submicrometer sulfuric acid aerosol on particle clearance from ciliated human lung airways. *Am. ind. Hyg. Assoc. J.*, **45**, 285–292

Levy, B.S.B. (1976) *Health Hazard Evaluation Determination, Cooper Union School of Art, New York, NY* (Report No. 75-12-321), Cincinnati, OH, National Institute for Occupational Safety and Health

Lewis, F.A. (1980) *Health Hazard Evaluation Determination, Wheeling–Pittsburgh Steel Corporation Coke Plant, Follansbee, WV* (Report HHE 79-65/98-748), Cincinnati, OH, National Institute for Occupational Safety and Health

Lippmann, M., Schlesinger, R.B., Leikauf, G., Spektor, D. & Albert, R.E. (1982) Effects of sulphuric acid aerosols on respiratory tract airways. *Ann. occup. Hyg.*, **26**, 677–690

Lippmann, M., Gearhart, J.M. & Schlesinger, R.B. (1987) Basis for a particle size-selective TLV for sulfuric acid aerosols. *Appl. ind. Hyg.*, **2**, 188–199

Lucas, A.D. & Cone, J. (1982) *Health Hazard Evaluation, General Motors, McCook, IL* (Report No. HETA 80-251/252-1099), Cincinnati, OH, National Institute for Occupational Safety and Health

Lucas, A.D & Schloemer, J.R. (1982) *Health Hazard Evaluation, PVC Container Corporation, Eatontown, NJ* (Report No. TA 80-104-1158), Cincinnati, OH, National Institute for Occupational Safety and Health

Lynch, J., Hanis, N.M., Bird, M.G., Murray, K.J. & Walsh, J.P. (1979) An association of upper respiratory cancer with exposure to diethyl sulfate. *J. occup. Med.*, **21**, 333–341

Malcolm, D. & Barnett, H.A.R. (1982) A mortality study of lead workers 1925–76. *Br. J. ind. Med.*, **39**, 404–410

Malcolm, D. & Paul, E. (1961) Erosion of the teeth due to sulphuric acid in the battery industry. *Br. J. ind. Med.*, **18**, 63–69

Mannsville Chemical Products (1987) *Chemical Products Synopsis: Sulfuric Acid*, Asbury Park, NJ

Mappes, R. (1980) TLV for hydrochloric acid in pickling plants (Ger.). *Zbl. Arbeitsmed.*, **30**, 172–173

Markel, H.L., Jr & Ruhe, R. (1981) *Health Hazard Evaluation, US Border Crossing Stations, El Paso, TX* (Report No. TA 79-027-979), Cincinnati, OH, National Institute for Occupational Safety and Health

Martonen, T.B., Barnett, A.E. & Miller, F.J. (1985) Ambient sulfate aerosol deposition in man: modeling the influence of hydroscopicity. *Environ. Health Perspectives*, **63**, 11–24

Mazumdar, S., Lerer, T. & Redmond, C.K. (1975) Long-term mortality study of steelworkers. IX. Mortality patterns among sheet and tin mill workers. *J. occup. Med.*, **17**, 751–755

McGlothlin, J.D., Schulte, P. & Van Wagenen, H. (1982) *Health Hazard Evaluation, American Cyanamid Company, Kalamazoo, MI* (Report No. HETA 80-190-1135), Cincinnati, OH, National Institute for Occupational Safety and Health

Meng, Z. & Zhang, L. (1990a) Chromosomal aberrations and sister-chromatid exchanges in lymphocytes of workers exposed to sulphur dioxide. *Mutat. Res.*, **241**, 15–20

Meng, Z. & Zhang, L. (1990b) Observation of frequencies of lymphocytes with micronuclei in human peripheral blood cultures from workers in a sulphuric acid factory. *Environ. mol. Mutag.*, **15**, 218–220

Morita, T., Watanabe, Y., Takeda, K. & Okumura, K. (1989) Effects of pH in the in vitro chromosomal aberration test. *Mutat. Res.*, **225**, 55–60

Morris, P.D., Koepsell, T.D., Daling, J.R., Taylor, J.W., Lyon, J.L., Swanson, G.M., Child, M. & Weiss, N.S. (1986) Toxic substance exposure and multiple myeloma: a case–control study. *J. natl Cancer Inst.*, **76**, 987–994

Morse, K. (1983) Pickling. In: Parmeggiani, L., ed., *Encyclopedia of Occupational Health and Safety*, 3rd rev. ed., Vol. 2, Geneva, International Labour Office, pp. 1702–1704

Mortimer, V.D., Sheehy, J.W., Jones, J.H. & Kemme, D.R. (1982) *In Depth Survey Report of Valley Chrome Platers, Bay City, MI, April 27–May 1, 1981* (Report No. PB83-181032), Cincinnati, OH, National Institute for Occupational Safety and Health

Moseley, C.L. (1983) *Health Hazard Evaluation, Siemens Components, Inc., Broomfield, CO* (Report No. HETA 83-164-1377), Cincinnati, OH, National Institute for Occupational Safety and Health

Moseley, C.L., Melius, J., Garabrant, D.H. & Fine, L.J. (1980) *Health Hazard Evaluation, RMI Metals Reduction Plant, Ashtabula, OH* (Report No. 79-17-751), Cincinnati, OH, National Institute for Occupational Safety and Health

Muravyeva, L.M., Mishunina, A.A. & Kolotilova, T.V. (1987) Hygienic assessment of working conditions of galvanic workers in instrument-manufacturing plants (Russ.). *Gig. Tr. Prof. Zabol.*, **5**, 11–14

Murray, F.J., Schwetz, B.A., Nitschke, K.D., Crawford, A.A., Quast, J.F. & Staples, R.E. (1979) Embryotoxicity of inhaled sulfuric acid aerosol in mice and rabbits. *J. environ. Sci. Health*, **C13**, 251–266

Nanni, N., Bauer, C., Cundari, E., Corsi, C., Del Carratore, R., Nieri, R., Paolini, M., Crewshaw, J. & Bronzetti, G. (1984) Studies of genetic effects in the D7 strain of *Saccharomyces cerevisiae* under different conditions of pH. *Mutat. Res.*, **139**, 189–192

Newman, D.J. (1981) Nitric acid. In: Mark, H.F., Othmer, D.F., Overberger, C.G., Seaborg, G.T. & Grayson, N., eds, *Kirk–Othmer Encyclopedia of Chemical Technology*, 3rd ed., Vol. 15, New York, John Wiley & Sons, pp. 853–871

Özkaynak, H. & Thurston, G.D. (1987) Associations between 1980 US mortality rates and alternative measures of airborne particle concentration. *Risk Anal.*, 7, 449–461

Pagano, G., Cipollaro, M., Corsale, G., Esposito, A., Ragucci, E. & Giordano, G.G. (1985a) pH-Induced changes in mitotic and developmental patterns in sea urchin embryogenesis. I. Exposure of embryos. *Teratog. Carcinog. Mutag.*, 5, 101–112

Pagano, G., Cipollaro, M., Corsale, G., Esposito, A., Ragucci, E. & Giordano, G.G. (1985b) pH-Induced changes in mitotic and developmental patterns in sea urchin embryogenesis. II. Exposure of sperm. *Teratog. Carcinog. Mutag.*, 5, 113–121

Papa, A.J. (1982) Isopropyl alcohol. In: Mark, H.F., Othmer, D.F., Overberger, C.G., Seaborg, G.T. & Grayson, M., eds, *Kirk–Othmer Encyclopedia of Chemical Toxicology*, 3rd ed., Vol. 12, New York, John Wiley & Sons, pp. 198–220

Petrov, B.A. (1987) Sanitation of working conditions and environment for the process of sulfuric acid manufacture from metallurgical gases (Russ.). *Gig. Sanit.*, 10, 70–71

Price, J.H. (1977) *Health Hazard Evaluation Determination, Inland Steel Corporation, East Chicago, IN* (Report No. 77-31-432), Cincinnati, OH, National Institute for Occupational Safety and Health

Pryor, P. (1987) *Health Hazard Evaluation, Nutech Corporation, Denver, CO* (Report No. HETA 84-401-1784), Cincinnati, OH, National Institute for Occupational Safety and Health

Remijn, B., Koster, P., Houthuijs, D., Boleij, J., Willems, H., Brunekreef, B., Biersteker, K. & van Loveren, C. (1982) Zinc chloride, zinc oxide, hydrochloric acid exposure and dental erosion in a zinc galvanizing plant in the Netherlands. *Ann. occup. Hyg.*, 25, 299–307

Rencher, A.C., Carter, M.W. & McKee, D.W. (1977) A retrospective epidemiological study of mortality at a large Western copper smelter. *J. occup. Med.*, 19, 754–758

Rivera, R. (1976) *Health Hazard Evaluation Determination, Adolph Coors Company Brewery Warehouse, Golden, CO* (Report No. 76-26-320), Cincinnati, OH, National Institute for Occupational Safety and Health

Roto, P. (1980) Asthma, symptoms of chronic bronchitis and ventilatory capacity among cobalt and zinc production workers. *Scand. J. Work Environ. Health*, 6 (Suppl. 1), 1–49

Ruhe, R.L. (1976) *Health Hazard Evaluation Determination, The Foxboro Company, Highland Plant, East Bridgewater, MA* (Report No. 75-180-311), Cincinnati, OH, National Institute for Occupational Safety and Health

Ruhe, R.L. & Andersen, L. (1977) *Health Hazard Evaluation Determination, The Hayes and Albion Company, Spencerville, OH* (Report No. 76-17-395), Cincinnati, OH, National Institute for Occupational Safety and Health

Ruhe, R.L. & Donohue, M. (1979) *Health Hazard Evaluation Determination, Cities Service Company, Miami, AZ* (Report HE 79-10-576), Cincinnati, OH, National Institute for Occupational Safety and Health

Ruhe, R.L. & Donohue, M. (1980) *Health Hazard Evaluation Determination, Duralectra, Inc., Natick, MA* (Report No. HE 79-147-702), Cincinnati, OH, National Institute for Occupational Safety and Health

Schlesinger, R.B. (1990) Exposure–response pattern for sulfuric acid-induced effects on particle clearance from the respiratory region of rabbit lungs. *Inhal. Toxicol.*, 2, 21–27

Schlesinger, R.B. & Gearhart, J.M. (1986) Early alveolar clearance in rabbits intermittently exposed to sulfuric acid mist. *J. Toxicol. environ. Health*, 17, 213–220

Schlesinger, R.B., Chen, L.C., Finkelstein, I. & Zelikoff, J.T. (1990) Comparative potency of inhaled acidic sulfates: speciation and the role of hydrogen ion. *Environ. Res.*, **52**, 210–224

Schneberger, G.L. (1981) Metal surface treatments (cleaning). Pickling. In: Mark, H.F., Othmer, D.F., Overberger, C.G., Seaborg, G.T. & Grayson, M., eds, *Kirk–Othmer Encyclopedia of Chemical Technology*, Vol. 15, New York, John Wiley & Sons, pp. 300–303

Scott, D., Galloway, S.M., Marshall, R.R., Ishidate, M., Jr, Brusick, D., Ashby, J. & Myhr, B.C. (1991) Genotoxicity under extreme culture conditions. *Mutat. Res.*, **257**, 147–204

Sheehy, J.W., Spottswood, S., Hurley, D.E., Amendola, A.A. & Cassinelli, M.E. (1982a) *In-depth Survey Report, Honeywell, Incorporated, Minneapolis, MN* (Report No. ECTB 106-11a), Cincinnati, OH, National Institute for Occupational Safety and Health

Sheehy, J.W., Frede, J.C. & Schroer, D.E. (1982b) *In-depth Survey Report of US Chrome, Fond Du Lac, WI* (Report No. CT 106-19A), Cincinnati, OH, National Institute for Occupational Safety and Health

Sheehy, J.W., Hurley, D.E. & Frede, J.F. (1982c) *In-depth Survey Report of Sodus Hardchrome, Inc., Sodus, MI* (Report No. CT 106-13a), Cincinnati, OH, National Institute for Occupational Safety and Health

Siemiatycki, J., ed. (1991) *Risk Factors for Cancer in the Workplace*, Boca Raton, FL, CRC Press

Singal, M., Zey, J.N. & Arnold, S.J. (1985) *Health Hazard Evaluation, Johnson Controls, Inc., Owosso, MI* (Report No. HETA 84-041-1592), Cincinnati, OH, National Institute for Occupational Safety and Health

Singer, B. & Grunberger, D. (1983) *Molecular Biology of Mutagens and Carcinogens*, New York, Plenum Press, pp. 16–19

Sinha, A., Gollapudi, B.B., Linscombe, V.A. & McClintock, M.L. (1989) Utilization of rat lymphocytes for the in vitro chromosomal aberration assay. *Mutagenesis*, **4**, 147–153

Skyttä, E. (1978) *Tilasto Työhygieenisistä Mittauksista v. 19710–1976* [Statistics of Industrial Hygiene Measurements in 1971–1976], Helsinki, Institute of Occupational Health

Soskolne, C.L., Zeighami, E.A., Hanis, N.M., Kupper, L.L., Herrmann, N., Amsel, J., Mausner, J.S. & Stellman, J.M. (1984) Laryngeal cancer and occupational exposure to sulfuric acid. *Am. J. Epidemiol.*, **120**, 358–369

Soskolne, C.L., Jhangri, G.S., Siemiatycki, J., Lakhani, R., Dewar, R., Burch, J.D., Howe, G.R. & Miller, A.B. (1992) Occupational exposure to sulfuric acid associated with laryngeal cancer, southern Ontario, Canada. *Scand. J. Work Environ. Health* (in press)

Soule, R.D. (1982) Electroplating. In: Cralley, L.V. & Cralley, L.J., eds, *Industrial Hygiene Aspects of Plant Operations*, New York, Macmillan Publishing Co., pp. 293–319

Speizer, F.E. (1989) Studies of acid aerosols in six cities and in a new multi-city investigation: design issues. *Environ. Health Perspectives*, **79**, 61–67

Spottswood, S.E., Sheehy, J.W., Kercher, S. & Martinez, K. (1983) *In-depth Survey Report of Greensboro Industrial Plating, Greensboro, NC* (Report No. PB83-187807), Cincinnati, OH, National Institute for Occupational Safety and Health

Stayner, L.T., Meinhardt, T., Lemen, R., Bayliss, D., Herrick, R., Reeve, G.R., Smith, A.B. & Halperin, W. (1985) A retrospective cohort mortality study of a phosphate fertilizer production facility. *Arch. environ. Health*, **40**, 133–138

Steenland, K. & Beaumont, J. (1989) Further follow-up and adjustment for smoking in a study of lung cancer and acid mists. *Am. J. ind. Med.*, **16**, 347–354

Steenland, K., Schnorr, T., Beaumont, J., Halperin, W. & Bloom, T. (1988) Incidence of laryngeal cancer and exposure to acid mists. *Br. J. ind. Med.*, **45**, 766–776

Stephenson, F., Cassady M., Donaldson, H. & Boyle, T. (1977a) *Industrial Hygiene Survey. IMC, Phosphate Chemical Complex, New Wales, FL* (Report No. PB-278804), Cincinnati, OH, National Institute for Occupational Safety and Health

Stephenson, F., Donaldson, H., Boyle, T., Crandall, M., Sandusky, T. & Cohen, H. (1977b) *Industrial Hygiene Survey, CF Chemicals, Inc., Bartow, FL, August 9–12, 1976* (Report No. IWS 57-10B), Cincinnati, OH, National Institute for Occupational Safety and Health

Stern, F.B., Beaumont J.J., Halperin, W.E., Murthy, L.I., Hills, B.W. & Fajen, J.M. (1987) Mortality of chrome leather tannery workers and chemical exposures in tanneries. *Scand. J. Work Environ. Health*, **13**, 108–117

Tadzhibaeva, N.S. & Gol'eva, I.V. (1976) Industrial hygiene and condition of the upper respiratory tract of people working in the production of superphosphate in Uzbekistan (Russ.). *Med. Zh. Uzb.*, **4**, 57–59

Tanner, R.L. (1987) State-of-the-art review. The measurement of strong acids in atmospheric samples. In: Lodge, J.P., Jr, ed., *Methods of Air Sampling and Analysis*, 3rd ed., Chelsea, MI, Lewis Publishers, pp. 703–714

Teta, M.J., Perlman, G.D. & Ott, M.G. (1992) Mortality study of ethanol and isopropanol production workers at two facilities. *Scand. J. Work Environ. Health* (in press)

Thiess, A.M., Oettel, H. & Uhl, C. (1969) Occupational lung cancers. Long-term observations at BASF, Ludwigshafen am Rhein, 2nd Communication (Ger.). *Zbl. Arbeitsmed. Arbeitsschutz*, **19**, 97–113

Thurston, G.D., Ito, K., Lippmann, M. & Hayes, C. (1989) Reexamination of London, England, mortality in relation to exposure to acidic aerosols during 1963–1972 winters. *Environ. Health Perspectives*, **79**, 73–82

Tomlinson, C.R. (1980) Effects of pH on the mutagenicity of sodium azide in *Neurospora crassa* and *Salmonella typhimurium. Mutat. Res.*, **70**, 179–191

Tuominen, M., Tuominen, R., Ranta, K. & Ranta, H. (1989) Association between acid fumes in the work environment and dental erosion. *Scand. J. Work Environ. Health*, **15**, 335–338

United Nations Industrial Development Organization (1978) *Process Technologies for Phosphate Fertilizers* (Development and Transfer of Technology Series No. 8), New York, pp. 1–19

US Environmental Protection Agency (1989a) *Review of New Source Performance Standards for Lead–Acid Battery Manufacture* (Preliminary Draft), Research Triangle Park, NC, Office of Air Quality, pp. 3-1-3-25

US Environmental Protection Agency (1989b) *An Acid Aerosols Issue Paper: Health Effects and Aerometrics* (EPA Report No. EPA-600/8-88-005F), Washington DC, Office of Health and Environmental Assessment

US National Institute for Occupational Safety and Health (1974) *Criteria for a Recommended Standard...Occupational Exposure to Sulfuric Acid* (DHEW (NIOSH) Publication No. 74-128), Cincinnati, OH

US National Institute for Occupational Safety and Health (1976) *Criteria for a Recommended Standard...Occupational Exposure to Nitric Acid* (HEW (NIOSH) Publication No. 76-141), Cincinnati, OH

US National Institute for Occupational Safety and Health (1990) *National Occupational Exposure Survey 1981–83*, Cincinnati, OH

US Occupational Safety and Health Administration (1989) Air contaminants—permissible exposure limits. *Code fed. Regul.*, **Title 29**, Part 1910.1000

Utell, M.J. (1985) Effects of inhaled acid aerosols on lung mechanics: an analysis of human exposure studies. *Environ. Health Perspectives*, **63**, 39–44

Utell, M.J., Mariglio, J.A., Morrow, P.E., Gibb, F.R. & Speers, D.M. (1989) Effects of inhaled acid aerosols on respiratory function: the role of endogenous ammonia. *J. Aerosol Med.*, **2**, 141–147

Weast, R.C., ed. (1989) *CRC Handbook of Chemistry and Physics*, 70th ed., Boca Raton, FL, CRC Press, pp. B-84, B-85, B-94, B-111–113, B-135, B-136, C-203, C-266, C-279, C-351, D-165, D-197

Weil, C.S., Smyth, H.F., Jr & Nale, T.W. (1952) Quest for a suspected industrial carcinogen. *Arch. ind. Hyg.*, **5**, 535–547

West, J.R. & Duecker, W.W. (1974) Sulfuric acid and sulfur. In: Kent, J.A., ed., *Riegel's Handbook of Industrial Chemistry*, 7th ed., New York, Van Nostrand Reinhold, pp. 62–74

West, J.R. & Smith, G.M. (1983) Sulfuric acid and sulfur. In: Kent, J.A., ed., *Riegel's Handbook of Industrial Chemistry*, 8th ed., New York, Van Nostrand Reinhold, pp. 130–142

WHO (1987) *Air Quality Guidelines for Europe*, Copenhagen, Regional Office for Europe, pp. 338–360

WHO Working Group (1986) Health impact of acidic deposition. *Sci. total Environ.*, **52**, 157–187

Whong, W.-Z., Ong, T.-M. & Brockman, H.E. (1985) Effect of pH on the mutagenic and killing potencies of ICR-170 in *ad-3* tests of *Neurospora crassa*. *Mutat. Res.*, **142**, 19–22

Wolf, F. & Cassady, M.E. (1976) *Industrial Hygiene Survey, Stauffer Chemical Company, Salt Lake City, UT, July 16–25, 1975* (Report No. IWS 57-14), Cincinnati, OH, National Institute for Occupational Safety and Health

Xu, P. & Zhang, R. (1985) Control of hydrochloric acid fumes in strip pickling by the ultra-high-voltage electrostatic technique (Chin.). *Gangtie*, **20**, 69–73

Young, M. (1979a) *Walk-through Survey Report as Part of the Sulfuric Acid Study at Bethlehem Steel Company, Johnstown, PA* (Report No. IWS 62-16), Cincinnati, OH, National Institute for Occupational Safety and Health

Young, M. (1979b) *Walk-through Survey Report as Part of the Sulfuric Acid Study at Jones and Laughlin Steel Corporation, Pittsburgh, PA* (Report No. IWS 62-17), Cincinnati, OH, National Institute for Occupational Safety and Health

Young, M. (1979c) *Walk-through Survey Report of Standard Industries, Inc. (Reliable Battery Company), San Antonio, TX* (Report No. IWS 62-14), Cincinnati, OH, National Institute for Occupational Safety and Health

Young, M. (1979d) *Walk-through Survey Report of Electric Storage Battery, Inc., Dallas, TX* (Report No. IWS 62-13), Cincinnati, OH, National Institute for Occupational Safety and Health

Young, M. (1979e) *Walk-through Survey Report of General Battery and Ceramic Corporation, Dallas, TX* (Report No. IWS 62-15), Cincinnati, OH, National Institute for Occupational Safety and Health

Young, M., Beaumont, J. & Leveton, J. (1979) *Walk-through Survey Report as Part of the Sulfuric Acid Study at United States Steel Corporation, Dravosburg, PA* (Report No. IWS 62-18), Cincinnati, OH, National Institute for Occupational Safety and Health

Zemla, B., Day, N., Swiatnicka, J. & Banasik, R. (1987) Larynx cancer risk factors. *Neoplasma*, **34**, 223–233

Zengtai, Z. (1984) Major trades of chemical industry in China: sulfuric acid. In: Guangqi, Y., ed., *China Chemical Industry* (World Chemical Industry Yearbook), English ed., Beijing, Scientific & Technical Information, Research Institute of the Ministry of Chemical Industry of China, pp. 46–50

Zey, J.N. & Richardson, F. (1989) *Health Hazard Evaluation, North Riverside Fire Department, North Riverside, IL* (Report No. HETA-87-109-1950), Cincinnati, OH, National Institute for Occupational Safety and Health

Zura, K.D. & Grant, W.F. (1981) The role of the hydronium ion in the induction of chromosomal aberrations by weak acid solutions. *Mutat. Res.*, **84**, 349–364

ANNEX: CHEMICAL AND PHYSICAL PROPERTIES AND USES OF SULFURIC ACID AND SULFUR TRIOXIDE

1. Synonyms

Sulfuric acid

    Chem. Abstr. Serv. Reg. No.: 7664-93-9
    Replaced CAS Reg. Nos.: 119540-51-1; 127529-01-5
    Chem. Abstr. Name: Sulfuric acid
    IUPAC Systematic Name: Sulfuric acid
    Synonyms: Battery acid; BOV; dihydrogen sulfate; dipping acid; electrolyte acid; hydrogen sulfate; matting acid; mattling acid; Nordhausen acid; oil of vitriol; sulphuric acid; vitriol brown oil

Sulfur trioxide

    Chem. Abstr. Serv. Reg. No.: 7446-11-9
    Chem. Abstr. Name: Sulfur trioxide
    IUPAC Systematic Name: Sulfur trioxide
    Synonyms: Sulfan; sulfuric anhydride; sulfuric oxide; sulfur oxide (SO_3); sulphur trioxide

Oleum

    Chem. Abstr. Serv. Reg. No.: 8014-95-7
    Chem. Abstr. Name: Sulfuric acid mixture with sulfur trioxide
    Synonyms: Fuming sulfuric acid; sulfuric acid fuming

2. Structural and molecular data

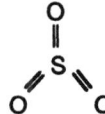

H_2SO_4 Mol. wt.: 98.08

SO_3 Mol. wt.: 80.07

3. Chemical and physical properties

3.1 Sulfuric acid

Sulfuric acid is a strong acid with characteristic hygroscopic and oxidizing properties. The dehydrating effect of concentrated sulfuric acid is due to the formation of hydrates. Several hydrates have been identified in solid sulfuric acid; their presence explains the irregular variation with concentration of some of the physical properties of sulfuric acid. Known hydrates are $H_2SO_4 \cdot H_2O$ (corresponding to 84.5 wt% H_2SO_4); $H_2SO_4 \cdot 2H_2O$ (71.3 wt% H_2SO_4); $H_2SO_4 \cdot 3H_2O$ (64.5 wt% H_2SO_4); $H_2SO_4 \cdot 4H_2O$ (57.6 wt% H_2SO_4); and $H_2SO_4 \cdot 6H_2O$ (47.6 wt% H_2SO_4). Pure sulfuric acid is ionized to only a small extent, in accordance with the following equations:

$$2 H_2SO_4 \rightleftharpoons H_3SO_4^+ + HSO_4^-$$

and

$$2 H_2SO_4 \rightleftharpoons H_3O^+ + HS_2O_7^-.$$

The electrical conductivity therefore has its lowest value at about 100% H_2SO_4. When pure sulfuric acid is diluted with water, dissociation occurs increasingly, by the mechanism shown in the following equation:

$$H_2SO_4 + H_2O \rightleftharpoons H_3O^+ + HSO_4^-.$$

Conductivity increases accordingly. At between 92 and 84.5 wt% H_2SO_4, the monohydrate, $H_2SO_4 \cdot H_2O$, predominates in equilibrium with the ionic species, and conductivity therefore decreases slightly. At lower concentrations of H_2SO_4, the degree of both dissociation and conductivity increases. At high water contents, a second stage of dissociation becomes of increasing importance:

$$HSO_4^- + H_2O \rightleftharpoons H_3O^+ + SO_4^{2-}.$$

Because of the decreasing total concentration of sulfuric acid, however, conductivity reaches a maximum at about 30 wt% H_2SO_4 (the exact value depends on the temperature) and decreases steeply down to 0 wt% H_2SO_4. Diluted sulfuric acid is the preferred electrolyte for industrial metal electrowinning and electroplating because of its high conductivity and because of the chemical stability of the sulfate ion. To take advantage of maximal electrical conductivity, sulfuric acid of about 33 wt% is used in lead–acid (accumulator) batteries (Sander et al., 1984).

The density (specific gravity) of sulfuric acid and of mixtures of sulfuric acid and sulfur trioxide (oleum) is dependent on the H_2SO_4 and SO_3 concentrations, the temperature and the pressure. At constant temperature, the density of sulfuric acid increases steeply with rising H_2SO_4 concentration, reaching a maximum at about 98%. From 98 to 100%, the density decreases slightly but rises again in the oleum range up to a concentration of about 60% free SO_3.

- (*a*) *Description*: Clear, colourless, odourless, oily liquid (Budavari, 1989; Weast, 1989)
- (*b*) *Boiling-point*: 330 °C; can vary over a range of 315–338 °C owing to loss of sulfur trioxide during heating to 300 °C or higher (Sax & Lewis, 1987; Weast, 1989)
- (*c*) *Melting-point*: 10.36 °C (100%); 3.0 °C (98%); −32 °C (93%); −38 °C (78%); −44 °C (74%); −64 °C (65%) (Budavari, 1989; Weast, 1989)

(d) *Density*: See Table 1 for specific gravity at various acid strengths.
(e) *Solubility*: Miscible with water, with generation of much heat and with reduction in volume; decomposes in ethanol (Budavari, 1989; Weast, 1989)
(f) *Volatility*: Vapour pressure, 1 mm Hg (133 Pa) at 145.8 °C (Weast, 1989)
(g) *Stability*: Decomposes at 340 °C into sulfur trioxide and water (Budavari, 1989)
(h) *Reactivity*: Very corrosive; has great affinity for water, absorbing it from air and from many organic substances; dissolves most metals; concentrated acid oxidizes, dehydrates or sulfonates many organic compounds (Sax & Lewis, 1987; Budavari, 1989).
(i) *Conversion factor*: mg/m^3 = 4.0 × ppm[a]

3.2 Sulfur trioxide

Sulfur trioxide is the anhydride of sulfuric acid. It can exist as a gas, liquid or solid. In the gaseous and liquid phases, an equilibrium exists between the monomer, SO_3, and the cyclic trimer, S_3O_9. In the presence of slight traces of moisture (approximately 100 ppm H_2O), liquid sulfur trioxide (below about 27 °C) and solid sulfur trioxide are transformed to solid polymers, which form intergrown crystal needles. They consist of the α and β forms which are currently believed to correspond to long sulfur trioxide chains with water saturation at the chain ends. Pure, solid sulfur trioxide, referred to as γ-SO_3, forms silky orthorhombic (ice-like) crystals. The melting-points of the polymeric α and β forms given below indicate the temperatures at which these solid forms depolymerize to form liquid sulfur trioxide. Discrepancies in reported values for various physical properties of sulfur trioxide reflect, in part, the extreme sensitivity of these values to trace contamination with moisture (Sander *et al.*, 1984).

(a) *Description*: Colourless liquid that fumes in air, at room temperature and atmospheric pressure (Donovan & Salamone, 1983)
(b) *Boiling-point*: 44.8 °C (liquid) (Sander *et al.*, 1984)
(c) *Melting-point*: 62.3 °C (α), 32.5 °C (β), 16.8 °C (γ) (solid) (Donovan & Salamone, 1983)
(d) *Density*: 3.57 g/l at 0 °C (gaseous); 1.92 g/cm^3 at 20 °C (liquid); 2.29 g/cm^3 at −10 °C (γ, solid) (Donovan & Salamone, 1983; Sander *et al.*, 1984)
(e) *Volatility*: Vapour pressure (solid, at 25 °C), 73 mm Hg (10 kPa) (α), 344 mm Hg (46 kPa) (β), 433 mm Hg (58 kPa) (γ) (Budavari, 1989); liquid: 195 mm Hg (26 kPa) at 20 °C, 353 mm Hg (47 kPa) at 30 °C (Sander *et al.*, 1984); relative vapour density (air = 1), 2.003 (Anon., 1972)
(f) *Stability*: The α form appears to be the stable form (Sax & Lewis, 1987).
(g) *Reactivity*: Unreactive towards most metals in absolutely dry conditions; reacts with metal oxides at moderately high temperatures to form the respective metal sulfates; reacts instantaneously and violently with water to form sulfuric acid and with water vapour to form sulfuric acid mists; reacts readily with organic compounds, which may be sulfonated, oxidized or dehydrated (Sander *et al.*, 1984; Budavari, 1989).

---

[a]Calculated from: mg/m^3 = (molecular weight/24.45) × ppm, assuming normal temperature (25 °C) and pressure (760 mm Hg [101.3 kPa])

(h) *Conversion factor*: mg/m^3 = 3.27 × ppm^a

4. Technical products and impurities

Two commercial designations of acid strength are used for sulfuric acid: percentage sulfuric acid (% H$_2$SO$_4$) and degrees Baumé (°Bé) (Olin Chemicals, 1979). Degrees Baumé is defined as: °Bé = 145 − (145/specific gravity) (Sax & Lewis, 1987). For acid concentrations up to 93.2% H$_2$SO$_4$, the specific gravity of a solution is related to its concentration; at acid concentrations above that level, there is no consistent mathematical relationship, and these are referred to simply in terms of percentage sulfuric acid. The strength of oleum (fuming sulfuric acid) can be designated by the percentage of free dissolved sulfur trioxide or as the equivalent percentage of 100% H$_2$SO$_4$ (Olin Chemicals, 1979). Table 1 displays these relationships and the typical concentrations of sulfuric acid produced commercially, with some common uses.

Table 1. Acid strengths and end uses

H$_2$SO$_4$ (%)	°Bé	Oleum (% free SO$_3$)	Specific gravity	Uses
35.67	30.8	–	1.27	Storage batteries
62.18–69.65	50–55	–	–	Normal superphosphate and other fertilizers
77.67	60.0	–	1.7059	Normal superphosphate and other fertilizers; isopropyl and *sec*-butyl alcohol production
80.00	61.3	–	1.7323	Copper leaching
93.19	66.0	–	1.8354	Phosphoric acid, titanium dioxide production
98.99	–	–	–	Alkylation, phosphoric acid, boric acid production
104.50^a	–	20	1.9056	
106.75^a	–	30	1.9412	
109.00^a	–	40	1.9737	Caprolactam, nitrations and sulfonations, dehydration, blending with weaker acids
111.25^a	–	50	1.9900	
113.50^a	–	60	1.9919	
114.63^a	–	65	1.9842	

From West & Smith (1983); Sander *et al.* (1984)
^{a}Percentage equivalent H$_2$SO$_4$

Originally, sulfuric acid was marketed in four grades, known as chamber acid, 50 °Bé; tower acid, 60 °Bé; oil of vitriol, 66 °Bé; and fuming acid. Today, sulfuric acids are commonly specified as commercial, electrolyte (high purity for batteries), textile (low organic content) and chemically pure or reagent grades (West & Smith, 1983; US Environmental Protection Agency, 1985). Sulfuric acid is produced in grades of exacting purity for use in storage batteries and for the rayon, dye and pharmaceutical industries and to less exacting

---

^{a}Calculated from: mg/m^3 = (molecular weight/24.45) × ppm, assuming normal temperature (25°C) and pressure (760 mm Hg [101.3 kPa])

specifications for use in the steel, heavy chemical and fertilizer industries (West & Duecker, 1974).

The range of specifications of impurities in several grades and concentrations are (ppm, max.): ammonium, 10; antimony, 0.03–1.0; arsenic (see IARC, 1987), 0.3–50.0; bismuth, 0.1; cadmium (see IARC, 1987), 0.05–1.0; chlorides, 0.5–10; copper, 0.2–50; iron, 25–200; lead (see IARC, 1987), < 1.0–4.0; manganese, 0.2–0.3; mercury, 1; nickel (see IARC, 1990), 0.3–1.0; nitrates, 5–150; selenium (see IARC, 1975), 0.1–20; sulfurous acid (as SO_2), 40; and zinc, 0.3–40 (American Smelting and Refining Co., 1988; Du Pont Co., 1988; Akzo Chemicals, undated; Boliden Intertrade, undated; Koch Sulfur Products, undated a,b).

In many processes in which sulfuric acid is used, waste or 'spent' sulfuric acid must be disposed of. In some cases, the spent acid is returned to the manufacturer, who then reprocesses it for captive consumption or resale (see also pp. 48–49). Spent sulfuric acid is available at a purity range of 70.0–75.0% with the following allowable impurities (ppm, max.): free chlorine, 500; iron, 100; organics, 50; fluorides, 10; calcium, 5; sodium, 10; mercury, 0.15; lead, 50; and chloride, 100 (Occidental Chemical Corp., 1983).

Oleum is available in several grades (free SO_3 ranging from 20 to 99.9% and the corresponding percentage H_2SO_4 equivalents ranging from 104.5 to 122.5%), with the following specifications for impurities (ppm, max.): arsenic, 0.05; chlorides, < 1; iron, 1–40; and lead, < 1 (Du Pont Co., 1987, 1988; Boliden Intertrade, undated).

Sulfur trioxide is available as technical-grade stabilized (with a proprietary stabilizer) and unstabilized liquids with a minimal purity of 99.5%, a maximal sulfuric acid content of 0.4% and a maximal iron content of 5.0 ppm (Du Pont Co., 1980).

5. Analysis

Selected methods for the analysis of sulfuric acid in air and stack gases are presented in Table 2.

6. Use

Sulfuric acid is one of the most widely used of all industrial chemicals. Most of its uses may be considered indirect, because it is used as a reagent rather than an ingredient; little of it appears in end products and most finishes as spent acid or some kind of sulfate waste. A number of products contain sulfur derived from sulfuric acid, but nearly all of them are low-volume, specialty products (Sander et al., 1984).

The principal use of sulfuric acid is in the manufacture of fertilizers (both phosphate and ammonium sulfate types). Other significant applications include rayon and other fibres, pigments and colours, explosives, plastics, coal-tar products such as dyes and drugs, storage batteries, synthetic detergents, natural and synthetic rubber, pulp and paper, cellophane and catalysts. It is also used to make inorganic chemicals such as hydrochloric acid, hydrofluoric acid, aluminium sulfate, copper sulfate and chromium chemicals. It is used in petroleum refining, in pickling iron, steel and other metals and in ore concentration (Sander et al., 1984; Mannsville Chemical Products, 1985).

Table 2. Methods for the analysis of sulfuric acid

Sample matrix	Sample preparation	Assay procedure	Limit of detection	Reference
Air	Pass through heater (120°C); then through a diffusion denuder; then through detector	FPD	1–2 μg/m^3	Appel et al. (1987)
	Draw through silica gel tube; desorb with sodium bicarbonate/sodium carbonate and heat	IC	4 μg/sample (~0.5 mg/m^3)	Eller (1984)
	Collect on cellulose filter paper; heat for 72 h; compare charring coloration to standard	Colorimetric	15 μg (~0.2 mg/m^3)	Taylor (1979)
	Absorb in water in midget impinger; precipitate as barium sulfate; measure turbidity at 420 nm	Turbidimetry	10 μg (0.1 mg/m^3)	Taylor (1977a)
	Collect on cellulose membrane; extract with distilled water and isopropanol; titrate using 0.005 M barium perchlorate and Thorin indicator	Titration	0.5 mg/m^3 (lower validated value)	Taylor (1977b)
Stack gases	Collect via impinger (using controlled condensation method); titrate using sodium hydroxide and bromophenol blue indicator	AT	40 mg/m^3	Knapp et al. (1987)
	Extract isokinetically; separate sulfuric acid mist (including sulfur trioxide) and sulfur dioxide; add isopropanol; titrate using 0.01 M barium perchlorate and Thorin indicator	Titration	NR 0.05 mg/m^3 (SO$_3$) 1.2 mg/m^3 (SO$_2$)	US Environmental Protection Agency (1989)
Water, wastes	Add solid barium chloranilate; measure colour intensity	Colorimetric	NR 10–400 mg/l	US Environmental Protection Agency (1986a)
	Pass through a sodium-form cation-exchange column; react with ethanol solution of barium chloride and methylthymol blue at pH 2.5–3.0; raise to pH 12.5–13.0; measure colour intensity	Colorimetric	NR 0.5–300 mg/l	US Environmental Protection Agency (1986b)
	Convert sulfate ion to a barium sulfate suspension; compare turbidity to a standard curve	Turbidimetry	1 mg/l	US Environmental Protection Agency (1986c)

Abbreviations: AT, alkalimetric titration; FPD, flame photometric detection; IC, ion chromatography; NR, not reported

In the production of fertilizers, sulfuric acid is used to digest phosphate rock (chiefly calcium phosphate) to produce superphosphate. In the manufacture of phosphoric acid, calcium sulfate (gypsum) is a by-product. Ammonium sulfate fertilizers are made directly from ammonia, as a by-product of caprolactam manufacture or by recovery from coke oven gases. Substantial quantities of sulfuric acid are used as a medium for acidic dehydrating reactions in organic chemical and petrochemical processes involving reactions such as nitration, condensation and dehydration. In the petroleum industry, sulfuric acid is used as an alkylation catalyst and in the refining of lubricating oil; recently, it has been replaced by hydrofluoric acid in this use. Sulfuric acid is also used extensively in the manufacture of catalytic cracking catalysts. In the steel industry, it is used in 'pickling', in which steel is freed of the oxide coating that forms during heating for casting, forging, rolling or annealing. Pickling is used in the surface treatment of other metals, including cadmium, chromium, copper, gold, nickel, silver, tin and zinc. Sulfuric acid is also used in other processes requiring the acid treatment of metals, such as electroplating and etching (Sander et al., 1984; Mannsville Chemical Products, 1985). (See the monograph on occupational exposure to mists and vapours from sulfuric acid and other strong inorganic acids for details of some of these processes.)

Under certain conditions, sulfuric acid is used directly in agriculture for rehabilitating extremely alkaline soils; this is, however, not a widespread use. Probably the largest use of sulfuric acid in which its sulfur becomes incorporated in the final product is organic sulfonation, particularly for the production of detergents. Other, minor organic chemicals and pharmaceuticals are made by sulfonation. One of the most familiar consumer products that contains sulfuric acid, the lead–acid (accumulator) battery, accounts for only a tiny fraction of total sulfuric acid consumption (Sander et al., 1984).

In the production of fibres such as viscose rayon, the viscous alkaline solution is run through spinnerettes and forms filaments which are coagulated as they pass through a sulfuric acid spinning bath. In the sulfate process for producing titanium dioxide, sulfuric acid is used to digest titanium ore; however, this use is declining because of environmental problems and the greater efficiency of the chloride process. Other uses for sulfuric acid include pharmaceuticals, pesticides, dyes and electronic etchants. Fuming sulfuric acid (oleum) is used as the sulfonating agent in synthetic detergents (Mannsville Chemical Products, 1985).

Sulfur trioxide is used primarily as a sulfating or sulfonating agent. The reactivity of sulfur trioxide eliminates the need for excess sulfonating agent, so neutralization of excess sulfonating agent is not required, and salt-free products can be produced. Unlike sulfuric acid and some other sulfonating agents, sulfur trioxide is miscible in a number of solvents, such as liquid sulfur dioxide and various halogenated organic solvents. Pyridine, dioxane, trimethylamine, dimethylformamide and other Lewis bases are used as complexing agents and moderate the reactivity of sulfur trioxide. Vaporized sulfur trioxide, diluted with dry air or nitrogen, is often used in place of liquid sulfur trioxide (Du Pont Co., 1980).

In the detergent industry, sulfur trioxide sulfonation is used to produce alkyl–aryl sulfonates, and particularly dodecylbenzene sulfonate. Alkylated benzene produced from straight-chain, normal paraffins may be sulfonated with sulfur trioxide to produce linear alkylated sulfonates. These materials are widely used in industrial detergents and are highly biodegradable under aerobic conditions. Sulfation of long-chain primary alcohols, such as lauryl alcohol, produces alkylsulfates, which are used in detergent powders, in dishwashing formulations and as shampoo ingredients. These products are biodegradable, as are the ethoxylated alcohol sulfates produced from ethoxylated alcohols and sulfur trioxide. Fats and oils such as castor, lard, soya bean and peanut, may be sulfonated with sulfur trioxide to produce wetting agents, detergents and emulsifiers (Du Pont Co., 1980).

In the chemical industry, sulfur trioxide is used to prepare linear, water-soluble, sulfonated polystyrenes which are used as ion-exchange resins and dispersing agents. Sulfur trioxide is also incorporated to sulfonate benzene in the preparation of benzene sulfonic acid, which is used in the manufacture of phenol by the alkali fusion method (Du Pont Co., 1980).

Substituted benzenes sulfonated with sulfur trioxide are involved in the synthesis of a number of intermediates for dyestuffs, drugs and insecticides. Sulfur trioxide is used to convert long-chain alkylated benzenes to oil-soluble sulfonates for lubricant additives, emulsifiers and rust preventives. Addition of low levels of sulfur trioxide to off-gases improves the efficiency of electrostatic fume precipitators. Surface sulfonating of a number of polymers with sulfur trioxide increases their resistance to permeation by gases and hydrocarbons (Du Pont Co., 1980).

The annual estimated patterns of use of sulfuric acid in the USA over several years are presented in Table 3. Patterns of use may vary from country to country. For example, whereas in most countries 60–70% of the sulfuric acid is used in the manufacture of fertilizers, in Germany in 1978 the fertilizer industry accounted for only about 14% of sulfuric acid consumption, owing to the historical predominance of other processes (Sander *et al.*, 1984; Zengtai, 1984).

Table 3. Annual estimated patterns of use (%) of sulfuric acid in the USA

Use	1970	1978	1983	1984	1985	1987	1988
Phosphate fertilizers	54	67	72	70	70	67	68
Petroleum refining	8	5	7	5	5	8	7
Mining and metallurgy	6	6	–	5	–	4	–
Inorganic chemicals and pigments	6	4	4	4	4	4	4
Ore processing (mostly copper leaching)	1	2	2	–	3	–	3.5
Industrial organic chemicals	6	4	3	3	2.5	4	3.5
Synthetic rubber and plastics	–	–	3	3	2.5	2	2.5
Pulp and paper	–	–	2	2	2	2	2.5
Soap and detergents	–	–	–	1	–	1	–
Water treatment chemicals	–	–	1	1	–	1	–
Cellulose fibres and films (including rayon and cellophane)	2	1	–	1	–	1	–
Inorganic pigments and paints	6	2	1	–	–	–	–
Other	11	9	5	5	11	6	9

From West & Smith (1983); Anon. (1985); Mannsville Chemical Products (1985); US Environmental Protection Agency (1985); Mannsville Chemical Products (1987); Anon. (1988)

7. References

Akzo Chemicals (undated) *Data Sheet: Sulfuric Acid—Electrolyte Grade*, Chicago, IL

American Smelting and Refining Co. (1988) *Typical Specifications: 93% and 98% Technical Grade Sulfuric Acid (East Helena, Hayden, and El Paso Plants)*, Tucson, AZ

Anon. (1972) Hygienic Guide Series: sulfur trioxide. *Am. ind. Hyg. Assoc. J.*, **33**, 53–55

Anon. (1985) Chemical profile: sulfuric acid. *Chem. Mark. Rep.*, **228**, 49–50

Anon. (1988) Chemical profile: sulfuric acid. *Chem. Mark. Rep.*, **234**, 44, 50

Appel, B.R., Tanner, R.L., Adams, D.F., Dasgupta, P.K., Knapp, K.T., Kok, G.L., Pierson, W.R. & Reiszner, K.D. (1987) Semi-continuous determination of atmospheric particulate sulfur, sulfuric acid and ammonium sulfates (Method 713). In: Lodge, J.P., Jr, ed., *Methods of Air Sampling and Analysis*, 3rd ed., Chelsea, MI, Lewis Publishers, pp. 529–532

Boliden Intertrade (undated) *Table of Typical Analyses and Properties—Sulfuric Acid*, Atlanta, GA

Budavari, S., ed. (1989) *The Merck Index*, 11th ed., Rahway, NJ, Merck & Co., pp. 1417–1418

Donovan, J.R. & Salamone, J.M. (1983) Sulfuric acid and sulfur trioxide. In: Mark, H.F., Othmer. D.F., Overberger, C.G., Seaborg, G.T. & Grayson, N., eds, *Kirk–Othmer Encyclopedia of Chemical Technology*, 3rd ed., Vol. 22, New York, John Wiley & Sons, pp. 190–232

Du Pont Co. (1980) *Data Sheet: Sulfur Trioxide—Stabilized Liquid, Technical*, Wilmington, DE

Du Pont Co. (1987) *Sulfur Trioxide and Oleum—Storage and Handling*, Wilmington, DE

Du Pont Co. (1988) *Data Sheet: Sulfuric Acid and Oleum—Technical*, Wilmington, DE

Eller, P.M., ed. (1984) *NIOSH Manual of Analytical Methods*, Method 7903, 3rd ed., Vol. 1 (DHHS (NIOSH) Publ. No. 84-100), Washington DC, US Government Printing Office, pp. 7903-1–7903-6

IARC (1975) *IARC Monographs on the Evaluation of Carcinogenic Risk of Chemicals to Man*, Vol. 9, *Some Aziridines, N-, S- & O-Mustards and Selenium*, Lyon, pp. 245–260

IARC (1987) *IARC Monographs on the Evaluation of Carcinogenic Risks to Humans*, Suppl. 7, *Overall Evaluations of Carcinogenicity: An Updating of* IARC Monographs *Volumes 1 to 42*, Lyon, pp. 100–106, 139–142, 230–232

IARC (1990) *IARC Monographs on the Evaluation of Carcinogenic Risks to Humans*, Vol. 49, *Chromium, Nickel and Welding*, Lyon, pp. 257–445

Knapp, K.T., Pierson, W.R., Dasgupta, P.K., Adams, D.F., Appel, B.R., Farwell, S.O., Kok, G.L., Reiszner, K.D. & Tanner, R.L. (1987) Determination of gaseous sulfuric acid and sulfur dioxide in stack gases. In: Lodge, J.P., Jr, ed., *Methods of Air Sampling and Analysis*, 3rd ed., Chelsea, MI, Lewis Publishers, pp. 523–528

Koch Sulfur Products (undated a) *Laboratory Specification Sheet: Electrolytic Grade Sulfuric Acid (H_2SO_4)*, Wilmington, NC

Koch Sulfur Products (undated b) *Laboratory Specification Sheet: Sulfuric Acid (H_2SO_4)*, Wilmington, NC

Mannsville Chemical Products (1985) *Chemical Products Synopsis: Sulfuric Acid*, Cortland, NY

Mannsville Chemical Products (1987) *Chemical Products Synopsis: Sulfuric Acid*, Asbury Park, NJ

Occidental Chemical Corp. (1983) *Spent Sulfuric Acid 70–75% H_2SO_4* (Data Sheet No. 748), Niagara Falls, NY

Olin Chemicals (1979) *Sulfuric Acid*, Stamford, CT

Sander, U.H.F., Rothe, U. & Kola, R. (1984) Sulphuric acid. In: Sander, U.H.F., Fischer, H., Rothe, U. & Kola, R., eds, *Sulphur, Sulphur Dioxide and Sulphuric Acid. An Introduction to Their Industrial Chemistry and Technology*, London, The British Sulphur Corporation, pp. 257–415

Sax, N.I. & Lewis, R.J., Sr (1987) *Hawley's Condensed Chemical Dictionary*, 11th ed., New York, Van Nostrand Reinhold, pp. 83, 125, 1108–1109

Taylor, D.G. (1977a) *NIOSH Manual of Analytical Methods*, 2nd ed., Vol. 1 (DHEW (NIOSH) Publ. No. 77-157-A), Washington DC, US Government Printing Office, pp. 187-1–187-5

Taylor, D.G. (1977b) *NIOSH Manual of Analytical Methods*, 2nd ed., Vol. 3 (DHEW (NIOSH) Publ. No. 77-157-C), Washington DC, US Government Printing Office, pp. S174-1–S174-8

Taylor, D.G. (1979) *NIOSH Manual of Analytical Methods*, 2nd ed., Vol. 5 (DHEW (NIOSH) Publ. No. 79-141), Washington DC, US Government Printing Office, pp. 267-1–267-5

US Environmental Protection Agency (1985) *Review of New Source Performance Standards for Sulfuric Acid Plants* (EPA-450/3-85-012; US NTIS PB85-249787), Research Triangle Park, NC, Office of Air Quality Planning and Standards

US Environmental Protection Agency (1986a) Method 9035. Sulfate (colorimetric, automated, chloranilate). In: *Test Methods for Evaluating Solid Waste—Physical/Chemical Methods*, 3rd ed., Vol. 1C (EPA No. SW-846), Washington DC, Office of Solid Waste and Emergency Response, pp. 9035-1–9035-6

US Environmental Protection Agency (1986b) Method 9036. Sulfate (colorimetric, automated, methylthymol blue, AA II). In: *Test Methods for Evaluating Solid Waste—Physical/Chemical Methods*, 3rd ed., Vol. 1C (EPA No. SW-846), Washington DC, Office of Solid Waste and Emergency Response, pp. 9036-1–9036-7

US Environmental Protection Agency (1986c) Method 9038. Sulfate (turbidimetric). In: *Test Methods for Evaluating Solid Waste—Physical/Chemical Methods*, 3rd ed., Vol. 1C (EPA No. SW-846), Washington DC, Office of Solid Waste and Emergency Response, pp. 9038-1–9038-6

US Environmental Protection Agency (1989) Method 8—Determination of sulfuric acid mist and sulfur dioxide emissions from stationary sources. *US Code fed. Regul.*, Title 40, Part 60, Appendix A, pp. 731–739

Weast, R.C., ed. (1989) *CRC Handbook of Chemistry and Physics*, 70th ed., Boca Raton, FL, CRC Press, pp. B-84, B-85, B-94, B-111–113, B-135–136, C-203, C-266, C-279, C-351, D-165, D-197

West, J.R. & Duecker, W.W. (1974) Sulfuric acid and sulfur. In: Kent, J.A., ed., *Riegel's Handbook of Industrial Chemistry*, 7th ed., New York, Van Nostrand Reinhold, pp. 62–74

West, J.R. & Smith, G.M. (1983) Sulfuric acid and sulfur. In: Kent, J.A., ed., *Riegel's Handbook of Industrial Chemistry*, 8th ed., New York, Van Nostrand Reinhold, pp. 130–142

Zengtai, Z. (1984) Major trades of chemical industry in China: sulfuric acid. In: Guangqi, Y., ed., *China Chemical Industry* (World Chemical Industry Yearbook), English ed., Beijing, Scientific & Technical Information, Research Institute of the Ministry of Chemical Industry of China, pp. 46–50

SULFUR DIOXIDE AND SOME SULFITES, BISULFITES AND METABISULFITES

1. Exposure Data

1.1 Chemical and physical data

1.1.1 *Synonyms and structural and molecular data*

Sulfur dioxide

Chem. Abstr. Serv. Reg. No.: 7446-09-5
Replaced CAS Nos.: 8014-94-6; 12396-99-5; 83008-56-4; 89125-89-3
Chem. Abstr. Name: Sulfur dioxide
IUPAC Systematic Name: Sulfur dioxide
Synonyms: Sulfurous acid anhydride; sulfurous anhydride; sulfurous oxide; sulfur oxide (SO_2); sulfur superoxide; sulphur dioxide

$$O=S=O$$

SO_2 Mol. wt: 64.07

Sodium sulfite

Chem. Abstr. Serv. Reg. No.: 7757-83-7
Alternate CAS No.: 10579-83-6
Replaced CAS No.: 68135-69-3
Chem. Abstr. Name: Sulfurous acid, disodium salt
IUPAC Systematic Name: Sulfurous acid, disodium salt
Synonyms: Anhydrous sodium sulfite; disodium sulfite; sodium sulphite

$$\text{Na} \cdot \text{O} - \overset{\overset{\displaystyle O}{\|}}{\text{S}} - \text{O} \cdot \text{Na}$$

Na_2SO_3 Mol. wt: 126.04

Sodium bisulfite

Chem. Abstr. Serv. Reg. No.: 7631-90-5
Replaced CAS Nos.: 57414-01-4; 69098-86-8; 89830-27-3; 91829-63-9
Chem. Abstr. Name: Sulfurous acid, monosodium salt
IUPAC Systematic Name: Sulfurous acid, monosodium salt

Synonyms: Hydrogen sulfite sodium; monosodium sulfite; sodium acid sulfite; sodium bisulphite; sodium hydrogen sulfite; sodium sulfite (NaHSO$_3$)

$$HO-\overset{\overset{O}{\|}}{S}-O \cdot Na$$

NaHSO$_3$ Mol. wt: 104.06

Sodium metabisulfite

Chem. Abstr. Serv. Reg. No.: 7681-57-4
Alternate CAS No.: 7757-74-6
Replaced CAS No.: 15771-29-6
Chem. Abstr. Name: Disulfurous acid, disodium salt
IUPAC Systematic Name: Pyrosulfurous acid, disodium salt
Synonyms: Disodium disulfite; disodium metabisulfite; disodium pyrosulfite; sodium disulfite; sodium metabisulphite; sodium pyrosulfite

$$Na \cdot O-\overset{\overset{O}{\|}}{S}-O-\overset{\overset{O}{\|}}{S}-O \cdot Na$$

Na$_2$S$_2$O$_5$ Mol. wt: 190.11

Potassium metabisulfite

Chem. Abstr. Serv. Reg. No.: 16731-55-8
Alternate CAS No.: 4429-42-9
Chem. Abstr. Name: Disulfurous acid, dipotassium salt
IUPAC Systematic Name: Pyrosulfurous acid, dipotassium salt
Synonyms: Dipotassium disulfite; dipotassium metabisulfite; dipotassium pyrosulfite; potassium disulfite; potassium metabisulphite; potassium pyrosulfite

$$K \cdot O-\overset{\overset{O}{\|}}{S}-O-\overset{\overset{O}{\|}}{S}-O \cdot K$$

K$_2$S$_2$O$_5$ Mol. wt: 222.33

1.1.2 Chemical and physical properties

The chemistry of sulfur dioxide in aqueous solutions involves complex equilibria among a number of species of sulfur oxidation state IV, including sulfite, bisulfite, metabisulfite and sulfurous acid. The composition of the mixture depends on the concentration of sulfur dioxide in the water, the pH and the temperature (Weil, 1983).

Sulfur dioxide

(a) *Description*: Colourless gas or liquid with sharp pungent (suffocating) odour (Sax & Lewis, 1987; Budavari, 1989; Weast, 1989)
(b) *Boiling-point*: −10 °C (Weast, 1989)
(c) *Melting-point*: −72.7 °C (Weast, 1989)

(d) *Density*: 1.434 g/ml (pressurized liquid at 0 °C); 2.927 g/l (gas) (Weast, 1989)
(e) *Solubility*: Soluble in water (g/100 g water at 760 mm Hg [101.3 kPa]): 23.0 at 0 °C, 11.6 at 20 °C and 5.9 at 40 °C; in ethanol, 25 g/100 g; in methanol, 32 g/100 g. Liquid sulfur dioxide is only slightly miscible with water; miscible in all proportions with liquid sulfur trioxide; readily dissolves in most organic liquids: acetone, benzene, carbon tetrachloride and formic acid; completely miscible in diethyl ether, carbon disulfide and chloroform (Weil, 1983; Sander et al., 1984; Budavari, 1989). The solubility of sulfur dioxide in sulfuric acid first decreases with rising sulfuric acid concentration, reaching a minimum at a sulfuric acid concentration of about 85%; beyond this concentration, it increases again (Sander et al., 1984).
(f) *Volatility*: Vapour pressure, 2477 mm Hg [330 kPa] at 20 °C; relative vapour density at 0 °C (air = 1), 2.263 (Weil, 1983)
(g) *Stability*: Extremely stable to heat, even up to 2000 °C; not explosive or inflammable in admixture with air (Weil, 1983)
(h) *Reactivity*: Oxidized by air and pure oxygen; can also be reduced by hydrogen and hydrogen sulfide. With hot metals, usually forms both metal sulfides and metal oxides (Weil, 1983)
(i) *Conversion factor*: mg/m^3 = 2.62 × ppm[a]

Sodium sulfite
(a) *Description*: White powder or hexagonal prisms (Weast, 1989)
(b) *Melting-point*: Decomposes (Weast, 1989)
(c) *Density*: 2.633 g/ml at 15.4 °C (Weast, 1989)
(d) *Solubility*: Very soluble in water (12.54 g/100 ml at 0 °C; 28.3 g/100 ml at 80 °C); slightly soluble in ethanol; insoluble in acetone and most other organic solvents (Weil, 1983; Weast, 1989)
(e) *Stability*: Stable in dry air at ambient temperatures or at 100 °C; undergoes rapid oxidation to sodium sulfate in moist air; on heating to 600 °C, disproportionates to sodium sulfate and sodium sulfide; above 900 °C, decomposes to sodium oxide and sulfur dioxide (Weil, 1983)

Sodium bisulfite
(a) *Description*: White, monoclinic crystals, yellow in solution (Weast, 1989)
(b) *Melting-point*: Decomposes (Weast, 1989)
(c) *Density*: 1.48 g/ml (Weast, 1989)
(d) *Solubility*: Very soluble in cold and hot water; slightly soluble in ethanol (Weast, 1989)
(e) *Stability*: Unstable with respect to metabisulfite (Weil, 1983)

Sodium metabisulfite
(a) *Description*: White powder or crystal (Weast, 1989)
(b) *Melting-point*: Decomposes at > 150 °C (Weast, 1989)

---

[a]Calculated from: mg/m^3 = (molecular weight/24.45) × ppm, assuming normal temperature (25 °C) and pressure (760 mm Hg [101.3 kPa])

(c) *Density*: 1.4 g/ml (Weast, 1989)
(d) *Solubility*: Soluble in water (54 g/100 ml at 20 °C; 81.7 g/100 ml at 100 °C) and glycerine; slightly soluble in ethanol (Weast, 1989)
(e) *Stability*: Decomposes in moist air with loss of part of its sulfur dioxide content and by oxidation to sodium sulfate; forms hydrates with water at low temperatures (Weil, 1983)

Potassium metabisulfite
(a) *Description*: Colourless, monoclinic plates (Weast, 1989)
(c) *Melting-point*: Decomposes at 190 °C (Weast, 1989)
(d) *Density*: 2.34 g/ml (Weast, 1989)
(e) *Solubility*: Slightly soluble in water and ethanol; insoluble in diethyl ether (Weast, 1989)

1.1.3 Technical products and impurities

The main grade of liquid sulfur dioxide (pressurized gas) is known as the technical, industrial or commercial grade. This grade contains a minimum of 99.98 wt% sulfur dioxide and is a water-white liquid, free of sulfur trioxide and sulfuric acid. It contains only a trace at most of nonvolatile residue. Its most important specification is the moisture content, which is generally set at a maximum of 100 ppm. The only other grade of liquid sulfur dioxide sold is the refrigeration grade, which is a premium grade of the same purity and specifications as the industrial grade but with a maximal moisture content specified as 50 ppm (Weil, 1983).

Sodium sulfite is available commercially in several grades (Catalyzed SULFTECH®, Catalyzed SULFTECH® with sodium metabisulfite, reagent ACS [American Chemical Society]), with the following ranges of specifications: purity, 94.5–98.5%; sodium chloride, 0.01–0.02%; iron (Fe), 0.001–< 0.002%; arsenic (see IARC, 1987), 1 ppm (mg/kg); heavy metals (as lead), 0.001%; and additives (cobalt salts (see IARC, 1991), 0.01%; anti-caking agent, 0.07%) (General Chemical Corp., undated a,b).

Sodium bisulfite is not sufficiently stable in the solid state to be marketed for commercial use. The 'sodium bisulfite' of commerce consists chiefly of sodium metabisulfite. A technical-grade aqueous solution is available commercially, with the following specifications: concentration, 40.0 wt%; sulfate, 0.7 wt% max; and iron, 15.0 ppm (mg/l) max (Weil, 1983; Calabrian Corp., undated).

Sodium metabisulfite is available commercially in several grades—food and non-food, photographic, technical and industrial—with the following ranges of specifications: purity, 95–98.7%; sodium sulfite, 0.6% max; sulfur dioxide, 65.5–66.5%; iron, 0.0005–0.0015%; selenium (see IARC, 1975), < 0.0005%; heavy metals (as lead), < 0.001–0.002%; chloride, < 0.02%; thiosulfate, < 0.01%; arsenic, < 2.0 ppm (mg/kg); and lead (see IARC, 1987), < 2.0 ppm (mg/kg) (Calabrian Corp., 1990a,b; Virginia Basic Chemicals Co., 1991; General Chemical Corp., undated c,d).

No data were available on technical products and impurities of potassium metabisulfite.

1.1.4 Analysis

Techniques for the detection and measurement of sulfur dioxide have been reviewed (Karchmer, 1970; Snell & Ettre, 1973). This compound can be recognized even at extreme dilutions by its pungent smell. Solutions of sulfur dioxide, sulfites or bisulfites decolourize iodine and permanganate by reducing them. Sulfur dioxide and sulfites are reduced by zinc in a hydrochloric acid solution to hydrogen sulfide, which is readily detected by its smell. Sulfur dioxide can be determined chemically by iodometry, titrimetry, gravimetry or colorimetry (Sander *et al.*, 1984).

Routine monitoring of performance in plants usually entails continuous measurement of the sulfur dioxide content of, for instance, roaster gases, contact gases and tail gases in a sulfuric acid plant by automatic recording, based on some physical property, such as spectroscopic absorption in the infrared or ultraviolet range or electrical conductivity (Sander *et al.*, 1984).

The classical, manual method of iodometric determination (Reich, 1961) is still widely used in industrial practice. A partial stream of sulfur dioxide-containing gas is drawn through an iodide solution, and the sulfur dioxide concentration in the stream is calculated from the gas volume and the titrated iodine released. For titrimetric or gravimetric determination of sulfur dioxide, the gases to be analysed are passed through a hydrogen peroxide solution, which oxidizes sulfur dioxide to sulfuric acid; the sulfuric acid is either titrated with caustic soda solution against bromophenol blue or precipitated as barium sulfate and weighed (Sander *et al.*, 1984).

Typical methods for the analysis of sulfur dioxide in various matrices are summarized in Table 1.

1.2 Production and use

1.2.1 *Production*

Sulfur dioxide has been produced commercially from the following raw materials: elemental sulfur; pyrites; sulfide ores of non-ferrous metals; waste sulfuric acid and sulfates; gypsum and anhydrite; hydrogen sulfide-containing waste gases; and flue gases from the combustion of sulfurous fossil fuels (Sander *et al.*, 1984).

Elemental sulfur is the most important raw material for sulfur dioxide production worldwide. It is the raw material of choice in the production of 100% sulfur dioxide and of commercially important sulfites, such as calcium hydrogen sulfite solution used in cellulose production. The proportion of industrial sulfur dioxide production that is based on elemental sulfur varies in different countries. Of the total amount of sulfur in all forms used for producing sulfur dioxide-containing gases for sulfuric acid production in 1979, the share of elemental sulfur was about 80% in the USA, about 50% in Germany and probably less than 25% in the USSR (Sander *et al.*, 1984).

Sulfur dioxide is produced by burning molten sulfur in a special burner with a controlled amount of air. The burner gas, free of dust and cooled, is dissolved in water in two towers in series. In a third tower, the solution is sprayed at the top and flows down while steam is injected at the base. The gas issuing from the third tower is then cooled to remove most moisture and passed up a fourth tower against a countercurrent of sulfuric acid. The dried gas is liquefied by compression (Mannsville Chemical Products Corp., 1985).

Pyrites and other iron sulfide ores still constitute the main raw material for sulfur dioxide production in some countries, especially in the primary stage of sulfuric dioxide manufacture.

Table 1. Methods for the analysis of sulfur dioxide

Sample matrix	Sample preparation	Assay procedure[a]	Limit of detection	Reference
Air	Collect on cellulose filter saturated with KOH preceded by a cellulose ester membrane; oxidize sulfite to sulfate with 30% w/v H_2O_2; elute with $NaHCO_3/Na_2CO_3$	IC	0.01 mg/ sample	Eller (1987)
	Absorb in 0.3N H_2O_2; titrate using bromocresol green and methyl red solution	Titration	Range, 0.01–10 ppm [0.026–26 mg/m^3]	Taylor (1977)
	Absorb in potassium or sodium tetrachloromercurate; complex heavy metals with EDTA; treat with 0.6% sulfamic acid; treat with formaldehyde and para-rosaniline; adjust pH to 1.6 with 3M H_3PO_4; read maximal absorbance at 548 nm	Colorimetry	0.01 ppm (26 $\mu g/m^3$)	Taylor (1977); Kok et al. (1987a)
	Absorb in buffered formaldehyde solution; treat with 0.6% sulfamic acid; treat with NaOH and para-rosaniline; read maximal absorbance at 580 nm	Colorimetry	26 $\mu g/m^3$	Kok et al. (1987b)
	Draw air through bubbler containing 0.3N H_2O_2; add isopropanol; adjust pH with dilute $HClO_4$; titrate using 0.005M $Ba(ClO_4)_2$ and Thorin indicator	Titration	Range, 6.55–26.8 mg/m^3	Taylor (1978)
	Adsorb onto Molecular Sieve 5A; desorb with heat	MS	2 mg/m^3	Taylor (1977)
Stack gases	Collect on impinger; absorb with 3% H_2O_2; titrate using NaOH and bromophenol blue indicator	AT	Range, 26–15 600 mg/m^3	Knapp et al. (1987)
	Irradiate sample with pulsed ultraviolet light; pass emitted fluorescent light through broad-band optical filter; detect by photomultiplier tube	PFD	Range 2.6–13 000 mg/m^3	Adams et al. (1987)
Beer	Add mercury stabilizing solution and 0.1N H_2SO_4; add 0.1N NaOH; add para-rosaniline and formaldehyde solutions	Colorimetric	Not reported	Helrich (1990)
Food[b]	Heat in refluxing 1N HCl; add nitrogen gas stream; condense gas into 3% H_2O_2 solution; titrate with NaOH and methyl red indicator	Titration	10 ppm	US Food and Drug Administration (1987)

[a]Abbreviations: AT, alkalimetric titration; IC, ion chromatography; MS, mass spectrometry; PFD, pulsed fluorescence detection
[b]Method is also applicable to the following sulfiting preservative agents: potassium metabisulfite, sodium bisulfite, sodium metabisulfite and sodium sulfite

The most important iron sulfide minerals are pyrite and marcasite, both FeS_2. The sulfur content of pyrite concentrates may be as high as 50%. In Japan and some other countries, all the pyrite ores produced are processed domestically; whereas other countries, especially Norway, Spain and the countries of the ex-USSR, still export pyrites as raw materials for sulfuric acid production (Sander et al., 1984).

Non-ferrous metal sulfide ores are also important raw materials for sulfur dioxide production, as in the pyrometallurgical processing of sulfide ores for extraction of copper, nickel, zinc and lead, waste gases containing sulfur dioxide are inevitably produced (Sander et al., 1984).

Sulfur dioxide is normally recovered from waste sulfuric acid and sulfates, from hydrogen sulfide-containing industrial waste gases and from power station flue gases only for environmental reasons. Industrial and public utility boilers can be significant sources of sulfur dioxide, which is a by-product of the combustion of fuel oil and coal. The concentration of sulfur dioxide in these gases is often low and difficult to recover economically. US government regulations restrict the emissions of sulfur dioxide from the stacks of utilities to 10.2 pounds [4.6 kg] per million British thermal units [1 055 055 kJ] of fuel burned (Sander et al., 1984; Mannsville Chemical Products Corp., 1985).

Sulfur dioxide is also recovered commercially by liquefying gas obtained during smelting of non-ferrous metals such as lead, copper and nickel. Much of this smelter by-product is recovered and oxidized to sulfur trioxide for producing sulfuric acid (Sander et al., 1984; Mannsville Chemical Products Corp., 1985).

Calcium sulfate, in the form of natural gypsum or anhydrite, was formerly used in a few small plants as a raw material for sulfur dioxide and sulfuric acid production; owing to the high energy consumption of such plants, however, they have been shut down or modified to process waste gypsum (for example, from phosphoric acid manufacture) (Sander et al., 1984).

In a typical sodium sulfite manufacturing process, a solution of sodium carbonate is allowed to percolate downwards through a series of absorption towers through which sulfur dioxide is passed countercurrently. The solution leaving the towers is chiefly sodium bisulfite of, typically, 27 wt% combined sulfur dioxide content. The solution is then run into a stirred vessel, where aqueous sodium carbonate or sodium hydroxide is added until the bisulfite is entirely converted to sulfite. The solution may be filtered to attain the required product grade. A pure grade of anhydrous sodium sulfite can be crystallized at above 40 °C, since its solubility decreases with increasing temperature (Weil, 1983).

Sodium metabisulfite is produced by reacting an aqueous sodium hydroxide, sodium bicarbonate, sodium carbonate or sodium sulfite solution with sulfur dioxide. The solution is cooled, and the precipitated sodium metabisulfite is removed by centrifugation or filtration. Rapid drying, in a steam-heated shelf dryer or a flash dryer, avoids the excessive decomposition or oxidation to which moist sodium metabisulfite is susceptible. Potassium metabisulfite can be produced by a similar process (Weil, 1983).

Sulfur dioxide was produced for sale in the USA at a level of 64 thousand tonnes in 1960, 99 thousand in 1970, 124 thousand in 1980 and 118 thousand in 1985 (Mannsville Chemical Products Corp., 1985). Demand rose to 227 thousand tonnes in 1987 (Anon., 1988) and to 290 thousand tonnes in 1990 (Anon., 1991). Most of the sulfur dioxide produced worldwide is for captive use in the sulfuric acid and wood pulp industries (Weil, 1983; Sander *et al.*, 1984). The numbers of companies producing sulfur dioxide, sodium sulfite, sodium bisulfite, sodium metabisulfite and potassium bisulfite in various countries and regions are given in Table 2.

Table 2. Numbers of companies producing sulfur dioxide, sodium sulfite, sodium bisulfite, sodium metabisulfite and potassium bisulfite in different countries in 1988–90

Country or region	SO_2	Na_2SO_3	$NaHSO_3$	$Na_2S_2O_5$	$K_2S_2O_5$
Argentina	–	1	1	1	–
Australia	1	–	–	–	–
Austria	1	1	–	–	1
Belgium	1	–	–	–	–
Brazil	2	3	2	1	–
Canada	4	1	–	–	–
Chile	1	–	–	–	–
China	–	4	–	2	–
Colombia	1	1	–	1	–
Czechoslovakia	–	1	–	–	1
Finland	1	–	–	–	–
France	2	–	1	–	–
Germany	6	4	3	–	1
Greece	1	–	–	–	–
India	2	3	4	3	1
Israel	–	–	1	–	–
Italy	2	3	4	2	3
Japan	3	17	2	3	1
Mexico	3	2	1	–	–
Netherlands	1	–	–	–	–
New Zealand	–	–	1	–	–
Norway	1	–	–	–	–
Philippines	1	–	–	–	–
Poland	1	1	–	1	–
South Africa	1	–	1	–	–
Spain	4	3	2	2	4
Sweden	3	–	–	–	–
Switzerland	2	1	2	–	–
Taiwan	3	2	–	1	–
Turkey	1	1	–	1	–
United Kingdom	3	5	3	2	2
USA	7	5	4	3	1
USSR	–	1	–	–	–
Yugoslavia	–	1	–	–	1

From Anon. (1988, 1990); Chemical Information Services (1988); –, not known to be produced

1.2.2 Use

The commercial uses of sulfur dioxide are based on its function as an acid, as a reducing or oxidizing agent or as a catalyst (Mannsville Chemical Products Corp., 1985).

The dominant uses of sulfur dioxide are as a captive intermediate in the production of sulfuric acid and in the pulp and paper industry for sulfite pulping (see p. 145); it is also used as an intermediate for on-site production of bleaches, e.g., chlorine dioxide, by the reduction of sodium chlorate in sulfuric acid solution, and of sodium hydrosulfite (sodium dithionite) ($Na_2S_2O_4$), by the reaction of sodium borohydride with sulfur dioxide. Sulfur dioxide is often used in water treatment to reduce residual chlorine after chlorination and in filter bed cleaning (Weil, 1983; Sander *et al.*, 1984; Mannsville Chemical Products Corp., 1985).

In food processing, sulfur dioxide has a wide range of applications as a fumigant, preservative, bleach and steeping agent for grain. In the production of high-fructose corn syrup, sulfur dioxide is used to steep corn and remove the husks as the corn is prepared for processing. In the manufacture of wine, a small amount of sulfur dioxide is added to the must to destroy bacterial moulds and wild yeasts without harming the yeasts that produce the desired fermentation (Weil, 1983; Sander *et al.*, 1984; Mannsville Chemical Products Corp., 1985).

In petroleum technology, sulfur, most commonly as sodium sulfite, is used as an oxygen scavenger. Sulfur dioxide is used in oil refining as a selective extraction solvent in the Edeleanu process, in which aromatic components are extracted from a kerosene stream with sulfur dioxide, leaving a purified stream of saturated aliphatic hydrocarbons, which are relatively insoluble in sulfur dioxide. Sulfur dioxide acts as a cocatalyst or catalyst modifier in certain processes for oxidation of *ortho*-xylene or naphthalene to phthalic anhydride (Weil, 1983).

In mineral technology, sulfur dioxide and sulfites are used as flotation depressants for sulfide ores. In electrowinning of copper from leach solutions containing iron, sulfur dioxide is used to pre-reduce ferric to ferrous ions to improve current efficiency and copper cathode quality. Sulfur dioxide also initiates precipitation of metallic selenium from selenous acid, a by-product of copper metallurgy (Weil, 1983). In chrome waste disposal, it is used to reduce hexavalent chromium (Mannsville Chemical Products Corp., 1985).

Sulfur dioxide is also used to reduce coloured impurities in clay processing. In the bromine industry, it is used as an antioxidant in spent brine to be reinjected underground. In agriculture, it increases water penetration and the availability of soil nutrients by virtue of its ability to acidulate saline–alkali soils. In glass container manufacture, it is used as a surface alkali neutralizer which improves resistance to scratching and prepares leach-resistant bottles for medicinals, blood plasma and detergents (Weil, 1983).

Sodium sulfite is used in neutral semi-chemical pulping, in acid sulfite pulping, in high-yield sulfite cooling and in some kraft pulping processes; in the chemical industry as a reducing agent and source of sulfite ion; as an antioxidant in water treatment chemicals; in the food industry as an antioxidant and enzyme inhibitor in the processing of fruit and vegetables; in the photographic industry as a film and stain preservative during developing; in the textile industry as a bleach and antichlor; and to remove oxygen from water used in boilers, oil-well flooding, oil-well drilling muds and other situations in which it is important to remove oxygen to reduce corrosion (Weil, 1983; General Chemical Corp., undated a,b).

Estimated uses of sulfur dioxide in 1988 and of sodium sulfite in 1990 in the USA are presented in Table 3.

Table 3. Estimated percentage uses of sulfur dioxide and sodium sulfite in the USA

Use	Sulfur dioxide 1988[a]	Sodium sulfite 1990[b]
Hydrosulfites and other chemicals	40	-
Pulp and paper	20	59
Food and agriculture (mainly corn processing)	16	-
Textile bleaching, food preservatives, chemical intermediate, ore flotation, oil recovery	-	10
Water treatment	10	11
Photography	-	5
Metal and ore refining	6	-
Petroleum refining	4	-
Export	-	15
Miscellaneous	4	-

-, not used or not exported
[a]From Anon. (1988)
[b]From Anon. (1990)

Sodium metabisulfite is used in chemical processing to activate polymerization of acrylonitrile and in waste treatment to reduce chrome wastes; in fruit and vegetable processing as a bleach and preservative; in photoprocessing as a preservative for thiosulfate fixing baths and as a reductant for reversal developing; in tanneries to accelerate the depilatory action of lime for unhairing hides; in the textile industry as an antichlor following chlorine bleaching of cotton and following shrink proofing of wool and as a mordant; in dye manufacture to inhibit oxidation of sensitive amine groups, to replace chlorine groups with the sulfite radical and as an aid in the formation of naphthylamine derivatives; in water treatment as an antichlor; and in the manufacture of explosives and detergents (Weil, 1983; Virginia Basic Chemicals Co., 1991; General Chemical Corp., undated c,d).

The uses of potassium metabisulfite are similar to those of sodium metabisulfite; it is used especially in the processing and preserving of foods and beverages (Sax & Lewis, 1987).

1.3 Occurrence

1.3.1 *Air*

Anthropogenic activities result in a significant contribution to the atmospheric burden of sulfur compounds regionally and on a global scale. By 1976, it was estimated that global gaseous sulfur emissions from anthropogenic combustion sources were about 90 million tonnes per year. This estimate may be compared with the 90 million tonnes per year contributed by all natural sources of gaseous sulfur compounds, principally biogenic, in addition to 40 million tonnes per year as sulfate in sea-spray particles (Winchester, 1983). In another study, it was estimated that approximately 65 million tonnes of sulfur, mostly as sulfur dioxide, are released into the global atmosphere yearly from the burning of fossil fuels and the roasting of metal sulfide ores; the same authors estimated that the total natural releases of sulfur to the atmosphere were approximately 80 million tonnes per year (Turner & Liss, 1983).

Sulfur occurs in a variety of compounds in the atmosphere, many of which participate in the sulfur cycle. Hydrogen sulfide is believed to be emitted into the atmosphere in large but uncertain quantities, mainly from natural sources such as swamps and estuaries; most of it is rapidly oxidized to sulfur dioxide and sulfuric acid by a number of reactions involving reactive oxygen species. Sulfur dioxide is not only a product of hydrogen sulfide oxidation, it constitutes about 95% of the sulfur compounds produced by the burning of sulfur-containing fossil fuels. The major anthropogenic sources of sulfur dioxide are the combustion of coal and fuel oil; production, refining and use of petroleum and natural gas; industries using and manufacturing sulfuric acid and other sulfur products; and smelting and refining of ores (Krupa, 1980).

Natural sources of sulfur include sea spray, volcanic activity, decay of animal and plant tissue, marine algae, anaerobic microbiological activity and other soil processes. Biogenic sulfur compounds originate from nonspecific bacterial reduction of organic sulfur, i.e., plant decomposition, and from specific sulfate-reducing bacteria. Sulfated sea spray accounts for approximately 10% of the natural sulfur emissions, volcanic activity for another 10% and biogenic activity for the balance (Aneja et al., 1982).

Because all sulfur species are eventually oxidized to sulfur dioxide and sulfates, the concentration of atmospheric sulfur dioxide gives a general indication of the original total concentration of other sulfur compounds. In a remote, moist equatorial forest in the Ivory Coast, the atmospheric sulfur dioxide concentration was approximately 30 $\mu g/m^3$. Such levels of sulfur dioxide are secondary reaction products from the decomposition of organic litter and humus. The concentration is comparable to that in industrial zones and higher than those reported for rural areas in the USA and Europe. In comparison, marine concentrations of sulfur dioxide in the air near the Ivory Coast were 0.1–0.5 $\mu g/m^3$ (Aneja et al., 1982).

The average concentration of sulfur dioxide in the dry, unpolluted atmosphere is generally in the range of 10^{-5}–10^{-4} ppm (0.03–0.3 $\mu g/m^3$), with an approximate residence time in the atmosphere of 10 days (Harrison, 1990).

Sulfur dioxide in the atmosphere can contribute to environmental corrosion and can influence the pH of precipitation both by acting as a weak acid itself and by its conversion to the strong acid, sulfuric acid. Sulfur dioxide is a stronger acid than carbon dioxide and at a concentration of only 5 ppb (13 $\mu g/m^3$) in air will, at equilibrium, decrease the pH of rainwater to 4.6 at 15 °C. In many instances, however, low pH is not attained, owing to severe kinetic constraints upon achievement of equilibrium, as is the case with many atmospheric trace gases. Dissolved sulfur dioxide may contribute appreciably to measured total sulfate and acidity in urban rainwater (Harrison, 1990).

The mechanisms by which sulfur dioxide is oxidized to sulfates are important because they determine the rate of formation of sulfate, the influence of the concentration of sulfur dioxide on the reaction rate and, to some extent, the final form of sulfate. Because atmospheric oxidation of sulfur dioxide proceeds *via* a range of mechanisms, depending upon the concentrations of the responsible oxidants, the oxidation rate is extremely variable with space and time; typically, it is 1–5% per hour (Wilson, 1978; Harrison, 1990).

Several mechanisms have been investigated for the gas-phase oxidation of sulfur dioxide. The major pathway appears to involve the hydroxy radical, and gives rise to sulfur trioxide and ultimately sulfuric acid (Wilson, 1978; Harrison, 1990).

In the presence of water droplets, in the form of fog, clouds, rain or hygroscopic aerosols, sulfur dioxide dissolves, so that aqueous-phase oxidation can give rise to bisulfite and sulfite. These equilibria are sensitive to pH, and HSO_3^- is the predominant species over the pH range of 2–7. The other consequence of these equilibria is that the more acidic the droplet, the greater the degree to which the equilibria move towards gaseous sulfur dioxide and limit the concentrations of dissolved sulfur[IV] species (Harrison, 1990).

Estimated sulfur dioxide emissions in 22 countries in 1980 are shown in Table 4. In the United Kingdom, it was estimated that sulfur dioxide contributes 71% of the total atmospheric acidity, compared to 25% from nitrogen oxides and 4% from hydrochloric acid. In the rest of western Europe, sulfur dioxide is estimated to contribute 68%, nitrogen oxides, 30% and hydrochloric acid, 2% (Lightowlers & Cape, 1988). It should be noted, however, that production quantities or emission inventories are not reliable indicators of atmospheric concentrations for a region or country, due to cross-boundary air transport of sulfur dioxide (US Environmental Protection Agency, 1986).

It was estimated that, in 1985, anthropogenic sources contributed approximately 21 million tonnes of sulfur dioxide in the USA, while emissions in Canada were approximately 4 million tonnes. Contributions from different emission sources in the USA and Canada, respectively, were: electric utilities, 69% and 19%; industrial and manufacturing processes, 13% and 69%; industrial combustion, 11% and 8%; transportation, 4% and 3%; and commercial, residential and other combustion, 3% and 1%. Most emissions of sulfur dioxide come from large utility and industrial sources (Placet, 1990).

Between 1900 and 1970, annual estimated sulfur dioxide emissions in the USA increased from 9 to 28 million tonnes; in 1970–87, emissions decreased by an estimated 28%. Natural sources have been estimated to contribute 1–5% of total US sulfur dioxide emissions; they do not appear to make a significant contribution to the sulfate component of acidic deposition in the USA or Canada (Placet, 1990). Total US sulfur dioxide emissions from electric utilities decreased by 16% between 1973 and 1982, from almost 17 million tonnes to slightly under 14.5 million tonnes. Of the sulfur dioxide emissions from utilities in 1982, more than 93% came from coal-fired utilities and less than 7% from oil-fired utilities (Pechan & Wilson, 1984).

Concentrations of sulfur dioxide in ambient air have been measured in many different locations worldwide. Some examples are given in Table 5. Average concentrations of sulfur dioxide have generally been found to be highest in and around large cities (WHO, 1979).

Table 4. Sulfur dioxide emissions in 1980

Country or region	Emission (thousand tonnes)
USSR	25 500
USA	23 000 (21 200 in 1984)
United Kingdom	4 680
Italy	3 800
Germany (western)	3 580
France	3 270
Czechoslovakia	3 100
Yugoslavia	3 000
Poland	2 755
Hungary	1 663
Bulgaria	1 000
Belgium	809
Greece	700
Finland	600
The Netherlands	487
Sweden	450
Austria	440
Denmark	399
Romania	200
Portugal	149
Norway	137
Switzerland	119

From US Environmental Protection Agency (1986)

Table 5. Sulfur dioxide concentrations in ambient air

Location	Year	SO_2 concentration ($\mu g/m^3$)	Reference
Rural NY, USA	1984–86	3.38–7.44	Kelly et al. (1989)
PA, USA	1983	26–31	Pierson et al. (1989)
Rural PA, USA	1984	3–131	Lewin et al. (1986)
Bermuda	1982–83	0–1.67	Wolff et al. (1986)
Coastal DE, USA	1985	13.4	Hastie et al. (1988)
Bermuda (mid-ocean)	1985	0.7	Hastie et al. (1988)
Northwest Territories, Canada	Nov–Dec 1981	0.33–0.69	Hoff et al. (1983)
Northwest Territories, Canada	Feb 1982	2.3–4.3	
Ontario, Canada	1982	8.4–16.2	Anlauf et al. (1985)
Ontario, Canada	1984	0.1–62.8	Barrie (1988)
Near H_2SO_4 producer, United Kingdom	1981	0.5–120	Harrison (1983)

1.3.2 Occupational exposure

The uses of sulfur dioxide described above indicate its widespread occurrence in the work place. It also occurs in the work environment as a result of oxidation (e.g., burning) of sulfuric ores, sulfur-containing fuels and other materials. Table 6 is a list of occupations entailing frequent exposure to sulfur dioxide. The number of workers exposed to sulfur dioxide in the USA in 1974 was estimated to be about 500 000 (US National Institute for Occupational Safety and Health, 1974), which is 0.2% of the total population. The corresponding figure in Finland in 1991 was 10 000 (Kangas, 1991), which is similarly 0.2% of the population. On the basis of these estimates and of the characteristics of the populations and industrial development on the five continents, the global number of exposed workers is probably several million.

Table 6. Occupations in which there is potential exposure to sulfur dioxide

Beet sugar bleaching	Oil bleaching
Blast furnace tending	Oil processing
Brewery work	Ore smelting
Diesel engine operation	Organic sulfonate manufacture
Diesel engine repair	Papermaking
Disinfectant manufacture	Petroleum refinery work
Disinfection	Preservative manufacture
Fire-fighting	Refrigeration
Flour bleaching	Straw bleaching
Food bleaching	Sugar refining
Food protein manufacture	Sulfite manufacture
Foundry work	Sulfur dioxide work
Fruit bleaching	Sulfuric acid manufacture
Fumigant manufacture	Sulfuryl chloride manufacture
Fumigation	Tannery work
Furnace operation	Textile bleaching
Gelatin bleaching	Thermometer manufacture
Glass making	Thionyl chloride manufacture
Glue bleaching	Wickerware bleaching
Grain bleaching	Winemaking
Ice making	Wood bleaching
Industrial protein manufacture	Wood pulp bleaching
Meat preserving	

From US National Institute for Occupational Safety and Health (1974)

Sulfur dioxide has been measured in many industries, but most of the data come from pulp manufacture by the acidic (sulfite) process (see IARC, 1987) and the manufacture of basic metals. Some data are available from the chemical industry (e.g., sulfuric acid manufacture), oil refining and the petrochemical industry, textile processing, refrigerator production, food preparation, the rubber industry (see IARC, 1987), the glass industry, the brick industry, mineral fibre production (see IARC, 1988), photography, silicon carbide production, power plants and fire fighting. Exposure may occur also in the pharmaceutical industry, in mining, in water treatment, in chrome-waste treatment and during fumigation and other operations (US National Institute for Occupational Safety and Health, 1974; US National Institute for Occupational Safety and Health/Occupational Safety and Health Administration, 1981), but no data on levels of exposure were available to the Working Group, nor was any information available on occupational exposure to sulfites, bisulfites or metabisulfites.

The methods used to take occupational hygiene measurements have varied over the years. Detector tubes showing the crude concentration of sulfur dioxide in work-room air during measurement, which usually lasts 1-2 min, were used commonly in the 1950s and 1960s. An older method that allows longer sampling is based on liquid absorption of sulfur dioxide and determination by titration. More recently, long-term detector tubes, passive dosimeters and other methods have been used. Most samples have been collected from static sampling points at sites that workers visit occasionally or regularly; some measurements are made during relatively brief episodes when high-peak exposures are expected to occur. Long-term personal sampling has rarely been done because liquid absorption sampling is difficult under these conditions and because the aim of measurements has traditionally been to identify acute risks of exposure to sulfur dioxide. Therefore, many of the reported results reflect mainly short-term exposure and are overestimates of the exposure levels experienced by workers during longer periods (Smith *et al.*, 1978; Broder *et al.*, 1989).

(a) Pulp industry

Large amounts of sulfur dioxide are used in the preparation of cooking liquor in sulfite pulp mills. Sulfur dioxide gas is reacted with water and calcium carbonate or other carbonate minerals in an absorption tower ('acid' tower), where the cooking liquor containing sulfurous acid, bisulfites and sulfur dioxide is formed. The cooking acid and wood chips are charged into a continuous or batch-type digester where the lignin of the wood dissolves in liquor during cooking under raised temperature and pressure. Pulp is dropped or 'blown' from the digester into covered or uncovered pits to be washed. This operation often releases large amounts of sulfur dioxide into the work-room air; in addition, the raw pulp contains residues of cooking liquor, which contribute to the emissions. Sulfur dioxide is thus a major air contaminant in sulfite pulp mills, and nearly all process workers involved in the preparation of cooking liquor or cooking, washing and other operations are exposed. Work in acid plants is usually continuous, and exposure occurs during the whole work day. In other areas, exposure varies, being relatively low in control rooms (where most time is spent) but high episodically during certain operations and during leakages of the process equipment (Feiner & Marlowe, 1956; Jäppinen, 1987). Sulfur dioxide may also be used in the bleaching departments of pulp and paper plants to neutralize residual chemicals and during final acidification to remove metallic ions from the pulp. Occasionally, mechanically produced pulp is bleached with sodium dithionite, which may release sulfur dioxide (Kangas, 1991). Occupational exposure measurements in the pulp industry are given in Table 7.

Sulfite pulp workers were exposed for shorter or longer periods in the 1950s to measured concentrations of sulfur dioxide well above 26 mg/m^3. The scarce data available on daily mean exposures suggest levels of 13 mg/m^3 or more; but these data represent only the situation in digesting and pulp storage in one mill at one period of time. Measurements in the

Table 7. Measurements of sulfur dioxide in the pulp industry

Industry, operation	No. of samples	Concentration of sulfur dioxide (mg/m^3)^a		Year of measurement	Country	Reference
		Mean	Range			
Five sulfite pulp mills				1954–67	Finland	FIOH (1990)
Burning of pyrite, acid plants, digesting, blow pits	156	68.1	ND–560			
Sulfite pulp mills				1972–74	Finland	Skyttä (1978)
Acid departments	3		7.1–66			
Blow pits	2		12.6–37			
Digesting departments	2		20–34			
Filtering	1		<0.3			
Burning of sulfur	2		6.6–13.6			
Power plants	2		2.4–3.4			
Chimney sweeping	1		17.0			
Four sulfite pulp mills				1978–85	Finland	Kangas (1991)
Acid departments	31					
Control rooms	NR	<1.3	0.3–2.6			
Other sites	NR	12.6	2.1–86.5			
Digesting, washing	196					
Control rooms	NR	2.1	NR–16.5			
Digesters, blow pits	NR	5.8	NR–60.3			
Evaporation						
Winter			5.5			
Summer			3.9			
Bleaching		<5.2	NR			
Four sulfite pulp mills				NR	USA	Feiner & Marlow (1956)
Sulfur burner rooms	3	13.1	5.2–31.4			
Blow valve floors	5	NR	13.1–>131			
Blow pit floors	3	79	52.4–131			
Digester loading floors	4	NR	5.2–>131			
Acid plant	1		52.4			
Four sulfite pulp mills				NR	Norway	Skalpe (1964)
Acid towers	6	46.3	26.2–94.3			
Digester plants						
Top floors	4	17.2	3.1–31.4			
Middle floors	2	20	3.1–36.7			
Bottom floors	5	27	13.1–49.8			
Sulfite pulp mill				1958–63	USA	Ferris et al. (1967)
Digester loading room	13	14.2	ND–29			
Blow pit floor	2		ND			
Recovery boiler	2	8.5	3.9–13			
Washer operating floor	2	0.7	ND–1.31			
Evaporators	1		10.5			
Dryers	1		<0.3			
Lower floor	6	9.2	2.6–15.7			
Pyrite plant	3	1.5	ND–4.45			
Acid room	5	15.1	Traces–26.2			
Bleaching plant	1		3.7			
Blower house	2	85.2	83.8–86.5			

Table 7 (contd)

Industry, operation	No. of samples	Concentration of sulfur dioxide (mg/m^3)^a		Year of measurement	Country	Reference
		Mean	Range			
Sulfite pulp mill				NR	Sweden	Stjernberg et al. (1984)
Digester room and wood pulp storage						
> 50% of daily means	NR	14.28 (TWA)	NR			
Maximal daily means	NR	NR	114–140			
Semichemical pulp mill	NR	< 3	NR	NR	Finland	Kangas (1991)
Sulfate pulp mill				1963	USA	Ferris et al. (1967)
Digester loading room	1	2.6				
Washer operating floor	3	2.0	ND–4.7			
Evaporators	1	3.7				
Other sites	2		ND			
Mechanical pulp mills				NR	Finland	Kangas (1991)
Dosing of dithionite in bleaching departments	12	3.34	0.8–39.3			
Pulp mill, general plant				1963	USA	Ferris et al. (1967)
Wood chipper room	1		ND			
Barker drum plant	1		ND			
Power plant	1		0.3			

ND, not detected; NR, not reported
^{a}Measurements based on long-term sampling and given as the average concentration over about one working day or longer are indicated as TWA (time-weighted average concentration).

1980s suggested lower levels, especially in control rooms (Table 7). Other agents present in the work environment of sulfite pulp mills include sulfur, ammonia, limestone, sulfurous acid, calcium bisulfite, calcium oxide, carbon monoxide, lignosulfonates, methanol, acetic acid, formic acid, formaldehyde (see IARC, 1987), furaldehyde and cymene (Jäppinen, 1987).

(b) Metallurgy

In the basic metal industries, in which steel, copper, nickel, zinc, cobalt, aluminium and other metals are produced, sulfur dioxide occurs when sulfidic ores or sulfuric impurities of the ores are sintered, roasted or melted. Impurities of coal, coke, heavy fuel oils and other materials used in the processes may also contribute to emissions of sulfur dioxide. The exposure level in a specific mill depends on many factors, including the composition of the raw materials, temperatures and other parameters of the processes, intensity of the production, tightness of the furnaces and other process equipment, ventilation and use of respirators. The concentration of sulfur dioxide in the air also varies over time, with the operations carried out and possible leakages of the process equipment. Occupational exposure measurements in metallurgy are given in Table 8.

Table 8. Measurements of sulfur dioxide in metallurgy

Industry, operation	No. of samples	Concentration of sulfur dioxide (mg/m³)[a]		Year of measurement	Country	Reference
		Mean	Range			
Copper smelter (furnaces, converters, etc.)	36	17.5	1.57–100	1951–57	Finland	FIOH (1990)
Copper smelter				NR	Sweden	Lundgren (1954)
Roaster	NR	~222	66–550			
Reverberatory furnace	NR	~152	0–500			
Converter hall	NR	~24	0–52.4			
Copper smelter				1972	USA	US National Institute for Occupational Health (1974)
Reverberatory furnaces	3	16	2.6–26.3			
Other sites	8	<3	NR			
Reverberatory furnaces, chargers floor	20	60	4.2–118			
Main floor opposite skimming end	20	6.6	0.8–23.6			
Skimmers' platforms	21	25.1	2.1–68			
Copper smelter				1940–74	USA	Smith et al. (1978)
Reverberatory furnace						
Area measurements, 1940–74	NR	20.5[b] TWA	2.0–75.4[b,c] TWA			
Stationary measurements, 1972–74	181	10.6[b] TWA	1.1–62.0[c] TWA			
Personal monitoring, 1973–74	NR	3.1[b] TWA	2.7–3.5[c] TWA			
Converter						
Area measurements, 1940–74	NR	7.0[b] TWA	1.2–30.9[c] TWA			
Stationary measurements, 1972–74	198	3.7[b] TWA	1.5–14[c] TWA			
Personal monitoring, 1973–74	NR	2.6[b] TWA	2.6[c] TWA			
Reverberatory furnace and converter area						
Personal monitoring, 1973–74						
Supervisors	NR	2.6 TWA	NR			
Maintenance workers	NR	1.7 TWA	NR			
Anode plant						
Area measurements, 1959–74	NR	3.2[b] TWA	1.4–4.2[c] TWA			
Stationary measurements, 1972–74	100	3.9 TWA	NR–7.3 (SD, 1.8)			
Personal monitoring, 1973–74	NR	2.5 TWA	NR			

Table 8 (contd)

Industry, operation	No. of samples	Concentration of sulfur dioxide (mg/m³)[a]		Year of measurement	Country	Reference
		mean	range			
Copper smelter (contd)						Smith et al. (1978) (contd)
Acid plant						
Area measurements, 1940–74	NR	3.5[b] TWA	0.4–9.4[c] TWA			
Stationary measurement, 1972–74	53	5.4 TWA	NR (SD, 3.6)			
Personal monitoring, 1973–74	NR	4.2 TWA	NR			
Truck shop						
Area measurements, 1973–74	91	<0.2 TWA	NR			
Unspecified smelter area						
Personal monitoring, 1973–74	NR	2.1 TWA	NR			
Copper smelter					USA	Rom et al. (1986)
Old plant		4.5 TWA	0.5–17.6 TWA	1976		
New plant		6.0 TWA	0.5–14.7 TWA	1982		
Copper/nickel mill (furnaces, converters)	23	5.9	0.3–34.1	1968	Finland	FIOH (1990)
Copper/nickel mill				NR	Finland	Kangas (1991)
Reverberatory furnaces		~3	NR–10.5			
Converters		~3	NR–7.9			
Casting of copper anodes		<3	NR–5.2			
Pretreatment of precious metal ores		<3	NR–13.1			
Nickel smelter	NR	1.8 TWA	0.05–9.4 TWA	1985	Canada	Broder et al. (1989)
Steel mill				1968	Finland	FIOH (1990)
Blast furnace	4	0.3	0.3			
Steel smelter	4	1.1	0.26–1.8			
Rolling mill						
Crane	4	9.4	0.26–19.1			
Other sites	3	0.8	0.3–1.8			
Two steel mills				1964–68	United Kingdom	Warner et al. (1969)
Blast furnace						
Mill 1	51	1.8 TWA	NR			
Mill 2	75	1.5 TWA	NR			

Table 8 (contd)

Industry, operation	No. of samples	Concentration of sulfur dioxide (mg/m³)[a] mean	range	Year of measurement	Country	Reference
Converters						Warner et al. (contd)
Mill 1	97	0.30 TWA	NR			
Mill 2	87	0.35 TWA	NR			
Open hearths						
Mill 1	37	0.18 TWA	NR			
Mill 2	96	0.33 TWA	NR			
Hot mill						
Mill 1	136	0.99 TWA	NR			
Mill 2	93	0.21 TWA	NR			
Cold mill						
Mill 1	217	1.50 TWA	NR			
Mill 2	75	0.28 TWA	NR			
Power plant						
Mill 1	26	0.84 TWA	NR			
Mill 2	38	0.06 TWA	NR			
Sinter, coke ovens, quarries, lime burning, central electrical workshops, engineering workshops, stores, laboratories, and offices (both mills)	338	0.08 TWA	NR			
Steel mills						
Sintering	NR	NR	0–26.2	NR	Finland	Kangas (1991)
Blast furnace						
Usually	NR	NR	1.05–2.6 TWA			
Occasionally	NR	NR	26.2–52.4			
Steelmaking, mixers						
Usually	NR	NR	0.3–2.4 TWA			
Occasionally	NR	NR	13.1–39.3			
Rolling mill 1						
Usually	NR	NR	1.31–2.1 TWA			
Rolling mills 2 & 3	47	4.2	1.31–42			

Table 8 (contd)

Industry, operation	No. of samples	Concentration of sulfur dioxide (mg/m³)[a]		Year of measurement	Country	Reference
		Mean	Range			
Zinc mill						
Roasting department						
Personal monitoring	NR	~ 3 TWA	NR	NR	Finland	Kangas (1991)
Static sampling	NR	~ 5 TWA	NR			
Cobalt mill						
Roasting department	14	12.8	0.6–44.5	1968	Finland	FIOH (1990)
Dissolving department	4	0.6	0.6			
Aluminium smelter						
Potroom workers (personal samples)	121	2.0 TWA	SD, 1.5	1979–80	Canada	Chan–Yeung et al. (1983)
Aluminium foundry (personal monitoring)	NR	2.6 TWA	0.5–7.9 TWA	NR	Sweden	Sorsa et al. (1982)
Foundries				NR	Finland	Kangas (1991)
Steel foundry using furan resins	14	5.8	< 1.3–2.1			
Other steel foundries	7	< 3	NR			
Light metal foundry	1	< 3	NR			
Brass/bronze foundry	7	12	NR			

NR, not reported; ND, not detected; SD, standard deviation
[a]Measurements based on long-term sampling and given as the average concentration over about one working day or longer are indicated as TWA (time-weighted average concentration).
[b]Mean of means
[c]Range of means

In copper smelters, the mean level of sulfur dioxide is often between 2.6 and 26 mg/m^3; high concentrations, well above 26 mg/m^3, may occur occasionally. In nickel, zinc and aluminium smelters, as well as in steel mills, lower mean concentrations have been measured (2.6 mg/m^3 or less) (Table 8). In most cases, sulfur dioxide is only one of the agents present in work-room air. Other agents that may occur simultaneously include iron, nickel, copper, aluminium, cobalt, zinc, lead, cadmium and arsenic and their compounds. Burning of raw materials and fuels also releases carbon monoxide, other combustion gases and particulates into the air. The airborne particulates may contain a complex mixture of polycyclic aromatic hydrocarbons and sometimes silica.

(c) *Other miscellaneous industries and operations* (see Table 9)

Sulfur dioxide is used as an intermediate in the production of sulfuric acid (see the monograph on occupational exposure to mists and vapours from sulfuric acid and other strong inorganic acids, p. 47). The mean levels of sulfur dioxide in long-term samples have varied between < 3 and 5 mg/m^3; peak exposure to a level of 26 mg/m^3 or more may occur occasionally (Table 9). Sulfur dioxide may in some cases be carried over to departments in which sulfuric acid is used as a raw material in the production of other chemicals, such as superphosphate fertilizers.

Workers manufacturing refrigerators in which sulfur dioxide was used as a refrigerant were reported to have experienced frequently brief but high (> 26 mg/m^3) exposures in the charging department and during the storage and distribution of sulfur dioxide. No other inhalatory exposure was mentioned (Kehoe *et al.*, 1932).

Crude oil contains varying amounts of sulfur compounds which are partly removed during petroleum refining. Even though oxidative processes are avoided, exposure to sulfur dioxide may occur during recovery of sulfur and in the vicinity of furnaces and flares. A wide variety of other agents including benzene (see IARC, 1987), asbestos (see IARC, 1987), 1,3-butadiene (see monograph, p. 237) and polycyclic aromatic compounds (see IARC, 1983) are present in oil refineries and related petrochemical plants (IARC, 1989).

Silicon carbide is produced by heating petroleum coke and silica sand in an electric furnace. The sulfur impurities of coke form sulfur dioxide during burning. Other agents present include dusts of raw materials (coke, silica (see IARC, 1987)) or products (silicon carbide) and furnace emissions (e.g., carbon monoxide and various hydrocarbons) (Smith *et al.*, 1984).

Vulcanization of rubber containing sulfur compounds as ingredients may also release sulfur dioxide. In addition, the air in the breathing zone of personnel working at vulcanization presses may contain a complex mixture of gases and vapours, including styrene, 1,3-butadiene, carbon monoxide, oil mist, acrylonitrile (see IARC, 1987), aromatic amines, formaldehyde, acrolein (see IARC, 1987), ammonia and methanol (Volkova & Bagdinov, 1969).

Sulfur dioxide, together with numerous other agents, is used in leather tanneries as a biocide in the beamhouses and as a chrome tanning chemical (IARC, 1981).

In the production of glass, porcelain, ceramics, bricks and mineral fibres, as well as in power plants, the source of sulfur dioxide is fuel that is burned in order to melt or dry raw materials or products. Occasionally, raw materials may also contain sulfur impurities (Kangas, 1991).

Fixing solutions for films usually contain sodium thiosulfate as an ingredient, which, under certain conditions, may release sulfur dioxide (Kangas 1991).

In addition to its limited use in the bleaching of pulp, sulfur dioxide has been used directly to bleach coir (coconut fibres) (Uragoda, 1981). Bisulfites that release sulfur dioxide are also used as finishing agents in the bleaching of wool.

1.3.3 *Food and beverages*

In food and beverage industries, sulfur dioxide may be used as a bleaching agent, preservative and sterilization agent. According to the few measurements of the Finnish Institute of Occupational Health (1990), the concentrations during some short-term tasks may be high (Table 9).

Sulfur dioxide and sulfite occur naturally in some foods and are added as preservatives. *Allium* and *Brassica* vegetables contain naturally occurring sulfur dioxide-producing components: The concentration of sulfur dioxide was 17 ppm (mg/kg) in fresh onions, 60 ppm in dried onions, 4 ppm in canned, boiled onions, 121 ppm in dried garlic, 7 ppm in dried leek soup mix and 10–30 ppm in dried onion soup mixes. Non-sulfited soya bean protein contained 20 ppm, sulfited soya bean proteins, 80–120 ppm, cherries, 24 ppm, white wine, 14 ppm, and 'burgundy' wine, 150 ppm of sulfur dioxide (Fazio & Warner, 1990). The concentrations of sulfite (measured by the Monier–Williams method and calculated as SO_2) were 173–197 ppm in mashed potatoes, 1977 ppm in dehydrated apricots, < 1–564 ppm in raisins, 1072 ppm in dried peaches, 5.2 ppm in corn syrup, < 1 ppm in frozen shrimps, 26 ppm in canned shrimps, 71 ppm in onion flakes, 126 ppm in garlic powder, 177 ppm in red wine, 138–218 ppm in white wine and 261 ppm in lemon juice (Lawrence & Chadha, 1988).

The total content of sulfur dioxide in wines from 12 countries ranged from 60 to 170 mg/l (Ough, 1986); 33–47 ppm were found in conventional corn syrups and 5–33 ppm in specialty starches (Coker, 1986). The US population has been estimated to consume an average of 10–15 mg/person of sulfiting agents daily. The daily intake varies widely depending on the diet and may be 120 mg or more (Allen, 1985; Emerson & Johnson, 1985).

1.4 Regulations and guidelines

Occupational exposure limits for sulfur dioxide in some countries are shown in Table 10.

WHO (1987) recommended ambient air quality guidelines for sulfur dioxide: Short-term exposures should not exceed 500 µg/m^3, based on a 10-min average, which corresponds to a 1-h maximal value of 350 µg/m^3. Guideline values for combined exposure to sulfur dioxide and particulate matter in a 24-h period should not exceed 126 µg/m^3 sulfur dioxide, 125 µg/m^3 black smoke, 120 µg/m^3 total suspended particulates and 70 µg/m^3 particles in the thorax. Guideline values for exposure to combined sulfur dioxide and particulate matter averaged over one year should not exceed 60 µg/m^3 sulfur dioxide and 60 µg/m^3 black smoke.

Table 9. Measurements of sulfur dioxide in miscellaneous industries and operations

Industry, operation	No. of samples	Concentration of sulfur dioxide (mg/m³)[a]		Year of measurement	Country	Reference
		Mean	Range			
Four sulfuric acid plants (furnaces, dilution, gas purification, tower room, etc.)	35	14.4	ND-79	1951-61	Finland	FIOH (1990)
Sulfuric acid plant	NR	NR	0.34-12.0		China	Meng & Zhang (1990a)
Sulfuric acid plant				1969-84	Sweden	Englander et al. (1988)
Stationary samples	NR	9.1[b] TWA	2.4-12.4			
Breathing zone samples	NR	3.6[b] TWA	1.1-2.3			
Sulfuric acid plants				NR	Finland	Kangas (1991)
Long-term samples	NR	< 3 TWA	NR			
Occasionally	NR	NR	NR-26.2			
Superphosphate plant (conveyors, mixing, etc.)	6	3.7	0.3-10.5	1951-62	Finland	FIOH (1990)
Refrigerator manufacturing plant				1929-30	USA	Kehoe et al. (1932)
Charging room	39	60	18-181			
Distribution and storage of sulfur dioxide	14	73	29-147	1930		
Oil refinery and special products plant				After 1945	Iran	Anderson (1950)
Usually	NR	NR	0-66			
Occasionally	NR	NR	157-262	1938-45		
Silicon carbide plant (furnace area)				1980	USA	Smith et al. (1984)
Personal samples	NR	2.0[c] TWA	<0.3-3.9[d] TWA			
Stationary samples	1	18.9				
Vulcanization of butadiene-styrene rubber				NR	USSR	Volkova & Bagdinov (1969)
Range	NR	NR	0.3-19			
Usual range	NR	NR	1-2			
Food production				1952	Finland	FIOH (1990)
Dosing of apple purée to a kettle	1	199				
Cooking of marmalade	1	16.2				
Beverage industry (sterilization of alcohol with sulfur dioxide gas)	5	7.7	2.4-17.8	1958	Finland	FIOH (1990)
Textile mill (finishing of bleached wool with hydrosulfite)	1	3.7		1954	Finland	FIOH (1990)

Table 9 (contd)

Industry, operation	No. of samples	Concentration of sulfur dioxide (mg/m³)[a]		Year of measurement	Country	Reference
		Mean	Range			
Power plants						
Boiler rooms	NR	< 1.3	NR	NR	Finland	Kangas (1991)
Boiler room, leakage	NR	NR	6.6–26.2			
Flame cutting of oil kettles	4	NR	21–65.5			
Close to diesel engines	4	< 2.6	NR	NR	Finland	Kangas (1991)
Nine photographic laboratories	29	< 2.6	NR	NR	Finland	Kangas (1991)
Glass, porcelain and ceramic products plants, close to furnaces	13	< 2.6	NR–44	NR	Finland	Kangas (1991)
Brick manufacturing plants, burning of bricks	27	< 2.6	NR–10	NR	Finland	Kangas (1991)
Mineral fibre plants, close to furnaces	9	< 2.6	NR	NR	Finland	Kangas (1991)
Paper mill, bleaching	6	0.4	ND–1.8	1963	Finland	FIOH (1990)
Paper mill				NR	Finland	IARC (1981)
Beating/refining	NR	0.2				
Wet end of paper machine	NR	0.01				
Two paper mills, recovery plant	2	2.4	1.1–3.6	1971	India	Gautam *et al.* (1979)
	3	0.5	Trace–0.8	1976–77		
Fire fighting at 14 sites during fires	26	6.0	0–109	1986	USA	Brandt-Rauf *et al.* (1988)

ND, not detected; NR, not reported
[a]Measurements based on long-term sampling and given as the average concentration over about one working day or longer are indicated as TWA (time-weighted average concentration).
[b]Median
[c]Mean of means
[d]Range of means

Table 10. Occupational exposure limits and guidelines for sulfur dioxide

Country	Year	Concentration (mg/m^3)	Interpretation[a]
Australia	1990	5	TWA
		10	STEL
Austria	1982	5	TWA
Belgium	1990	5.2	TWA
		13	STEL
Brazil	1978	10	TWA
Bulgaria	1984	10	TWA
Chile	1983	4	TWA
China	1981	13	TWA
Czechoslovakia	1990	5	TWA
		10	STEL
Denmark	1990	5	TWA
Finland	1990	5	TWA
		13	STEL
France	1990	5	TWA
		10	STEL
Germany	1990	5[b]	TWA
Hungary	1990	3[b]	TWA
		6[b]	STEL
India	1983	13	TWA
Indonesia	1978	13	TWA
Japan	1983	13	TWA
Mexico	1983	13	TWA
Netherlands	1986	13	TWA
Norway	1990	5	TWA
Poland	1984	10	TWA
Republic of Korea	1983	5	TWA
		10	STEL
Romania	1975	10	TWA
		15	Ceiling
Sweden	1990	5	TWA
		13	Ceiling
Switzerland	1990	5	TWA
		10	STEL
United Kingdom	1990	5	TWA
		13	STEL
USA			
ACGIH	1990	5.2	TWA
		13	STEL
OSHA	1989	5	TWA
		10	STEL
USSR	1990	10[b]	STEL

Table 10 (contd)

Country	Year	Concentration (mg/m^3)	Interpretation[a]
Venezuela	1978	13	TWA
		13	Ceiling
Yugoslavia	1971	10	TWA

From Arbeidsinspectie (1986); Cook (1987); US Occupational Safety and Health Administration (OSHA) (1989); American Conference of Governmental Industrial Hygienists (ACGIH) (1990); Direktoratet for Arbeidstilsynet (1990); International Labour Office (1991)
[a]TWA, 8-h time-weighted average; STEL, short-term exposure limit; MAC, maximum allowable concentration
[b]Skin notation

The Commission of the European Communities (1980) established limit values for sulfur dioxide (to become law on 1 April 1993) and for associated suspended particles, as follows. The annual median value should be no more than 80 $\mu g/m^3$ in the presence of > 40 $\mu g/m^3$ suspended particulates, or 120 $\mu g/m^3$ in association with $\geq$ 40 $\mu g/m^3$ particulates. The median value in winter (1 October–31 March) should not exceed 130 $\mu g/m^3$ with > 60 $\mu g/m^3$ particulates and 180 $\mu g/m^3$ with $\leq$ 60 $\mu g/m^3$ particulates. The 98th percentile of all daily mean values taken throughout the year should not exceed 250 $\mu g/m^3$ sulfur dioxide in the presence of > 150 $\mu g/m^3$ particulates and no more than 350 $\mu g/m^3$ with $\leq$ 150 $\mu g/m^3$ particulates.

The US national primary air quality standard for sulfur dioxide, set by the US Environmental Protection Agency, is 80 $\mu g/m^3$ (0.03 ppm) calculated as an annual arithmetic mean and 365 $\mu g/m^3$ (0.14 ppm) computed as a maximal 24-h concentration that is not to be exceeded more than once per year. Secondary standards, which protect the public from any known or anticipated adverse effects, allow 0.02 ppm (0.05 mg/m^3) as an annual arithmetic mean, 0.10 ppm (0.26 mg/m^3) as a 24-h maximum not to be exceeded more than once per year and 0.50 ppm (1.3 mg/m^3) as a 3-h maximum not to be exceeded more than once per year (Weil, 1983).

The US Environmental Protection Agency (1989) established sulfur dioxide emission standards for primary copper smelters, primary zinc smelters and primary lead smelters in which discharge of any gases that contain sulfur dioxide in excess of 0.065% by volume is prohibited. Sulfur dioxide emission standards also have been established for sulfuric acid plants: discharge into the atmosphere of gases that contain sulfur dioxide in excess of 2 kg/tonne of acid produced is prohibited, the production being expressed as 100% H_2SO_4. Stationary gas turbines are prohibited from discharging into the atmosphere gases that contain sulfur dioxide in excess of 0.015% by volume, at 15% oxygen and on a dry basis.

The standard for emissions of sulfur dioxide from municipal refuse-fired plants in the Federal Republic of Germany in 1981 was 34 ppm (90 mg/m^3) (Skizim, 1982).

The US Food and Drug Administration (1989) established that sulfur dioxide, sodium sulfite, sodium bisulfite, sodium metabisulfite and potassium metabisulfite are generally recognized as safe as chemical preservatives for foods, except that they must not be used in meats or in food recognized as a source of vitamin B_1, or on raw or fresh fruits and vegetables.

2. Studies of Cancer in Humans

Exposure to sulfur dioxide occurs in different occupational environments (see Section 1); however, the epidemiological studies that have specifically addressed cancer risks in relation to exposure to sulfur dioxide have been conducted primarily in smelter workers and in pulp and paper workers. These occupational groups are treated separately in view of the substantial differences in the exposure environments.

No epidemiological study was found on cancer risks in relation to exposure to sulfites, bisulfites or metabisulfites.

2.1 Smelting of nonferrous metals

A series of studies of both cohort and case–control design addressed cancer risks among workers at the Anaconda copper smelter in Montana, USA (Lubin et al., 1981; Welch et al., 1982; Lee-Feldstein, 1983). The studies focused mainly on exposure to arsenic (see IARC, 1987). Mortality was followed in 1938–77 for a cohort of 8045 white men who had been employed for 12 months or more before 1956 (Lee-Feldstein, 1983). Work areas were rated on a relative scale with respect to the level of sulfur dioxide (and arsenic). A total of 3522 workers died during the follow-up period, and 816 (10.1%) were lost. A total of 302 respiratory cancer deaths were seen, corresponding to standardized mortality ratios (SMR) of 2.09 [95% confidence interval (CI), 1.59–2.58] for men in the light exposure category for sulfur dioxide, 2.97 [2.00–3.95] for medium exposure and 3.17 [2.07–4.27] for heavy sulfur dioxide exposure in comparison with regional rates. The highest risks were seen in workers with high or medium exposure to both arsenic and sulfur dioxide, suggesting a positive interaction between the two exposures. Multivariate modelling (Lubin et al., 1981) suggested that respiratory cancer risks associated with work in the areas of medium and heavy sulfur dioxide exposure were not significantly increased when medium or heavy exposure to arsenic was controlled for. The authors noted that it was difficult to separate the effects of the two exposures since they often occurred together.

A follow-up of mortality through 1977 of a sample of 1800 men in the same cohort also included information on smoking habits for 81.6% of the sample (Welch et al., 1982). Telephone interviews or mailed questionnaires were used to obtain information on smoking from cases or next-of-kin. Although results were not reported on smoking habits in relation to sulfur dioxide exposure, few differences in smoking habits were reported between men in the different arsenic exposure categories; since arsenic and sulfur dioxide exposures were correlated, the finding suggests that smoking was not a confounder in relation to sulfur dioxide.

Another US copper smelter that has been investigated in many epidemiological studies was located in Tacoma, WA (USA). The studies also focused primarily on arsenic exposure; only one of them included data on risks in relation to exposure to sulfur dioxide (Enterline & Marsh, 1982). The mortality of 2802 men who had worked for one year or more at the smelter during the period 1940–64 was followed through to 1976. Only 1.8% could not be traced, and death certificates were obtained for 95.6% of deceased individuals. An overall SMR of 1.98 [95% CI, 1.60–2.36] was observed for cancer of the respiratory system in comparison with Washington State rates; no significant excess risk was seen for cancers at other sites. Two departments at the smelter (the cottrell area and the arsenic department) had high (> 0.5 mg/m^3) arsenic levels during 1938–47 but differed in sulfur dioxide concentrations. The levels of sulfur dioxide were reported to be 5–20 ppm (13–52 mg/m^3) in the cottrell area, where dust is eliminated by electrical precipitation, but very low in the arsenic department. For workers who had ever worked in the cottrell area, the SMR was 3.51 [95% CI, 1.75–6.27]; and for those who had ever worked in the arsenic department (and never at the cottrell), the SMR was 3.17 [1.97–4.36], suggesting that sulfur dioxide exposure did not play an important role in the respiratory cancer excess at the smelter.

A third copper smelter in the USA that has been investigated was located in Salt Lake City, Utah (Rencher et al., 1977). An attempt was made to include all deaths among the smelter workers occurring in 1959–69. [No detailed description of the cohort studied was given, and consequently the completeness of follow-up cannot be assessed.] Lung cancer constituted 7.0% of the deaths among the smelter workers compared with 2.7% for the state. A cumulative exposure index was computed for arsenic, sulfur dioxide and some other agents for each deceased worker from work histories and from estimated levels in different work areas. The workers who died of lung cancer had significantly higher indices of exposure to arsenic, lead and sulfur dioxide than workers who died of non-respiratory causes.

A combined analysis was performed on the mortality experience in 1949–80 of a cohort of 6078 white male workers who had been employed for at least three years between 1946 and 1976 at one or more of eight US copper smelters, including the Utah smelter described above (Enterline et al., 1987). Vital status was unknown for 1.6% at the end of follow-up; death certificates could be located for 94.1% of those known to be dead. Workers were assigned into different exposure categories on the basis of estimated levels of arsenic, sulfur dioxide and some other agents by job and year. Smoking histories were obtained through telephone interviews with the study subjects or next-of-kin for 76% of the lung cancer cases and for 85% of a 5% sample of the remaining members of the cohort. The relative risk for lung cancer increased with duration of exposure to sulfur dioxide at peak levels of 12 ppm (32 mg/m^3) and higher (p for trend, 0.03), without adjusting for exposure to arsenic and smoking. Exposure to sulfur dioxide at a level of more than 6 ppm (16 mg/m^3) did not, however, have a significant, independent effect in a logistic regression model that included age, arsenic, smoking and interaction terms.

A series of epidemiological studies was also performed at a smelter in northern Sweden which produces copper and other non-ferrous metals, mainly from arsenic-rich sulfide ores (Pershagen et al., 1977). Although increased rates were reported of cancers at a few sites, only lung cancer has been investigated in relation to sulfur dioxide exposure. A case–control study nested in a cohort of 3958 smelter workers, who had been employed for at least three months in 1928–66 and who were followed through to 1977, included 76 lung cancer cases and 152 age-matched, deceased controls (Pershagen et al., 1981). Assessment of exposure to arsenic and sulfur dioxide was based on estimations of levels in different departments; workers in the roaster department were most heavily exposed to both compounds. Few measurements were made, but, in 1954, sulfur dioxide concentrations of 15–300 mg/m^3 were reported in the departments with the highest levels. Information on smoking was obtained from next-of-kin of all study subjects. The relative risks for lung cancer were 6.5 for smokers in the 'high sulfur dioxide' departments, 14.7 for those in 'high arsenic' departments and 22.0 for workers in roaster departments, compared to nonsmoking workers with lowest exposure, indicating that arsenic is more important than sulfur dioxide in determining excess risk. [The Working Group noted that confidence intervals could not be estimated from the data presented.]

In a follow-up of mortality in the same cohort through 1981, 106 cases of lung cancer were identified; all but 0.4% of the workers were traced (Järup et al., 1989). Cumulative exposures to arsenic and sulfur dioxide were calculated on the basis of the work histories of each worker, and exposure levels during different time periods were estimated. The overall SMR for lung cancer was 3.72 (95% CI, 3.04–4.50). A positive dose–response relationship was found between cumulative exposure to arsenic and lung cancer risk ($p < 0.001$); no dose–response relationship was found for exposure to sulfur dioxide.

Lung cancer mortality was followed through 1982 in a cohort of 4393 men who had been employed for a minimum of one year in 1943–70 at a zinc–lead–cadmium smelter in the United Kingdom (Ades & Kazantzis, 1988). Only 0.7% of the cohort could not be traced; 182 men had died of lung cancer. Exposure to cadmium, zinc, sulfur dioxide, arsenic, lead and dust was assessed from job histories and from estimates of air concentrations in different work places, partly based on measurements and biological monitoring. The overall SMR for lung cancer was 1.25 (95% CI, 1.07–1.44) relative to regional rates. Although there were suggestions of increased relative risks with cumulative exposure for each of the factors under study, only the risks associated with exposures to arsenic and lead reached statistical significance ($p < 0.025$ and $p < 0.01$, respectively). The indices of cumulative exposure to sulfur dioxide, arsenic and lead were highly correlated.

2.2 Pulp and paper manufacture

Cancer risks in the pulp and paper industry have been evaluated previously (IARC, 1981, 1987). Here, only studies that specifically addressed exposures to sulfur dioxide or the sulfite process are addressed.

In a proportionate mortality analysis, the recorded causes of death of 2113 US and Canadian members of the Pulp, Sulfite and Paper Mill Workers' Union who died during 1935–64 were compared with corresponding US mortality rates (Milham & Demers, 1984). The proportionate mortality ratio (PMR) was increased ($p < 0.05$) for cancer of the stomach (PMR, 2.18; 33 deaths) and for lymphosarcoma and reticulum-cell sarcoma (PMR, 2.69; 7 deaths) in sulfite workers, when those who had also worked in the sulfate process were excluded. The PMR for lung cancer was 0.85 (21 deaths; $p > 0.05$).

Mortality in a cohort of 3572 men who had been employed for at least one year between 1945 and 1955 in one or more of five US pulp and paper mills in the states of Washington, Oregon and California was followed until 1977 (Robinson et al., 1986). Death certificates could not be retrieved for 1% of the deceased, and 1% was lost to follow-up. In a subcohort of 1779 sulfite process workers, cancer mortality was less frequent (SMR, 0.79; 90% CI, 0.66–0.95; 88 deaths) in comparison with national rates. For stomach cancer, lung cancer and lymphosarcoma and reticulosarcoma, the SMRs were 1.49 (90% CI, 0.83–2.46; 11 deaths),

0.81 (0.57–1.13; 26 deaths) and 1.33 (0.45–3.05; 4 deaths), respectively. After a 20-year latency, the SMR for stomach cancer was 1.76 [0.81–3.35], based on nine deaths.

Mortality was analysed until 1985 among 883 white men who had participated in a medical survey in 1961 and had worked for at least one year for a paper company in New Hampshire, USA (Henneberger et al., 1989). One percent was lost to follow-up, and 2.5% of the death certificates could not be traced. A total of 36 deaths from cancer were observed among 297 sulfite pulp mill workers, which corresponds to an SMR of 1.20 (95% CI, 0.84–1.66) in relation to national rates. The SMR for lung cancer was 1.13 (0.56–2.02, 11 deaths); one case each occurred of stomach cancer and leukaemia, compared with 1.4 and 1.1 expected, respectively; for cancer of the pancreas, the SMR was 3.05 (0.98–7.12, 5 deaths), and all five cases occurred after a latency of at least 20 years (mean latency, 51 years). The SMR for lung cancer was higher among workers with at least 20 years of latency and at least 20 years of duration of employment (SMR, 1.86 [95% CI, 0.74–3.80], 7 cases).

Cancer incidence was studied through 1980 in a cohort of 3545 workers who had been employed for at least one year in 1945–61 in one of three pulp and paper mills in south-eastern Finland (Jäppinen et al., 1987). Only 0.4% were lost to follow-up. Among the 248 men who had worked in the sulfite mill, there were 33 cases of cancer, corresponding to a standardized incidence ratio of 1.05 (95% CI, 0.72–1.47) compared with regional rates. The ratios were 1.29 (0.47–2.81; 6 cases) for cancer of the stomach and 0.90 (0.41–1.71; 9 cases) for cancer of the lung. One case of leukaemia was observed, with 0.7 expected.

2.3 Other industries

Occupational risk factors for cancers of the brain, kidney and lung were investigated in a series of case–control studies in a region of the USA where a large chemical plant was located (Bond et al., 1983, 1985, 1986). Industrial hygienists established chemical and physical agent-specific exposure profiles for the subjects employed at the plant on the basis of work histories and job functions. The plant produced many products, however, and the exposure environment included sulfur dioxide, chlorine, hydrogen chloride, carbon tetrachloride and heat.

In a study in four Texas counties in 1949–79, 28 former employees of the plant who had died of primary intracranial neoplasms were identified (Bond et al., 1983). One control group was matched on age and year of death and included 110 former employees who had died of causes other than cancer; the other control group consisted of 111 men matched on year and duration of employment, selected from a 5% random sample of people who had ever been employed at the plant. Odds ratios of 2.02 (90% CI, 0.99–4.11) and 1.19 (0.58–2.43) were reported for exposure to sulfur dioxide (11 cases) in relation to the first and second control groups, respectively. When the analysis was restricted to the 16 glioblastomas, an odds ratio of 1.40 (0.6–3.4; 7 cases) was seen in comparison with the second control group. No significant increase in risk was observed in subgroups with more than 20 years of service or first employment before 1945.

In another study, 26 former employees of the plant were identified who had died of renal cancer in 1958–80 in five nearby counties (Bond et al., 1985). Two matched control groups, selected according to the same criteria as in the previous study, comprised 92 and 98 men who had worked at the plant. The odds ratios for exposure to sulfur dioxide (five cases) were

0.31 (90% CI, 0.13–0.73) and 0.31 (0.13–0.76) in relation to the first and second control groups, respectively. The deficit was closely linked to a significantly decreased risk among workers who had been engaged in magnesium production and who were classified as having been exposed to sulfur dioxide.

A case–control study nested in a cohort of 19 608 men who had worked for at least one year between 1940 and 1980 at the same plant covered 308 who had died of lung cancer and an equal number of controls in each of two control groups of dead workers, matched on race, year of birth and year of hire (Bond *et al.*, 1986). Controls in the second group had each survived at least as long as the corresponding case. Information on potential confounding factors, including smoking, was obtained by telephone interviews with the study subjects or next-of-kin. Interviews were completed for 81.9% of 896 subjects—mostly with next-of-kin for cases and for the first control group and with the subjects themselves for the second control group. Workers who had been exposed to sulfur dioxide had an odds ratio of 1.40 (95% CI, 1.04–1.89; 126 cases) when the two control groups were considered together. When allowing for 15 years of latency, the odds ratio was 1.27 (95% CI, 0.93–1.73), based on 108 cases. In a multivariate analysis, with adjustment for cigarette use, vitamin A consumption, hot working conditions and socioeconomic status, the odds ratios for lung cancer were 0.48 (95% CI, 0.15–1.54) for low exposure to sulfur dioxide, 1.69 (0.88–3.22) for moderate exposure and 1.45 (0.67–3.17) for high exposure, as compared to the first control group (p for trend, 0.003). No trend was found in comparison with the second control group (p for trend, 0.32). Similar odds ratios were noted in relation to duration of exposure to heat.

A population-based case–control study carried out in Montréal (Siemiatycki, 1991), described in detail on p. 95, also examined exposure to sulfur dioxide (15% of the population). The only notable finding was an odds ratio of 1.5 for stomach cancer, restricted to the French-Canadian subset of the study population (30 exposed cases; 90% CI, 1.0–2.1), which increased to 3.5 with substantial exposure (4 cases; 90% CI, 1.3–9.2). Corresponding odds ratios for the whole population were 1.3 (90% CI, 0.9–1.7) for any exposure and 2.2 (0.9–5.6) for substantial exposure, based on 42 cases. The odds ratio for lung cancer was 1.0 (138 exposed cases; 90% CI, 0.8–1.3) for any exposure and 0.7 (8 cases; 90% CI, 0.3–1.6) for substantial exposure.

3. Studies of Cancer in Animals

3.1 Inhalation

Mouse: An experimental group of 35 male and 30 female LX mice and a control group of 41 males and 39 females, three months old, were exposed to 0 or 500 ppm [1310 mg/m^3] **sulfur dioxide** [purity unspecified] for 5 min per day on five days a week for life. Only mice that survived for 300 days or more were considered in the results [average survival time not shown], since lung tumours were not seen before that time. Female mice exposed to sulfur dioxide had an increased incidence of lung tumours: 13/30 adenomas and carcinomas *versus* 5/30 in controls, [p = 0.02; Peto's incidental test]; 4/30 lung carcinomas *versus* none in the controls. The incidence of lung neoplasias was higher in treated males (15/28 *versus* 11/35 in controls), but the difference was not significant; lung carcinomas occurred with equal frequency in treated and control males (2/28 and 2/35) (Peacock & Spence, 1967).

3.2 Oral administration

3.2.1 *Mouse*

Three groups of 50 male and 50 female ICR/ICL mice, aged eight weeks at the start of the experiment, were given 0, 1 or 2% **potassium metabisulfite** [purity unspecified] in distilled water as drinking-water *ad libitum* for 104 weeks. At least 94% of the mice in each group survived beyond 26 weeks. The incidences of various types of tumours were similar in the control and experimental groups: total tumour incidences were 14/99, 14/96 and 16/94 in the three groups, respectively (Tanaka *et al.*, 1979). [The Working Group noted that data on survival were incomplete.]

3.2.2 *Rat*

Six groups of 20 male and 20 female weanling Wistar rats were fed 0, 0.125, 0.25, 0.5, 1 or 2% **sodium metabisulfite** (95–99% pure [impurities unspecified]) in the diet for 104 weeks. More than 50% of controls and about 75% of each experimental group survived until the termination of experiment [average survival time unspecified]. Groups of five females and five males of the F_1 generation were fed the same concentrations in the diet for 104 weeks. Data on tumour incidence are given for the F_0 and F_1 generations combined. The incidences of thyroid and pituitary tumours were increased in treated males, but no dose–response relationship was observed. The authors reported that the incidences of these tumours in the concurrent controls were exceptionally low compared to those in historical controls and that the incidences found in treated animals represent the numbers normally found in this strain of rat (Til *et al.*, 1972).

3.3 Administration with known carcinogens

The Working Group was aware of studies in mice and hamsters involving combined administration of a carcinogen and mixtures of sulfur dioxide and nitrogen dioxide (Pott & Stöber, 1983; Heinrich *et al.*, 1989). These were not included in this monograph because the effect of sulfur dioxide alone could not be evaluated.

3.3.1 *Rat*

Six groups of rats [age, sex and strain unspecified] were exposed on five days per week for life to: Group 1, clean air (15 animals); Group 2, 10 ppm [26 mg/m^3] **sulfur dioxide** for 6 h per day (15 animals); Group 3, 10 mg/m^3 benzo[*a*]pyrene for 1 h per day (30 animals); Group 4, 10 ppm sulfur dioxide for 6 h per day plus 10 mg/m^3 benzo[*a*]pyrene for 1 h per day (30 animals); Group 5, 4 ppm [10.5 mg/m^3] sulfur dioxide plus 10 mg/m^3 benzo[*a*]pyrene for 1 h per day (45 animals); and Group 6, 10 ppm sulfur dioxide for 6 h per day followed by 4 ppm sulfur dioxide plus 10 mg/m^3 benzo[*a*]pyrene for 1 h per day (46 animals) [experimental time and survival not specified]. The following incidences of lung carcinomas were observed: Group 1, 0/15; Group 2, 0/15; Group 3, 1/30; Group 4, 2/30; Group 5, 4/45; and Group 6, 9/46 [no statistical analysis reported] (Laskin *et al.*, 1976). [The Working Group noted the incomplete reporting of the experiment, in particular, the lack of data on survival and the lack of clarity concerning hyperplastic changes in both control and treated animals.]

Seven groups of male Sprague-Dawley CD rats, aged nine weeks at the start of the experiment, were exposed by: Group 1, inhalation to clean air (46 animals); Group 2, inhalation to clean air plus intratracheal instillation of gelatin vehicle (0.05%) once weekly in weeks 4–19 (26 animals); Group 3, inhalation to 10 ppm [26 mg/m^3] **sulfur dioxide** for 6 h per day on five days a week for 21 weeks (20 animals); Group 4, inhalation to 30 ppm [79 mg/m^3] sulfur dioxide (20 animals) for 6 h per day on five days a week for 21 weeks; Group 5, inhalation to clean air plus intratracheal instillation of 1 mg benzo[a]pyrene once weekly in weeks 4–19 (74 animals); Group 6, inhalation to 10 ppm sulfur dioxide for 6 h per day on five days per week for 21 weeks plus 1 mg benzo[a]pyrene once weekly in weeks 4–19 (74 animals); and Group 7, inhalation to 30 ppm sulfur dioxide for 6 h per day on five days per week for 21 weeks plus intratracheal instillation of 1 mg benzo[a]pyrene once weekly in weeks 4–19 (74 animals). The experiment was terminated at 105 weeks [mean survival time unspecified]. The three groups treated with benz[a]pyrene had lower survival than other groups and a high incidence of squamous-cell carcinoma of the lung that was not enhanced by inhalation of sulfur dioxide: the incidences of squamous-cell carcinoma in groups 1–7 were 0/43, 0/26, 0/20, 0/18, 65/72, 65/72 and 69/74. Sulfur dioxide did not influence time to appearance of tumours. The authors noted that the high incidence of tumours in the group given benzo[a]pyrene alone precluded detection of a significant enhancing effect of sulfur dioxide on the incidence of benzo[a]pyrene-induced lung tumours (Gunnison *et al.*, 1988).

Groups of male Wistar rats, seven weeks of age, were treated as follows: Group 1 (10 animals) served as untreated controls; Group 2 (30 animals) was given *N*-methyl-*N*'-nitro-*N*-nitrosoguanidine in the drinking-water at 100 mg/l *ad libitum* for eight weeks; Group 3 (10 animals) was given tap water for eight weeks followed by 1% **potassium metabisulfite** in the drinking-water for 32 weeks; Group 4 (19 animals) was treated as Group 2 but was then given 1% potassium metabisulfite in the drinking-water for 32 weeks. All surviving animals were killed at 40 weeks [survival unspecified]. The incidence of adenocarcinoma of the gastric pylorus was 0/10, 1/30, 0/10 and 5/19 ($p < 0.05$, Fisher test) in the four groups, respectively (Takahashi *et al.*, 1986).

3.3.2 *Hamster*

In a study reported as a short communication, four groups of male Syrian golden hamsters [number of animals and age at start unspecified] were exposed for 104 weeks by nose inhalation only to: Group 1, 2 mg/m^3 benzo[a]pyrene; Group 2, 2 mg/m^3 benzo[a]pyrene plus 172 ppm [450 mg/m^3] **sulfur dioxide**; Group 3, 10 mg/m^3 benzo[a]pyrene; Group 4, 10 mg/m^3 benzo[a]pyrene plus 172 ppm sulfur dioxide [dosing schedule unspecified]. The mean survival times were: Group 1, 60 weeks; Group 2, 60 weeks; Group 3, 57 weeks; and Group 4, 45 weeks [no data on controls were given]. The authors stated, without presenting numerical data, that exposure to benzo[a]pyrene alone induced a few neoplastic alterations and that the addition of sulfur dioxide resulted in more tumours in the upper respiratory tract within a shorter time (Pauluhn *et al.*, 1985). [The Working Group noted the inadequate reporting.]

4. Other Relevant Data

4.1 Absorption, distribution, metabolism and excretion

Sulfur dioxide in aqueous solution is rapidly hydrated to sulfurous acid, which itself quickly dissociates to bisulfite and sulfite (Figure 1). The species that dominates among these rapidly interconvertible hydration products depends primarily upon pH but also on ionic strength and temperature (Gunnison & Jacobsen, 1987). At pH close to 7, the ratio of HSO_3^- to SO_2 concentrations is greater than 100 000:1. Therefore, sulfur dioxide is transported through aqueous systems at neutral pH almost totally in its hydrated form. Because of this rapid hydration, the interactions of sulfur dioxide with biological molecules in an aqueous medium are probably those of sulfite and bisulfite. Two alternative reaction pathways have been suggested, however, on the basis of observations *in vitro*: Eickenroht *et al.* (1975) suggested that sulfur dioxide itself acts directly as an electron receptor; Mottley *et al.* (1985) demonstrated anaerobic production of the SO_2 anion radical from sulfite by rat liver microsomes.

Figure 1. Interconversion of oxysulfur[IV] compounds

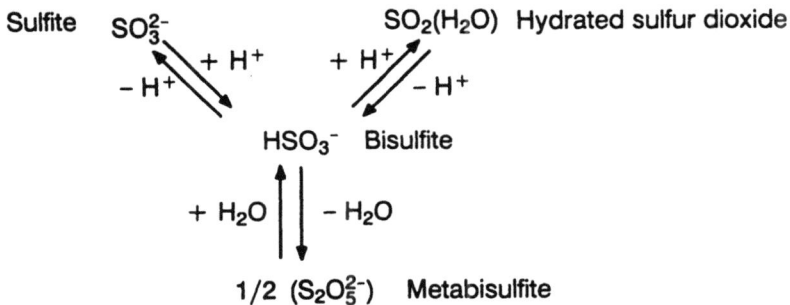

From Fazio & Warner (1990)

Except where specified to the contrary, the term 'sulfite' is used below to indicate the various rapidly interconvertible hydration products of sulfur dioxide.

4.1.1 *Humans*

Sulfur dioxide is a highly water-soluble gas and is thus rapidly absorbed in the moist upper respiratory tract. With quiet breathing through the nose, negligible quantities of sulfur dioxide reach the nasopharynx; deeper airway penetration can occur with oral inhalation, particularly when maximal deep breaths are taken, as in exercise. The fractional penetration increases at higher sulfur dioxide concentrations (Kleinman, 1984). Sulfur dioxide can also penetrate the airways by absorption on inhalable particulates, and especially deliquescent materials.

Plasma levels of S-sulfonates in humans exposed continuously under controlled conditions to sulfur dioxide at 0.3–6.0 ppm [0.8–15.7 mg/m^3] for up to 120 h were correlated positively with atmospheric levels of sulfur dioxide (Gunnison & Palmes, 1974). Human sulfite oxidase may have a protective effect in that it prevents sulfite from reacting with biological molecules by oxidizing it to sulfate (Gunnison & Jacobsen, 1987).

4.1.2 *Experimental systems*

The covalent reactions of sulfur dioxide and sulfite with cellular protein and non-protein sulfhydryl compounds have been reviewed (Menzel *et al.*, 1986). A central reaction is addition across disulfide bonds to form *S*-sulfonates (Gunnison & Benton, 1971). Sulfite can react with DNA (see Section 4.4.2).

Diffusion of sulfur dioxide, its solubility in aqueous solution and its irreversible reaction in tissue all appear to be linear processes in excised porcine trachea (Ben-Jebria *et al.*, 1990).

When dogs inhaled ^{35}S-sulfur dioxide through the nose and mouth, little of the label reached the lower airways; when the labelled sulfur dioxide was inhaled through a tracheostomy, however, it was absorbed rapidly through the lungs and trachea and radiolabel was found in all organs (Balchum *et al.*, 1960). Inhaled ^{35}S-sulfur dioxide was excreted primarily in the urine as sulfate by dogs (Yokoyama *et al.*, 1971).

Once absorbed, sulfur dioxide appears to be metabolized rapidly to sulfate by the widely distributed enzyme sulfite oxidase. After it has been oxidized to sulfate, it becomes part of the large sulfate pool within the body. Tejnorová (1978) reported relatively large differences in sulfite oxidase activity among five species: rats had the highest levels and rabbits the lowest. An inverse correlation was shown between enzyme activity and sensitivity to bisulfite toxicity. These results reflect species differences in rate of *S*-sulfonate formation (Gunnison & Palmes, 1978).

Ingested radiolabelled sulfite was reported to be excreted almost entirely in the urine of monkeys within 24 h, but no free sulfite was detected in rat urine. Seven days after dosing, mice retained < 1% and rats, 2% of the radiolabel (Gibson & Strong, 1973). In rabbits, sulfite was cleared predominantly by metabolism to sulfate (Gunnison & Palmes, 1976).

4.2 Toxic effects

4.2.1 *Humans*

Charan *et al.* (1979) reported acute accidental exposure of five subjects to very high concentrations of sulfur dioxide. The two with the highest exposure died immediately; histological examination of the lungs revealed acute pulmonary oedema and alveolar haemorrhage. Two of the survivors showed airway obstruction, which was irreversible in one and was mild in the other individual 116 days after the exposure. Pulmonary oedema, followed by the development of 'bronchiolitis obliterans', an obstructive, irreversible lung disease, was described in a nonsmoking man who was exposed accidentally to a high concentration of sulfur dioxide for 15–20 min when a canister of this compound ruptured beneath him (Woodford *et al.*, 1979). Two nonsmoking miners exposed to high concentrations of sulfur dioxide after a mine explosion also developed severe airway obstruction (Rabinovitch *et al.*, 1989).

Workplace standards (see Table 10) have been set to prevent local irritation of mucous membranes of the nose, throat and eyes (WHO, 1979).

The prevalence of chronic bronchitis was significantly increased over that in controls in workers exposed to sulfur dioxide while working in a sulfite pulp factory in Sweden. During the three years before the study was performed, more than 50% of the daily mean values for sulfur dioxide in the sulfite pulp mill were above 14 mg/m^3 (5 ppm), with occasional peak exposures up to 140 mg/m^3. The mean annual concentration of sulfur dioxide in the surrounding community was 6.5–40 μg/m^3 (Stjernberg et al., 1986).

In healthy individuals exposed to sulfur dioxide at levels below 1 ppm (2.6 mg/m^3), increased airway resistance is generally not observed; however, when young adult asthmatics were exposed while exercising to sulfur dioxide through a mouthpiece, increased airway resistance was reported with levels as low as 0.25 ppm [0.7 mg/m^3] (Sheppard et al., 1981). The effects were much less with unencumbered breathing (Linn et al., 1983). Bronchoconstriction due to sulfur dioxide appears to be mediated by a parasympathetic reflex reaction (Nadel et al., 1965).

Bronchoalveolar lavage of 12 healthy, nonsmoking subjects 24 h after exposure for 20 min to 4 or 8 ppm [10.5 or 21 mg/m^3] sulfur dioxide showed increased alveolar macrophage lysosomal activity; at the higher level, the numbers of macrophages and lymphocytes in the lavage fluid were increased. No effect on lung function was observed (Sandström et al., 1989a,b).

Many studies have linked sulfur dioxide levels in the general environment to a variety of adverse health consequences, including acute and chronic bronchitis, respiratory tract infections and mortality, particularly among people with pre-existing lung or heart disease. Sulfur dioxide is, however, only one component of gas–aerosol complexes including sulfate particulates of various toxicities (see p. 141). It has been suggested (WHO, 1987) that sulfur dioxide is not the most potent, direct cause of these effects but is a good surrogate for the components responsible for effects, as it is the most easily measured and is the atmospheric precursor of sulfuric acid and acid sulfates.

Ingestion of sulfites has been postulated to be a cause of rapid, acute allergic reactions, including fatal anaphylactic-like responses (Settipane, 1984). A sulfite-sensitive subpopulation of asthmatics has been postulated to exist who have a relative deficiency of sulfite oxidase (Stevenson & Simon, 1984). The possibility that sulfur dioxide may be generated from sulfite in the low pH of the stomach has been considered as a mechanism of sulfite sensitivity (Simon, 1986). Skin reactions have been noted rarely which have been suggested to result from allergy to inhaled sulfur dioxide (Pirilä et al., 1963).

4.2.2 Experimental systems

The extensive work of Amdur (1959, 1974) clearly demonstrated the bronchoconstrictive effects of sulfur dioxide in guinea-pigs. Cessation of tracheal ciliary activity was observed in rabbits that inhaled sulfur dioxide at concentrations above 200 ppm [524 mg/m^3] (Dalhamn & Strandberg, 1961). Only a relatively negligible amount of sulfur dioxide reached the trachea after nose inhalation, as 90–95% had been absorbed in the nasal cavities.

Increased bronchial hyperresponsiveness to acetylcholine has been observed in dogs following exposure to sulfur dioxide at 1 ppm [2.6 mg/m^3] (Islam et al., 1972).

Addition of sodium metabisulfite to the diet of rats at 0.5–8% for 10 days to 2 years induced hyperplastic and inflammatory changes in the forestomach and haemorrhagic microerosions, necrosis of epithelial cells, cellular inflammatory infiltration and atypical glandular hyperplasia in the glandular stomach (Feron & Wensvoort, 1972). Addition of this compound to the diet of groups of 20 male and 20 female rats at doses of 0.125–8% resulted in consumption levels of 0.098–1.91%. The no-effect level was established to be 0.44% over 48 weeks. At higher levels, several animals had mild inflammatory and hyperplastic changes to the gastric mucosa (Til *et al.*, 1972). These findings support the conclusion that dietary potassium metabisulfite promotes the carcinogenic activity of N-methyl-N'-nitro-N-nitrosoguanidine in rat stomach, as reported by Takahashi *et al.* (1986) (see p. 164).

4.3 Reproductive and developmental effects

4.3.1 *Humans*

A variety of environmental exposures involving sulfur dioxide have been related to human reproductive effects (Nordström *et al.*, 1978a,b, 1979a,b; Hemminki & Niemi, 1982; Sakai, 1984; Monteleone-Neto *et al.*, 1985). In none of these papers could a clear relationship be determined between sulfur dioxide concentrations and reproductive outcomes.

4.3.2 *Experimental systems*

(a) Sulfur dioxide

Groups of 10 female albino rats (weighing 165–185 g) were exposed for 12 h per day for three months to 0, 0.159 or 4.97 mg/m^3 sulfur dioxide (Shalamberidze & Tsereteli, 1971). An additional group was exposed to 2.52 mg/m^3 sulfur dioxide in combination with 1.20 mg/m^3 nitrogen dioxide. Oestrous cyclicity was determined for 24 days prior to exposure, during exposure and during a recovery period. Females with a normal oestrous cycle were tested for fertility. The ovaries, uterus and pituitary, thyroid and adrenal glands from four rats per group were examined by histopathology at the end of exposure. It was reported that the higher exposure level prolonged the interoestrual period (dioestrus) and the oestrus and that these females had fewer monthly oestrous cycles. Cycle length returned to normal within seven months after exposure. Circulatory changes were found in the ovaries and uteri of females in the high exposure group. In a second experiment, decreased litter sizes were found in similarly exposed groups of seven females. [The Working Group noted that it is not clear when the females were mated within the exposure period.] Body weights of the offspring were reduced at least through postnatal day 12 in these groups.

Groups of 40 or 32 CF-1 mice were exposed for 7 h per day to filtered air or to sulfur dioxide (purity, 99.98%) at 25 ppm [66 mg/m^3] on days 6–15 of gestation, and groups of 20 New Zealand white rabbits were exposed to filtered air or sulfur dioxide at 70 ppm [183 mg/m^3] on days 6–18 of gestation. In both species, less food was consumed during the first few days of exposure to sulfur dioxide; no other significant effect was seen in the dams. In mice, fetal weight was reduced by 5% by exposure to sulfur dioxide; ossification of the sternebrae and occipital was retarded [data not shown], but the incidence of malformations was not significantly increased. In rabbits, the incidence of a few minor skeletal variants was significantly increased [data not shown] in the group exposed to sulfur dioxide (Murray *et al.*, 1979).

Groups of 13–17 CD-1 mice were exposed to sulfur dioxide at 0, 32, 65, 125 or 250 ppm [0, 84, 170, 328 or 655 mg/m^3] on days 7–17 of gestation [presumably for 24 h]; pregnancy outcome was evaluated on day 18. No dose-related effect was seen on the dams, on fetal viability or on fetal morphology. Fetuses in the 65- and 125-ppm groups were smaller than controls; however, fetuses in the high-dose group weighed more than the controls (Singh, 1982). Additional females [numbers not stated] were exposed to sulfur dioxide at 0, 32 or 65 ppm on days 7–18 [presumably for 24 h] of gestation, and offspring were examined after birth for growth, viability and neurological development. Birth weight was reported to be significantly decreased at 65 ppm. The time required for the righting reflex on postnatal day 1 and negative geotaxic behaviour on postnatal day 10 were significantly increased at both exposure levels (Singh, 1989).

(b) Sulfite

Groups of 10–12 Wistar rats received 0, 0.32, 0.63, 1.25, 2.5 or 5.0% sodium sulfite heptahydrate (guaranteed grade) in the diet on days 8–20 of gestation. The average daily intakes in the exposed groups were 0.3, 1.1, 2.1 and 3.3 g/kg bw. Pregnancy outcome was examined on day 20. An additional four females that received 0.32 or 5.0% sodium sulfite heptahydrate on days 8–20 of gestation were allowed to give birth, and the growth and viability of the neonates was determined. The authors stated that food intake was low in the 0.32, 0.63 and 5.0% groups; maternal body weight gain during pregnancy was reduced in the 5.0% group. Fetal body weights were reduced in all treated groups but there was little evidence of a dose–response relationship. No external, skeletal or visceral malformation was observed in any group; fetal skeletal variations were not significantly affected by treatment. In the few litters examined postnatally, no effect was reported on viability or growth [weight data analysed on an individual basis] (Itami *et al.*, 1989).

An LD_{50} of 1.04 mg/egg was obtained when sodium sulfite was injected into the air cell of 0-h single-comb white Leghorn chickens. No teratogenic effect was observed (Verrett *et al.*, 1980).

(c) Bisulfite

Adult male Swiss mice were exposed by intraperitoneal injection to sodium bisulfite either at up to 1000 mg/kg bw acutely or for up to 40 times 400 mg/kg bw over a 56-day period. Dose-related mortality was observed at more than 700 mg/kg bw, but no effect on testicular histology was noted in survivors (Bhattacharjee *et al.*, 1980).

Pregnancy outcome was evaluated in groups of 14–29 female Wistar rats made deficient (1–2% of control level) in hepatic sulfite oxidase activity. A low-molybdenum diet and drinking-water with a high sodium tungstate level allowed systemic exposure to endogenous sulfite; administration of drinking-water supplemented with 25 or 50 mM sulfite (as sodium metabisulfite) beginning on day 21 of tungsten administration further increased sulfite exposure. Appropriate control groups were included in the design. Breeding began 42 days after initiation of treatment; fetuses were examined on day 21 of gestation. The authors paid particular attention to the induction of anophthalmia, the incidence of which was elevated in litters of sulfite oxidase-deficient rats in a pilot study. Controls given molybdenum gained less weight during pregnancy. The concentration of protein *S*-sulfonate in the aorta (an index of exposure to sulfite) was markedly elevated in the treated groups, but there was no significant effect on embryonic viability, fetal weight or fetal morphology (Dulak *et al.*, 1984).

(d) Metabisulfite

Groups of 13 female and five or six male, newly weaned rats [strain unspecified] received drinking-water containing sodium metabisulfite at doses equivalent to 0, 375 or 750 ppm sulfur dioxide [0, 983 or 1965 mg/m^3]. These animals produced two F$_1$ litters after 11 weeks of treatment; the F$_{1a}$ litters in turn produced an F$_2$ generation. Weights of females in the F$_{1b}$ and F$_2$ generations were lower than those of controls, but no effect was reported on fertility, general health, organ weight or histology (Lockett & Natoff, 1960).

In a multigeneration study, groups of 20 male and 20 female Wistar received diets (enriched with 50 ppm (mg/kg) thiamine and stored at −18 °C prior to feeding) containing 0, 0.125, 0.25, 0.5, 1.0 or 2.0% sodium metabisulfite (purity, 95–99%) beginning at weaning. F$_0$ rats were mated within their treatment group at 21 and 34 weeks. F$_{1a}$ rats were mated to produce F$_{2a}$ and F$_{2b}$ litters at 12 and 30 weeks of age, and F$_{2a}$ rats were mated at weeks 14 and 22 to produce an F$_3$ litter. The authors reported a marginal reduction in body weight gain in F$_1$ and F$_2$ generation rats given 2% metabisulfite. Litter size at birth was reduced only in the F$_{2a}$ generation in groups that had received more than 0.25% metabisulfite (Til *et al.*, 1972).

Groups of 18, 18, 13 and 20 Wistar rats received 0, 0.1, 1 and 10% potassium metabisulfite in the diet on days 7–14 of pregnancy. One-third of the control, low- and high-dose dams were allowed to deliver litters for evaluation of postnatal growth and viability; the remaining 12–13 females were examined for pregnancy outcome on day 20 of gestation. Dam body weight gain and fetal body weights were reduced in the group given 10%, as were neonatal survival and the survival rate of offspring on day 4 after birth. The incidences of several skeletal variations were elevated in the treated groups, but no significant difference was noted (Ema *et al.*, 1985).

A group of 40 male and 40 female Wistar rats, 28–32 days old, were given 1.2 g/l potassium metabisulfite (equivalent to about 700 mg/l of sulfur dioxide) in the drinking-water for about 20 months. A similar, untreated group served as controls. At nine months of age, 22 females from the control and 21 females from the treated group were mated; in the second generation, 23 control and 20 treated females were mated. In both generations, weaned young mice were given the same regimen as their parents. A 20% reduction ($p < 0.05$) in litter size was reported in the first generation of treated rats; a similar but not significant reduction in litter size was reported in the second generation. There were fewer males than females (21%) in the litter of the second generation than in controls (53%) ($p < 0.01$) (Cluzan *et al.*, 1965).

4.4 Genetic and related effects (see also Table 11 and Appendices 1 and 2)

4.4.1 *Humans*

Significant increases in the frequencies of sister chromatid exchange, micronuclei and chromosomal aberrations were observed in cultured lymphocytes from 40 workers exposed in a sulfuric acid factory in Taiyuan City, northern China, as described on p. 102. The workers were exposed to a variety of agents, including sulfur dioxide (Meng & Zhang, 1990a,b).

The frequency of chromosomal aberrations in cultured lymphocytes from seven workers exposed to sulfur dioxide in a sulfite pulp mill in Sweden was compared with that of 15 controls (Nordenson *et al.*, 1980). The exposed subjects had been employed for > 15 years at the mill, and one was a smoker. The controls were healthy men from Umeå, Sweden, five of whom were smokers. The mean numbers of breaks/100 cells were 3.72 ± 1.31 (standard deviation) for the sulfur dioxide-exposed workers and 0.66 ± 0.81 for the controls, analysed on the basis of individual values ($t = 5.79$; $p < 0.001$). The frequency of gaps was also increased in the exposed workers ($p < 0.01$). [The Working Group noted the lack of detail about the control subjects, in particular, about exposure conditions and other exposures.]

The frequencies of chromosomal aberrations and sister chromatid exchange in cultured lymphocytes from eight male workers exposed to sulfur dioxide in a light metal foundry in Scandinavia were compared with those of eight controls (Sorsa *et al.*, 1982). The controls were male clerical workers with an average age of 46.4; five of them were smokers. The exposed subjects were men with an average age of 47.9 and average length of employment of 19.5 years; three of them were smokers. Their average daily exposures to sulfur dioxide were estimated to vary between 0.2 and 3.0 ppm [0.52 and 7.9 mg/m^3], with individual mean time-weighted average exposures of 1.0 ± 0.85 (standard deviation) ppm [2.62 ± 2.23 mg/m^3]. The mean numbers of aberrations per 100 cells, excluding gaps, were 2.0 ± 1.3 in the exposed group and 2.25 ± 1.5 in the control group, and the mean numbers of sister chromatid exchanges per cell were 8.9 ± 0.9 in the exposed and 9.2 ± 1.8 in the control group. Thus, neither the low average level of sulfur dioxide to which the workers were exposed nor smoking had any effect on either parameter.

4.4.2 *Experimental systems*

At high concentrations (1 M), bisulfite deaminates cytosine to uracil in isolated DNA, the reaction rate being optimal between pH 5 and 6. If this reaction occurs in cells, there would be resulting cytosine-to-thymidine transition mutations. Lower concentrations of bisulfite can catalyse transaminations, which lead to protein–nucleic acid cross-linking and DNA damage as a result of bisulfite-generated radicals (Shapiro, 1977).

Bisulfite at very high concentrations induced clear plaque mutations in lambda phage but failed to induce mutations in T4 phage. In *Escherichia coli*, reverse mutations were induced at a number of loci containing cytosine–guanine bases (Mukai *et al.*, 1970); however, no mutation was induced in the *lacI* gene of repair-competent *E. coli*, which may also involve transitions of cytosine–guanine bases (Kunz & Glickman, 1983).

Bisulfite was mutagenic only to those strains of *Salmonella typhimurium* that contain the *his* G46 (base-pair substitution-sensitive) and *his* D6610 (frameshift-sensitive) mutations. These mutations occur preferentially under acidic conditions and at much lower concentrations of bisulfite than those required for addition to cystosine, which leads to deamination.

In *Saccharomyces cerevisiae*, bisulfite did not induce gene conversion, but sulfur dioxide and bisulfite induced mutation.

Sulfur dioxide and sulfite induced chromosomal aberrations in *Tradescantia paludosa* and *Vicia faba* and micronuclei in *T. paludosa*. Bisulfite induced chlorophyll mutations in *Hordeum vulgare*.

Bisulfite treatment did not affect DNA repair synthesis in Syrian hamster embryo (SHE) cells. It did not induce mutations at either the Na$^+$/K$^+$ ATPase or *hprt* locus in cultured Chinese hamster V79 or SHE cells. Sister chromatid exchange was induced in Chinese

Table 11. Genetic and related effects of sulfur dioxide, sodium bisulfite and metabisulfite

Test system	Result[a] Without exogenous metabolic system	Result[a] With exogenous metabolic system	Dose[b] LED/HID	Reference
BPF, Phage lambda, clear plaque mutation	+	0	192000.0000, pH 5.6	Hayatsu & Miura (1970)
BPF, Phage lambda, clear plaque mutation	(+)	0	64000.0000, pH 5	Hayatsu (1977)
BPR, Bacteriophage T4, reverse mutation	–	0	57600.0000, pH 5	Ripley & Drake (1984)
SA0, Salmonella typhimurium TA100, reverse mutation	–	0	64000.0000, pH 5.9	Münzner (1980)
SA0, Salmonella typhimurium TA100, reverse mutation	–	0	6400.0000	Pagano & Zeiger (1987)
SA5, Salmonella typhimurium TA1535, reverse mutation	–	0	64000.0000, pH 5.9	Münzner (1980)
SA5, Salmonella typhimurium TA1535, reverse mutation	–	0	12800.0000	Pagano & Zeiger (1987)
SA8, Salmonella typhimurium TA1538, reverse mutation	–	0	64000.0000, pH 5.9	Münzner (1980)
SA9, Salmonella typhimurium TA98, reverse mutation	–	0	64000.0000, pH 5.9	Münzner (1980)
SAS, Salmonella typhimurium G46, reverse mutation	+	0	64000.0000, pH 5.9	Münzner (1980)
SAS, Salmonella typhimurium G46, reverse mutation	+	0	32000.0000, pH 5.2	De Giovanni-Donnelly (1985)
SAS, Salmonella typhimurium G46, reverse mutation	(+)	0	5120.0000	Pagano & Zeiger (1987)
SAS, Salmonella typhimurium TA92, reverse mutation (G46)	+	0	64000.0000, pH 5.2	De Giovanni-Donnelly (1985)
SAS, Salmonella typhimurium TA92, reverse mutation (G46)	(+)	0	6400.0000	Pagano & Zeiger (1987)
SAS, Salmonella typhimurium TA1950, reverse mutation	+	0	64000.0000, pH 5.2	De Giovanni-Donnelly (1985)
SAS, Salmonella typhimurium TA2410, reverse mutation	+	0	64000.0000, pH 5.2	De Giovanni-Donnelly (1985)
SAS, Salmonella typhimurium TS24, reverse mutation	+	0	64000.0000, pH 5.2	De Giovanni-Donnelly (1985)
SAS, Salmonella typhimurium GW19, reverse mutation	+	0	64000.0000, pH 5.2	De Giovanni-Donnelly (1985)
SAS, Salmonella typhimurium SB2802, reverse mutation (G46)	+	0	2560.0000	Pagano & Zeiger (1987)
SAS, Salmonella typhimurium TR3243, reverse mutation (D6610)	+	0	6400.0000	Pagano & Zeiger (1987)
SAS, Salmonella typhimurium TA88, reverse mutation (D6610)	(+)	0	3840.0000	Pagano & Zeiger (1987)
SAS, Salmonella typhimurium TA110, reverse mutation (D6610)	(+)	0	2560.0000	Pagano & Zeiger (1987)
SAS, Salmonella typhimurium TA90, reverse mutation (D6610)	–	0	6400.0000	Pagano & Zeiger (1987)
SAS, Salmonella typhimurium TA97, reverse mutation (D6610)	+	0	640.0000, pH 5	Pagano & Zeiger (1987)
SAS, Salmonella typhimurium D3052, reverse mutation	–	0	38400.0000, pH 5	Pagano & Zeiger (1987)

Table 11 (contd)

Test system	Result[a]		Dose[b] LED/HID	Reference
	Without exogenous metabolic system	With exogenous metabolic system		
SAS, *Salmonella typhimurium* C3076, reverse mutation	–	0	19200.0000, pH 5	Pagano & Zeiger (1987)
SAS, *Salmonella typhimurium* TA97, reverse mutation	–	0	5120.0000, pH 7.0	Pagano et al. (1990)
SAS, *Salmonella typhimurium* TA97, reverse mutation	+	0	5120.0000, pH 5.0	Pagano et al. (1990)
ECK, *Escherichia coli* K12 (4 strains), reverse mutations (TA target)	–	0	64000.0000, pH 5.2	Mukai et al. (1970)
ECW, *Escherichia coli* WP2 uvrA, reverse mutation, *trp* locus	–	0	64000.0000	Mallon & Rossman (1981)
EC2, *Escherichia coli* WP2, reverse mutation, *trp* locus	–	0	64000.0000	Mallon & Rossman (1981)
EC2, *Escherichia coli* WP2 polA, reverse mutation, *trp* locus	–	0	64000.0000	Mallon & Rossman (1981)
EC2, *Escherichia coli* WP2 lexA, reverse mutation, *trp* locus	–	0	64000.0000	Mallon & Rossman (1981)
EC2, *Escherichia coli* WP2 recA, reverse mutation, *trp* locus	–	0	64000.0000	Mallon & Rossman (1981)
ECR, *Escherichia coli* K15 (9 strains) (TA or deletion targets)	–	0	64000.0000, pH 5.2	Mukai et al. (1970)
ECR, *Escherichia coli* K15 (13 strains) (CG targets)	+	0	64000.0000, pH 5.2	Mukai et al. (1970)
ECR, *Escherichia coli* LacI, reverse mutation	–	0	64000.0000, pH 5.2	Kunz & Glickman (1983)
SCG, *Saccharomyces cerevisiae* BZ34, gene conversion	–	0	6400.0000	Murthy et al. (1983)
SCR, *Saccharomyces cerevisiae*, reverse mutation, *ad* locus	+	0	128.0000, pH 3.6	Dorange & Dupuy (1972)
SCR, *Saccharomyces cerevisiae*, petite mutations, strains 626 & 5215	+	0	60.0000, pH 3	Guerra et al. (1981)
HSM, *Hordeum vulgare*, chlorophyll mutations	+	0	450.0000	Kak & Kaul (1979)
TSI, *Tradescantia paludosa*, micronuclei	+	0	1.0000, 2–6 h	Ma et al. (1984)
TSC, *Tradescantia paludosa*, chromosomal aberrations	+	0	0.0002	Ma et al. (1973)
VFC, *Vicia faba*, chromosomal aberrations	+	0	60.0000	Njagi & Gopalan (1982)
RIA, DNA repair synthesis, Syrian hamster embryo cells	–	0	3200.0000, pH 7	Doniger et al. (1982)
G9H, Gene mutation, Chinese hamster V79 cells, *hprt* locus	–	0	640.0000	Mallon & Rossman (1981)
GIA, Gene mutation, Chinese hamster V79 cells, Na$^+$/K$^+$ ATPase locus	–	0	1280.0000	Mallon & Rossman (1981)
GIA, Gene mutation, Syrian hamster embryo cells, *hprt* locus	–	0	1300.0000	Tsutsui & Barrett (1990)
GIA, Gene mutation, Syrian hamster embryo cells, Na$^+$/K$^+$ ATPase locus	–	0	1300.0000	Tsutsui & Barrett (1990)
SIC, Sister chromatid exchange, Chinese hamster ovary cells	+	0	6.0000	MacRae & Stich (1979)
SIS, Sister chromatid exchange, Syrian hamster embryo cells	+	0	30.0000	Tsutsui & Barrett (1990)
CIS, Chromosomal aberrations, Syrian hamster embryo cells	–	0	325.0000	Tsutsui & Barrett (1990)
TCS, Cell transformation, Syrian hamster embryo cells, focus assay	+	0	325.0000	DiPaolo et al. (1981)

Table 11 (contd)

Test system	Result[a]		Dose[b] LED/HID	Reference
	Without exogenous metabolic system	With exogenous metabolic system		
TCS, Cell transformation, Syrian hamster embryo cells, focus assay (confirmation by s.c. injection into *nu/nu* mice)	+	0	1280.0000	Wirth *et al.* (1986)
TCS, Cell transformation, Syrian hamster embryo cells, focus assay	+	0	30.0000	Tsutsui & Barrett (1990)
SHL, Sister chromatid exchange, human lymphocytes *in vitro*	+	0	25.0000	Beckman & Nordenson (1986)
CHL, Chromosomal aberrations, human lymphocytes *in vitro*	+	0	25.0000	Beckman & Nordenson (1986)
SVA, Sister chromatid exchange, NMRI mouse bone marrow *in vivo*	−	0	660.0000, × 1 oral	Renner & Wever (1983)
SVA, Sister chromatid exchange, NMRI mouse bone marrow *in vivo*	−	0	50.0000, × 12 s.c., over 3.7 h	Renner & Wever (1983)
SVA, Sister chromatid exchange, sulfite oxidase-deficient NMRI mouse bone marrow *in vivo*	−	0	165.0000, × 1 oral	Renner & Wever (1983)
SVA, Sister chromatid exchange, sulfite oxidase-deficient NMRI mouse bone marrow *in vivo*	−	0	50.0000, × 8 s.c., over 2.3 h	Renner & Wever (1983)
SVA, Sister chromatid exchange, Chinese hamster bone marrow *in vivo*	−	0	660.0000, × 1 oral	Renner & Wever (1983)
SVA, Sister chromatid exchange, Chinese hamster bone marrow *in vivo*	−	0	50.0000, × 12 s.c., over 3.7 h	Renner & Wever (1983)
SVA, Sister chromatid exchange, sulfite oxidase-deficient Chinese hamster bone marrow *in vivo*	−	0	330.0000, × 1 oral	Renner & Wever (1983)
SVA, Sister chromatid exchange, sulfite oxidase-deficient Chinese hamster bone marrow *in vivo*	−	0	50.0000, × 8 s.c., over 2.3 h	Renner & Wever (1983)
MVM, Micronuclei, NMRI mouse bone marrow *in vivo*	−	0	660.0000, × 2 oral	Renner & Wever (1983)
MVM, Micronuclei, sulfite oxidase-deficient NMRI mouse bone marrow	−	0	165.0000, × 2 oral	Renner & Wever (1983)
MVC, Micronuclei, Chinese hamster bone marrow *in vivo*	−	0	660.0000, × 2 oral	Renner & Wever (1983)
MVC, Micronucleus, sulfite oxidase-deficient Chinese hamster bone marrow *in vivo*	−	0	330.0000, × 2 oral	Renner & Wever (1983)
CBA, Chromosomal aberrations, NMRI mouse bone marrow *in vivo*	−	0	660.0000, × 2 oral	Renner & Wever (1983)

Table 11 (contd)

Test system	Result[a]		Dose[b] LED/HID	Reference
	Without exogenous metabolic system	With exogenous metabolic system		
CBA, Chromosomal aberrations, sulfite oxidase-deficient NMRI mouse bone marrow *in vivo*	–	0	165.0000, × 2 oral	Renner & Wever (1983)
CBA, Chromosomal aberrations, Chinese hamster bone marrow *in vivo*	–	0	660.0000, × 2 oral	Renner & Wever (1983)
CBA, Chromosomal aberrations, sulfite oxidase-deficient Chinese hamster bone marrow *in vivo*	–	0	330.0000, × 2 oral	Renner & Wever (1983)

[a] +, positive; (+), weakly positive; –, negative; 0, not tested; ?, inconclusive (variable response in several experiments within an adequate study)
[b] In-vitro tests, μg/ml; in-vivo tests, mg/kg bw, standardized to sulfur dioxide

hamster ovary and SHE cells, but chromosomal aberrations were not induced in SHE cells. Sulfur dioxide induced morphological transformation of SHE cells, but there was no synergism with ultra-violet light in the transformation process (DiPaolo *et al.*, 1981), such as was observed in V79 cells (Mallon & Rossman, 1981). Transformation occurred under conditions in which no change to DNA was observed, but consistent, qualitative polypeptide changes and quantitative changes were detected in these cells (Wirth *et al.*, 1986). In a single study, sulfur dioxide induced sister chromatid exchange and chromosomal aberrations in human lymphocytes *in vitro*.

After oral or parenteral administration, sodium metabisulfite did not induce bone-marrow cytogenetic damage in either hamsters or mice.

5. Summary of Data Reported and Evaluation

5.1 Exposure data

Sulfur dioxide is produced commercially by burning sulfur or various sulfides or by recovering it from flue gases or non-ferrous metal smelting gases. Large quantities are used as intermediates in the manufacture of sulfuric acid and sulfite pulp. It is also used in agriculture and in the food and beverage industries as, among other things, a biocide and a preservative. Sulfite pulp workers have been exposed to fluctuating levels of sulfur dioxide, often exceeding 10 ppm (26 mg/m^3), but levels have decreased with modernization of facilities and processes. In metal industries, the roasting of ores and the combustion of various sulfur-containing fuels have resulted in mean exposures to sulfur dioxide in the range of 1–10 ppm (2.6–26 mg/m^3) in copper smelters, but at about 1 ppm (2.6 mg/m^3) or less in other facilities. Mean levels exceeding 1 ppm (2.6 mg/m^3) have also been reported in the manufacture of sulfuric acid and of superphosphate fertilizers, as well as at certain fire sites during fire fighting. Levels of sulfur dioxide in ambient air do not usually exceed 0.05 ppm (0.1 mg/m^3), except in some urban areas.

Sodium sulfite is used mainly in the pulp industry. Both sodium and potassium metabisulfure are used in food processing, chemical industries, water treatment, photoprocessing and the textile industry. Levels of occupational exposure have not been reported.

5.2 Human carcinogenicity data

In four US and one Swedish cohort studies of copper smelters, increased lung cancer risks were observed in relation to exposure to arsenic, but no independent effect of sulfur dioxide was seen.

One proportionate mortality study from the USA and Canada, as well as two US and one Finnish cohort studies, analysed cancer risks among sulfite pulp mill workers. Three of them suggested an increase in risk for stomach cancer; however, potential confounding factors were not adequately controlled. Lung cancer risks were not elevated in any of these studies.

In case–control studies performed at a chemical facility in Texas with a complex exposure environment, increased risks for lung cancer and brain tumours were indicated in workers with high exposure to sulfur dioxide; however, the findings using two different control groups were not consistent.

A population-based case–control study from Canada suggested an increased risk for stomach cancer in men exposed to sulfur dioxide, but no excess was indicated for lung cancer.

No epidemiological studiy was available on cancer risks associated with exposure to sulfites, bisulfites or metabisulfites.

5.3 Carcinogenicity in experimental animals

Sulfur dioxide was tested for carcinogenicity in one study in mice by inhalation exposure. A significant increase in the incidence of lung tumours was observed in females.

Sulfur dioxide was tested for enhancement of carcinogenicity when administered with benzo[*a*]pyrene in two studies in rats and in one study in hamsters. One incompletely reported study found an increase in the incidence of lung tumours in rats exposed to sulfur dioxide in conjunction with benzo[*a*]pyrene. The other study in rats suffered from limitations owing to the high incidence of lung tumours in controls given benzo[*a*]pyrene. The study in hamsters was inadequately reported.

Potassium metabisulfite was tested for carcinogenicity in one study in mice by oral administration in the drinking-water and *sodium metabisulfite* in one study in rats by oral administration in the diet. No increase in tumour incidence was observed in mice, and there was no indication of a dose-related increase in tumour incidence in rats, but both studies had some inadequacies in reporting of data.

Potassium metabisulfite was tested for enhancement of carcinogenicity in one study in rats. It significantly increased the incidence of gastric adenocarcinoma after initiation with *N*-methyl-*N'*-nitro-*N*-nitrosoguanidine.

No data were available on the carcinogenicity in experimental animals of sulfites or bisulfites.

5.4 Other relevant data

At high concentrations, sulfur dioxide irritates the upper airways and can induce acute and chronic bronchitis. At lower levels (less than 0.25 ppm [0.65 mg/m^3]), no effect of sulfur dioxide is seen on the airways of sensitive individuals in the general population who take exercise, presumably since this relatively hygroscopic gas is removed by the nose and mouth.

Conflicting results for the induction of chromosomal aberrations in lymphocytes were obtained in two studies of workers exposed to sulfur dioxide, among other agents. In a single study, no increase was reported in the frequency of sister chromatid exchange in lymphocytes of exposed workers.

Sulfur dioxide and its aqueous forms did not induce sister chromatid exchange, chromosomal aberrations or micronucleus formation in bone marrow of mice or Chinese hamsters. In a single study, sister chromatid exchange and chromosomal aberrations were induced in human lymphocytes. In cultured mammalian cells, bisulfite induced transformation and sister chromatid exchange but not gene mutation, chromosomal aberrations or DNA repair synthesis. In plants, chromosomal aberrations, micronuclei and gene mutation were induced. Sulfur dioxide and bisulfite induced gene mutation but not gene conversion in yeast. Mutations were induced in bacteria and phage.

Bisulfite solutions at high concentrations caused deamination of cytosine in DNA *in vitro*.

5.5 Evaluation[1]

There is *inadequate evidence* for the carcinogenicity in humans of sulfur dioxide, sulfites, bisulfites and metabisulfites.

There is *limited evidence* for the carcinogenicity in experimental animals of sulfur dioxide.

There is *inadequate evidence* for the carcinogenicity in experimental animals of sulfites, bisulfites and metabisulfites.

Overall evaluation

Sulfur dioxide, sulfites, bisulfites and metabisulfites *are not classifiable as to their carcinogenicity to humans (Group 3)*.

6. References

Adams, D.F., Appel, B.R., Dasgupta, P.K., Farwell, S.O., Knapp, K.T., Kok, G.L., Pierson, W.R., Reiszner, K.D. & Tanner, R.L. (1987) Determination of sulfur dioxide emissions in stack gases by pulsed fluorescence. In: Lodge, J.P., Jr, ed., *Methods of Air Sampling and Analysis*, 3rd. ed., Chelsea, MI, Lewis Publishers, pp. 533-537

Ades, A.E. & Kazantzis, G. (1988) Lung cancer in a non-ferrous smelter: the role of cadmium. *Br. J. ind. Med.*, **45**, 435-442

Allen, D.H. (1985) Asthma induced by sulphites. *Food Technol. Aust.*, **37**, 506-507

Amdur, M.O. (1959) The physiological response of guinea pigs to atmospheric pollutants. *Int. J. Air Pollut.*, **1**, 170-183

Amdur, M.O. (1974) 1974 Cummings Memorial Lecture. The long road from Donora. *Am. ind. Hyg. Assoc. J.*, **35**, 589-597

Amer, S.M., Mikhael, E. & El-Ashry, Z.M. (1989) Cytogenetic effect of sulphur dioxide on *Vicia faba* plant I. *Cytologia*, **54**, 211-221

American Conference of Governmental Industrial Hygienists (1990) *1990-1991 Threshold Limit Values for Chemical Substances and Physical Agents and Biological Exposure Indices*, Cincinnati, OH, p. 34

Anderson, A. (1950) Possible long term effects of exposure to sulphur dioxide. *Br. J. ind. Med.*, **7**, 82-86

Aneja, P.V., Aneja, A.P. & Adams, D.F. (1982) Biogenic sulfur compounds and the global sulfur cycle. *J. Air Pollut. Control Assoc.*, **32**, 803-807

Anlauf, K.G., Bottenheim, J.W., Brice, K.A., Fellin, P., Wiebe, H.A., Schiff, H.I., Mackay, G.I., Braman, R.S. & Gilbert, R. (1985) Measurement of atmospheric aerosols and photochemical products at a rural site in SW Ontario. *Atmos. Environ.*, **19**, 1859-1870

Anon. (1988) Chemical profile: sulfur dioxide. *Chem. Mark. Rep.*, **234**, 54

Anon. (1990) Chemical profile: sodium sulfite. *Chem. Mark. Rep.*, **237**, 46

Anon. (1991) Chemical profile: sulfur dioxide. *Chem. Mark. Rep.*, **240**, 42

Arbeidsinspectie (Labour Inspection) (1986) *De Nationale MAC-Lijst 1986* (National MAC-List 1986), Voorburg, Netherlands, p. 23

---

[1]For definition of the italicized terms, see Preamble, pp. 26-29.

Balchum, O.J., Dybicki, J. & Meneely, G.R. (1960) Pulmonary resistance and compliance with concurrent radioactive sulfur distribution in dogs breathing $^{35}SO_2$. *J. appl. Physiol.*, **15**, 62–66

Barrie, L.A. (1988) Aspects of atmospheric pollutant origin and deposition revealed by multi-elemental observations at a rural location in eastern Canada. *J. geophys. Res.*, **93**, 3773–3788

Beckman, L. & Nordenson, I. (1986) Interaction between some common genotoxic agents. *Hum. Hered.*, **36**, 397–401

Ben-Jebria, A., Full, A.P., DeMaria, D.D., Ball, B.A. & Ultman, J.S. (1990) Dynamics of sulfur dioxide absorption in excised porcine tracheae. *Environ. Res.*, **53**, 119–134

Bhattacharjee, D., Shetty, T.K. & Sundaram, K. (1980) Effects on the spermatogonia of mice following treatment with sodium bisulfite. *J. environ. Pathol. Toxicol.*, **3**, 189–193

Bond, G.G., Cook, R.R., Wight, P.C. & Flores, G.H. (1983) A case–control study of brain tumor mortality at a Texas chemical plant. *J. occup. Med.*, **25**, 377–386

Bond, G.G., Shellenberger, R.J., Flores, G.H., Cook, R.R. & Fishbeck, W.A. (1985) A case–control study of renal cancer mortality at a Texas chemical plant. *Am. J. ind. Med.*, **7**, 123–139

Bond, G.G., Flores, G.H., Shellenberger, R.J., Cartmill, J.B., Fishbeck, W.A. & Cook, R.R. (1986) Nested case–control study of lung cancer among chemical workers. *Am. J. Epidemiol.*, **124**, 53–66

Brandt-Rauf, P.W., Fallon, L.F., Jr, Tarantini, T., Idema, C. & Andrews, L. (1988) Health hazards of fire fighters: exposure assessment. *Br. J. ind. Med.*, **45**, 606–612

Broder, I., Smith, J.W., Corey, P. & Holness, L. (1989) Health status and sulfur dioxide exposure of nickel smelter workers and civic laborers. *J. occup. Med.*, **31**, 347–353

Budavari, S., ed. (1989) *The Merck Index*, 11th ed., Rahway, NJ, Merck & Co., p. 1417

Calabrian Corp. (1990a) *Product Data Sheet: Technical Grade Sodium Bisulfite, Anhydrous (Sodium Metabisulfite)*, Houston, TX

Calabrian Corp. (1990b) *Product Data Sheet: Food Grade Sodium Bisulfite, Anhydrous (Sodium Metabisulfite)*, Houston, TX

Calabrian Corp. (undated) *Product Data Sheet: Sodium Bisulfite, Liquid*, Houston, TX

Chan-Yeung, M., Wong, R., MacLean, L., Tan, F., Schulzer, M., Enarson, D., Martin, A., Dennis, R. & Grzybowski, S. (1983) Epidemiologic health study of workers in an aluminum smelter in British Columbia. Effects on the respiratory system. *Am. Rev. respir. Dis.*, **127**, 465–469

Charan, N.B., Myers, C.G., Lakshminarayan, S. & Spencer, T.M. (1979) Pulmonary injuries associated with acute sulfur dioxide inhalation. *Am. Rev. respir. Dis.*, **119**, 555–560

Chemical Information Services (1988) *Directory of World Chemical Producers 1989/90 Edition*, Oceanside, NY

Cluzan, R., Causeret, J. & Hugot, D. (1965) Potassium metabisulfite. Long-term toxicity in the rat (Fr.). *Ann. Biol. Anim. Biochem. Biophys.*, **5**, 267–281

Coker, L.E. (1986) Uses and analysis of sulfites in the corn wet milling industry. *J. Assoc. off. anal. Chem.*, **69**, 8–10

Commission of the European Communities (1980) Council Directive of 15 July 1980 on air quality limit values and guide values for sulphur dioxide and suspended particulates. *Off. J. Eur. Commun.*, **L229**, 30–48

Cook, W.A. (1987) *Occupational Exposure Limits—Worldwide*, Akron, OH, American Industrial Hygiene Association, pp. 125, 153, 216

Dalhamn, T. & Strandberg, L. (1961) Acute effect of sulphur dioxide on the rate of ciliary beat in the trachea of rabbit, *in vivo* and *in vitro*, with studies on the absorptional capacity of the nasal cavity. *Int. J. Air Water Pollut.*, **4**, 154–167

De Giovanni-Donnelly, R. (1985) The mutagenicity of sodium bisulfite on base-substitution strains of *Salmonella typhimurium. Teratog. Carcinog. Mutag.*, 5, 195–203

DiPaolo, J.A., DeMarinis, A.J. & Doniger, J. (1981) Transformation of Syrian hamster embryo cells by sodium bisulfite. *Cancer Lett.*, 12, 203–208

Direktoratet for Arbeidstilsynet (Directorate of Labour Inspection) (1990) *Administrative Normer for Forurensning i Arbeidsatmosfaere 1990* [Administrative Norms for Pollution in Work Atmosphere 1990], Oslo, p. 18

Doniger, J., O'Neill, R. & DiPaolo, J.A. (1982) Neoplastic transformation of Syrian hamster embryo cells by bisulfite is accompanied with a decrease in the number of functioning replicons. *Carcinogenesis*, 3, 27–32

Dorange, J.-L. & Dupuy, P. (1972) Demonstration of a mutagenic action of sodium sulfite on yeast (Fr.). *C.R. Acad. Sci. Paris*, 274, 2798–2800

Dulak, L., Chiang, G. & Gunnison, A.F. (1984) A sulphite oxidase-deficient rat model: reproductive toxicology of sulphite in the female. *Food Chem. Toxicol.*, 22, 599–607

Eickenroht, E.Y., Gause, E.M. & Rowlands, J.R. (1975) The interaction of SO_2 with proteins. *Environ. Lett.*, 9, 265–277

Eller, P.M., ed. (1987) *NIOSH Manual of Analytical Methods*, 3rd ed., Suppl. 2, (DHHS (NIOSH) Publ. No. 84-100), Washington DC, US Government Printing Office, pp. 6004-1–6004-5

Ema, M., Itami, T. & Kanoh, S. (1985) Effect of potassium metabisulfite on pregnant rats and their offspring. *J. Food Hyg. Soc. Japan*, 26, 454–459

Emerson, J.G. & Johnson, J.L. (1985) Adverse reactions to sulphites. An overview. *Food Technol. Aust.*, 37 (Suppl.), i–iv

Englander, V., Sjöberg, A., Hagmar, L., Attewell, R., Schütz, A., Möller, T. & Skerfving, S. (1988) Mortality and cancer morbidity in workers exposed to sulphur dioxide in a sulphuric acid plant. *Int. Arch. occup. environ. Health*, 61, 157–162

Enterline, P.E. & Marsh, G.M. (1982) Cancer among workers exposed to arsenic and other substances in a copper smelter. *Am. J. Epidemiol.*, 116, 895–911

Enterline, P.E., Marsh, G.M., Esmen, N.A., Henderson, V.L., Callahan, C.M. & Paik, M. (1987) Some effects of cigarette smoking, arsenic and SO_2 on mortality among US copper smelter workers. *J. occup. Med.*, 29, 831–838

Fazio, T. & Warner, C.P. (1990) A review of sulphites in food: analytical methodology and reported findings. *Food Add. Contam.*, 7, 433–454

Feiner, B. & Marlow, S. (1956) Sulfur dioxide exposure and control. *Paper Ind.*, 38, 37–40

Feron, V.J. & Wensvoort, P. (1972) Gastric lesions in rats after the feeding of sulphite. *Pathol. Eur.*, 7, 103–111

Ferris, B.G., Jr, Burgess, W.A. & Worcester, J. (1967) Prevalence of chronic respiratory disease in a pulp mill and a paper mill in the United States. *Br. J. ind. Med.*, 24, 26–37

FIOH (Finnish Institute of Occupational Health) (1990) *Industrial Hygiene Measurements, 1950–69*, Data Base, Helsinki

Gautam, S.S., Venkatanarayanan, A.V. & Parthasarathy, B. (1979) Occupational environment of paper mill workers in south India. *Ann. occup. Hyg.*, 22, 371–382

General Chemical Corp. (undated a) *Technical Data: Catalyzed Sodium Sulfite, Anhydrous*, Parsippany, NJ

General Chemical Corp. (undated b) *Technical Data: Sodium Sulfite, Anhydrous, Reagent A.C.S.*, Parsippany, NJ

General Chemical Corp. (undated c) *Technical Data: Sodium Metabisulfite*, Parsippany, NJ

General Chemical Corp. (undated d) *Product Data: Met-tech(TM) Industrial Grade, Sodium Metabisulfite*, Parsippany, NJ

Gibson, W.B. & Strong, F.M. (1973) Metabolism and elimination of sulphite by rats, mice and monkeys. *Food Cosmet. Toxicol.*, 11, 185–198

Guerra, D., Romano, P. & Zambonelli, C. (1981) Mutagenic effects of sulfur dioxide on *Saccharomyces cerevisiae* diploid strains. *Experientia*, 37, 691–693

Gunnison, A.F. & Benton, A.W. (1971) Sulfur dioxide: sulfite. Interaction with mammalian serum and plasma. *Arch. environ. Health*, 22, 381–388

Gunnison, A.F. & Benton, A.W. (1972) Sulfur dioxide: sulfite. Interaction with mammalian serum and plasma. *Arch. environ. Health*, 22, 381–388

Gunnison, A.F. & Jacobsen, D.W. (1987) Sulfite hypersensitivity. A critical review. *CRC crit. Rev. Toxicol.*, 17, 185–214

Gunnison, A.F. & Palmes, E.D. (1974) S-Sulfonates in human plasma following inhalation of sulfur dioxide. *Am. ind. Hyg. Assoc. J.*, 35, 288–291

Gunnison, A.F. & Palmes, E.D. (1976) A model for the metabolism of sulfite in mammals. *Toxicol. appl. Pharmacol.*, 38, 111–126

Gunnison, A.F. & Palmes, E.D. (1978) Species variability in plasma S-sulfonate levels during and following sulfite administration. *Chem.-biol. Interactions*, 21, 315–329

Gunnison, A.F., Sellakumar, A., Snyder, E.A. & Currie, D. (1988) The effect of inhaled sulfur dioxide and systemic sulfite on the induction of lung carcinoma in rats by benzo(a)pyrene. *Environ. Res.*, 46, 59–73

Harrison, R.M. (1983) Ambient air quality in the vicinity of a works manufacturing sulphuric acid, phosphoric acid and sodium tripolyphosphate. *Sci. total Environ.*, 27, 121–131

Harrison, R.M. (1990) Chemistry of the troposphere. In: Harrison, R.M., ed., *Pollution: Causes, Effects, and Control*, 2nd ed., Boca Raton, FL, CRC Press, pp. 157–180

Hastie, D.R., Schiff, H.I., Whelpdale, D.M., Peterson, R.E., Zoller, W.H. & Anderson, D.L. (1988) Nitrogen and sulphur over the western Atlantic Ocean. *Atmos. Environ.*, 22, 2381–2391

Hayatsu, H. (1977) Co-operative mutagenic actions of bisulfite and nitrogen nucleophiles. *J. mol. Biol.*, 115, 19–31

Hayatsu, H. & Miura, A. (1970) The mutagenic action of sodium bisulfite. *Biochem. biophys. Res. Commun.*, 39, 156–160

Heinrich, U., Fuhst, R., Peters, L., Muhle, H., Dasenbrock, C. & Pott, F. (1989) Comparative long-term animal inhalation studies using various particulate matter: objectives, experimental design and preliminary results. *Exp. Pathol.*, 37, 27–31

Helrich, K. (1990) *Official Methods of Analysis of the Association of Official Analytical Chemists*, 15th ed., Vol. 2, Arlington, VA, Association of Official Analytical Chemists, p. 718

Hemminki, K. & Niemi, M.-L. (1982) Community study of spontaneous abortions: relation to occupation and air pollution by sulfur dioxide, hydrogen sulfide and carbon disulfide. *Int. Arch. occup. environ. Health*, 51, 55–63

Henneberger, P.K., Ferris, B.G., Jr & Monson, R.R. (1989) Mortality among pulp and paper workers in Berlin, New Hampshire. *Br. J. ind. Med.*, 46, 658–664

Hoff, R.M., Leaitch, W.R., Fellin, P. & Barrie, L.A. (1983) Mass size distributions of chemical constituents of the winter Arctic aerosol. *J. geophys. Res.*, 88, 10947–10956

IARC (1975) *IARC Monographs on the Evaluation of Carcinogenic Risk of Chemicals to Man*, Vol. 9, *Some Aziridines, N-, S- & O- Mustards and Selenium*, Lyon, pp. 245–260

IARC (1981) *IARC Monographs on the Evaluation of the Carcinogenic Risk of Chemicals to Humans*, Vol. 25, *Wood, Leather and Some Associated Industries*, Lyon, pp. 183, 191–197, 217, 219

IARC (1983) *IARC Monographs on the Evaluation of the Carcinogenic Risk of Chemicals to Humans*, Vol. 32, *Polynuclear Aromatic Compounds, Part 1, Chemical, Environmental and Experimental Data*, Lyon

IARC (1987) *IARC Monographs on the Evaluation of Carcinogenic Risks to Humans*, Suppl. 7, *Overall Evaluations of Carcinogenicity: An Updating of* IARC Monographs *Volumes 1–42*, Lyon, pp. 78, 79–80, 100–106, 106–116, 120–122, 211–216, 230–232, 341–345, 385–387

IARC (1988) *IARC Monographs on the Evaluation of Carcinogenic Risks to Humans*, Vol. 43, *Man-made Mineral Fibres and Radon*, Lyon

IARC (1989) *IARC Monographs on the Evaluation of Carcinogenic Risks to Humans*, Vol. 45, *Occupational Exposures in Petroleum Refining; Crude Oil and Major Petroleum Fuels*, Lyon, pp. 32–33, 60–62

IARC (1991) *IARC Monographs on the Evaluation of Carcinogenic Risks to Humans*, Vol. 52, *Chlorinated Drinking-water; Chlorination By-products; Some Other Halogenated Compounds; Cobalt and Cobalt Compounds*, Lyon, pp. 363–472

International Labour Office (1991) *Occupational Exposure Limits for Airborne Toxic Substances*, 3rd ed. (Occupational Safety and Health Series No. 37), Geneva, pp. 372–373

Islam, M.S., Vastag, E. & Ulmer, W.T. (1972) Sulphur dioxide-induced bronchial hyperreactivity against acetylcholine. *Int. Arch. Arbeitsmed.*, 29, 221–232

Itami, T., Ema, M., Kawasaki, H. & Kanoh, S. (1989) Evaluation of the teratogenic potential of sodium sulfite in rats. *Drug chem. Toxicol.*, 12, 123–135

Jäppinen, P. (1987) A mortality study of Finnish pulp and paper workers. *Br. J. ind. Med.*, 44, 580–587

Jäppinen, P., Hakulinen, T., Pukkala, E., Tola, S. & Kurppa, K. (1987) Cancer incidence of workers in the Finnish pulp and paper industry. *Scand. J. Work Environ. Health*, 13, 197–202

Järup, L., Pershagen, G. & Wall, S. (1989) Cumulative arsenic exposure and lung cancer in smelter workers: a dose-response study. *Am. J. ind. Med.*, 15, 31–41

Kak, S.N. & Kaul, B.L. (1979) Mutagenic activity of sodium bisulphite in barley. *Experientia*, 35, 739–741

Kangas, J. (1991) *Haihtuvat Rikkiyhdisteet* [Volatile Sulfur Compounds] (Altisteet Työssä—Series No. 11), Helsinki, Institute of Occupational Health, Work Environment Fund

Karchmer, J.H., ed. (1970) *The Analytical Chemistry of Sulphur and Its Compounds*, Part I, New York, Wiley-Interscience, pp. 183–283

Kehoe, R.A., Machle, W.F., Kitzmiller, K. & LeBlanc, T.J. (1932) On the effect of prolonged exposure to sulphur dioxide. *J. ind. Hyg.*, 14, 159–173

Kelly, T.J., McLaren, S.E. & Kadlecek, J.A. (1989) Seasonal variations in atmospheric SOx and NOy species in the Adirondacks. *Atmos. Environ.*, 23, 1315–1332

Kleinman, M.T. (1984) Sulfur dioxide and exercise: relationships between response and absorption in upper airways. *J. Air Pollut. Control. Assoc.*, 34, 32–37

Knapp, K.T., Pierson, W.R., Dasgupta, P.K., Adams, D.F., Appel, B.R., Farwell, S.O., Kok, G.L., Reiszner, K.D. & Tanner, R.L. (1987) Determination of gaseous sulfuric acid and sulfur dioxide in stack gases. In: Lodge, J.P., Jr, ed., *Methods of Air Sampling and Analysis*, 3rd ed., Chelsea, MI, Lewis Publishers, pp. 523–528

Kok, G.L., Dasgupta, P.K., Adams, D.F., Appel, B.R., Farwell, S.O., Knapp, K.T., Pierson, W.R., Reiszner, K.D. & Tanner, R.L. (1987a) Determination of sulfur dioxide content of the atmosphere (tetrachloromercurate absorber/para-rosaniline method). In: Lodge, J.P., Jr, ed., *Methods of Air Sampling and Analysis*, 3rd ed., Chelsea, MI, Lewis Publishers, pp. 493–493

Kok, G.L., Dasgupta, P.K., Adams, D.F., Appel, B.R., Farwell, S.O., Knapp, K.T., Pierson, W.R., Reiszner, K.D. & Tanner, R.L. (1987b) Determination of sulfur dioxide content of the atmosphere (formaldehyde absorber/para-rosaniline method). In: Lodge, J.P., Jr, ed., *Methods of Air Sampling and Analysis*, 3rd ed., Chelsea, MI, Lewis Publishers, pp. 499–502

Krupa, S.V. (1980) Atmospheric sulfur transformations: sulfur dioxide, sulfuric acid aerosols, acidic rain and their effects on vegetation. In: Raychaudhuri, S.P. & Gupta, D.S., eds, *Progress in Ecology: Proceedings of International Symposium on Environmental Pollution and Toxicology, 15 July 1980*, New Delhi, Today & Tomorrow's, pp. 11–31

Kunz, B.A. & Glickman, B.W. (1983) Absence of bisulfite mutagenesis in the *lacI* gene of *Escherichia coli*. *Mutat. Res.*, 119, 267–271

Laskin, S., Kuschner, M., Sellakumar, A. & Katz, G.V. (1976) Combined carcinogen–irritant animal inhalation studies. In: Aharonson, E.F., Ben David, A. & Klingberg, A.M., eds, *Air Pollution and the Lung*, New York, Wiley, pp. 190–213

Lawrence, J.F. & Chadha, R.K. (1988) Determination of sulfite in foods by head-space liquid chromatography. *J. Assoc. off. anal. Chem.*, 71, 930–933

Lee-Feldstein, A. (1983) Arsenic and respiratory cancer in humans: follow-up of copper smelter employees in Montana. *J. natl Cancer Inst.*, 70, 601–609

Lewin, E.E., de Pena, R.G. & Shimshock, J.P. (1986) Atmospheric gas and particle measurements at a rural northeastern US site. *Atmos. Environ.*, 20, 59–70

Lightowlers, P.J. & Cape, J.N. (1988) Sources and fate of atmospheric HCl in the UK and western Europe. *Atmos. Environ.*, 22, 7–15

Linn, W.S., Shamoo, D.A., Spier, C.E., Valencia, L.M., Anzar, U.T., Venet, T.G. & Hackney, J.D. (1983) Respiratory effects of 0.75 ppm sulfur dioxide in exercising asthmatics: influence of upper-respiratory defenses. *Environ. Res.*, 30, 340–348

Lockett, M.F. & Natoff, I.L. (1960) A study of the toxicity of sulphite. I. *J. Pharm. Pharmacol.*, 12, 488–496

Lubin, J.H., Pottern, L.M., Blot, W.J., Tokudome, S., Stone, B.J. & Fraumeni, J.F., Jr (1981) Respiratory cancer among copper smelter workers: recent mortality statistics. *J. occup. Med.*, 23, 779–784

Lundgren, K.D. (1954) Diseases of the respiratory organs of workers at a smelting plant (Swed.). *Nord. Hyg. Tidskr.*, 3, 66–82

Ma, T.-H., Isbandi, D., Khan, S.H. & Tseng, Y.-S. (1973) Low level of SO_2 enhanced chromatid aberrations in *Tradescantia* pollen tubes and seasonal variation of the aberration rates. *Mutat. Res.*, 21, 93–100

Ma, T.-H., Harris, M.M., Anderson V.A., Ahmed, I., Mohammad, K., Bare, J.L. & Lin, G. (1984) *Tradescantia*-micronucleus (Trad-MCN) tests on 140 health-related agents. *Mutat. Res.*, 138, 157–167

MacRae, W.D. & Stich, H.F. (1979) Induction of sister chromatid exchanges in Chinese hamster cells by the reducing agents bisulfite and ascorbic acid. *Toxicology*, 13, 167–174

Mallon, R.G. & Rossman, T.G. (1981) Bisulfite (sulfur dioxide) is a comutagen in *E. coli* and in Chinese hamster cells. *Mutat. Res.*, 88, 125–133

Mannsville Chemical Products Corp. (1985) *Chemical Products Synopsis: Sulfur Dioxide*, Cortland, NY

Meng, Z. & Zhang, L. (1990a) Chromosomal aberrations and sister-chromatid exchanges in lymphocytes of workers exposed to sulphur dioxide. *Mutat. Res.*, **241**, 15–20

Meng, Z. & Zhang, L. (1990b) Observation of frequencies of lymphocytes with micronuclei in human peripheral blood cultures from workers in a sulphuric acid factor. *Environ. mol. Mutag.*, **15**, 218–220

Menzel, D.B., Keller, D.A. & Leung, K.-H. (1986) Covalent reactions in the toxicity of SO_2 and sulfite. *Adv. exp. Med. Biol.*, **197**, 477–492

Milham, S., Jr & Demers, R.Y. (1984) Mortality among pulp and paper workers. *J. occup. Med.*, **26**, 844–846

Monteleone-Neto, R., Brunoni, D., Laurenti, R., de Mello Jorge, M.H., Gotlieb, S.L.D. & Lebrão, M.L. (1985) Birth defects and environmental pollution: the Cubatão example. In: Marios, M., ed., *Prevention of Physical and Mental Congenital Defects*, Part B, *Epidemiology, Early Detection and Therapy, and Environmental Factors*, New York, Alan R. Liss, pp. 65–68

Mottley, C., Harman, L.S. & Mason, R.P. (1985) Microsomal reduction of bisulfite (aqueous sulfur dioxide). Sulfur dioxide anion free radical formation by cytochrome P-450. *Biochem. Pharmacol.*, **34**, 3005–3008

Mukai, F., Hawryluk, I. & Shapiro, R. (1970) The mutagenic specificity of sodium bisulfite. *Biochem. biophys. Res. Commun.*, **39**, 983–988

Münzner, R. (1980) Investigations of the mutagenic effect of bisulfite (Ger.). *Lebensmittel-Wiss.-Technol.*, **13**, 219–220

Murray, F.J., Schwetz, B.A., Crawford, A.A., Henck, J.W., Quast, J.F. & Staples, R.E. (1979) Embryotoxicity of inhaled sulfur dioxide and carbon monoxide in mice and rabbits. *J. environ. Sci. Health*, **C13**, 233–250

Murthy, M.S.S., Deorukhakar, V.V. & Anjaria, K.B. (1983) A study of the induction of gene conversion in yeast by sodium bisulphite under radical reaction conditions. *Food chem. Toxicol.*, **21**, 499–501

Nadel, J.A., Salem, H., Tamplin, B. & Tokiwa, Y. (1965) Mechanism of bronchoconstriction during inhalation of sulfur dioxide. *J. appl. Physiol.*, **20**, 164–167

Njagi, G.D.E. & Gopalan, H.N.B. (1982) Cytogenetic effects of the food preservatives—sodium benzoate and sodium sulphite on *Vicia faba* root meristems. *Mutat. Res.*, **102**, 213–219

Nordenson, I., Beckman, G., Beckman, L., Rosenhall, L. & Stjernberg, N. (1980) Is exposure to sulphur dioxide clastogenic? Chromosomal aberrations among workers at a sulphite pulp factory. *Hereditas*, **93**, 161–164

Nordström, S., Beckman, L. & Nordenson, I. (1978a) Occupational and environmental risks in and around a smelter in northern Sweden. I. Variations in birth weight. *Hereditas*, **88**, 43–46

Nordström, S., Beckman, L. & Nordenson, I. (1978b) Occupational and environmental risks in and around a smelter in northern Sweden. III. Frequencies of spontaneous abortion. *Hereditas*, **88**, 51–54

Nordström, S., Beckman, L. & Nordenson, I. (1979a) Occupational and environmental risks in and around a smelter in northern Sweden. V. Spontaneous abortion among female employees and decreased birth weight in their offspring. *Hereditas*, **90**, 291–296

Nordström, S., Beckman, L. & Nordenson, I. (1979b) Occupational and environmental risks in and around a smelter in northern Sweden. VI. Congenital malformations. *Hereditas*, **90**, 297–302

Ough, C.S. (1986) Determination of sulfur dioxide in grapes and wines. *J. Assoc. off. anal. Chem.*, **69**, 5–7

Pagano, D.A. & Zeiger, E. (1987) Conditions affecting the mutagenicity of sodium bisulfite in *Salmonella typhimurium*. *Mutat. Res.*, **179**, 159–166

Pagano, D.A., Zeiger, E. & Stark, A.-A. (1990) Autoxidation and mutagenicity of sodium bisulfite. *Mutat. Res.*, **228**, 89–96

Pauluhn, J., Thyssen, J., Althoff, J., Kimmerle, G. & Mohr, U. (1985) Long-term inhalation study with benzo(*a*)pyrene and SO_2 in Syrian golden hamsters. *Exp. Pathol.*, **28**, 31

Peacock, P.R. & Spence, J.B. (1967) Incidence of lung tumours in LX mice exposed to (1) free radicals; (2) SO_2. *Br. J. Cancer*, **21**, 606–618

Pechan, E.H. & Wilson, J.H., Jr (1984) Estimates of 1973–1982 annual sulfur oxide emissions from electric utilities. *J. Air Pollut. Control Assoc.*, **34**, 1075–1078

Pershagen, G., Elinder, C.-G. & Belander, A.-M. (1977) Mortality in a region surrounding an arsenic emitting plant. *Environ. Health Perspectives*, **19**, 133–137

Pershagen, G., Wall, W., Taube, A. & Linnman, L. (1981) On the interaction between occupational arsenic exposure and smoking and its relationship to lung cancer. *Scand. J. Work Environ. Health*, **7**, 302–309

Pierson, W.R., Brachaczek, W.W., Gorse, R.A., Jr, Japar, S.M., Norbeck, J.M. & Keeler, G.J. (1989) Atmospheric acidity measurements on Allegheny Mountain and the origins of ambient acidity in the northeastern United States. *Atmos. Environ.*, **23**, 431–459

Pirilä, V., Kajanne, H. & Salo, O.P. (1963) Inhalation of sulfur dioxide as a cause of skin reaction resembling drug eruption. *J. occup. Med.*, **5**, 443–445

Placet, M. (1990) Emissions involved in acidic deposition processes: methodology and results. In: *Proceedings of the 83rd Annual Meeting and Exhibition of the Argonne National Laboratory* (Report No. CONF-900676-6; US NTIS DE90-011152), Washington DC, National Technical Information Service

Pott, F. & Stöber, W. (1983) Carcinogenicity of airborne combustion products observed in subcutaneous tissue and lungs of laboratory rodents. *Environ. Health Perspectives*, **47**, 293–303

Rabinovitch, S., Greyson, N.D., Weiser, W. & Hoffstein, V. (1989) Clinical and laboratory features of acute sulfur dioxide inhalation poisoning: two-year follow-up. *Am. Rev. respir. Dis.*, **139**, 556–558

Reich, A. (1961) *Analyse der Metalle* (Analysis of Metals), 2nd ed., Vol. 2, Part 1, Berlin, Springer, pp. 666–689

Rencher, A.C., Carter, M.W. & McKee, D.W. (1977) A retrospective epidemiological study of mortality at a large western copper smelter. *J. occup. Med.*, **19**, 754–758

Renner, H.W. & Wever, J. (1983) Attempts to induce cytogenetic effects with sulphite in sulphite oxidase-deficient Chinese hamsters and mice. *Food chem. Toxicol.*, **21**, 123–127

Ripley, L.S. & Drake, J.W. (1984) Bacteriophage T4 particles are refractory to bisulfite mutagenesis. *Mutat. Res.*, **129**, 149–152

Robinson, C.F., Waxweiler, R.J. & Fowler, D.P. (1986) Mortality among production workers in pulp and paper mills. *Scand. J. Work Environ. Health*, **12**, 552–560

Rom, W.N., Wood, S.D., White, G.L., Bang, K.M. & Reading, J.C. (1986) Longitudinal evaluation of pulmonary function in copper smelter workers exposed to sulfur dioxide. *Am. Rev. respir. Dis.*, **133**, 830–833

Sakai, R. (1984) Fetal abnormality in a Japanese industrial zone. *Int. J. environ. Res.*, **23**, 113–120

Sander, U.H.F., Rothe, U. & Kola, R. (1984) Sulphur dioxide. In: Sander, U.H.F., Fischer, H., Rothe, U. & Kola, R., eds, *Sulphur, Sulphur Dioxide and Sulphuric Acid. An Introduction to Their Industrial Chemistry and Technology*, London, The British Sulphur Corporation, pp. 151–254

Sandström, T., Stjernberg, N., Andersson, M.-C., Kolmodin-Hedman, B., Lundgren, R., Rosenhall, L. & Ångström, T. (1989a) Cell response in bronchoalveolar lavage fluid after exposure to sulfur dioxide: a time–response study. *Am. Rev. respir. Dis.*, **140**, 1828–1831

Sandström, T., Stjernberg, N., Andersson, M.-C., Kolmodin-Hedman, B., Lundgren, R. & Ångström, T. (1989b) Is the short term limit value for sulfur dioxide exposure safe? Effects of controlled chamber exposure investigated with bronchoalveolar lavage. *Br. J. ind. Med.*, **46**, 200–203

Sax, N.I. & Lewis, R.J., Sr (1987) *Hawley's Condensed Chemical Dictionary*, 11th ed., New York, Van Nostrand Reinhold, pp. 952, 1107

Settipane, G.A. (1984) Adverse reactions to sulfites in drugs and foods. *J. Am. Acad. Dermatol.*, **10**, 1077–1081

Shalamberidze, O.P. & Tsereteli, N.T. (1971) Effect of low concentrations of sulfur and nitrogen dioxides on the estrual cycles and reproductive functions of experimental animals. *Hyg. Sanit.*, **8**, 178–182

Shapiro, R. (1977) Genetic effects of bisulfite (sulfur dioxide). *Mutat. Res.*, **39**, 149–176

Sheppard, D., Saisho, A., Nadel, J.A. & Boushey, H.A. (1981) Exercise increases sulfur dioxide-induced bronchoconstriction in asthmatic subjects. *Am. Rev. respir. Dis.*, **123**, 486–491

Siemiatycki, J., ed. (1991) *Risk Factors for Cancer in the Workplace*, Boca Raton, FL, CRC Press

Simon, R.A. (1986) Sulfite sensitivity. *Ann. Allergy*, **56**, 281–291

Singh, J. (1982) Teratological evaluation of sulphur dioxide. *Proc. Inst. environ. Sci.*, **28**, 144–145

Singh, J. (1989) Neonatal development altered by maternal sulfur dioxide exposure. *Neurotoxicology*, **10**, 523–528

Skalpe, I.O. (1964) Long-term effects of sulphur dioxide exposure in pulp mills. *Br. J. ind. Med.*, **21**, 69–73

Skizim, D.T. (1982) Gaseous emission control is vital. *Solid Wastes Manag.*, **25**, 28–30, 61

Skyttä, E. (1978) *Tilasto Työhygieenisistä Mittauksista v. 1971–1976* [Statistics of Industrial Hygienic Measurements in 1971–1976] (Katsauksia Series No. 17), Helsinki, Institute of Occupational Health

Smith, T.J., Wagner, W.L. & Moore, D.E. (1978) Chronic sulfur dioxide exposure in a smelter. I. Exposure to SO_2 and dust: 1940–1974. *J. occup. Med.*, **20**, 83–87

Smith, T.J., Hammond, S.K., Laidlaw, F. & Fine, S. (1984) Respiratory exposures associated with silicon carbide production: estimation of cumulative exposures for an epidemiological study. *Br. J. ind. Med.*, **41**, 100–108

Snell, F.D. & Ettre, L.S., eds (1973) *Encyclopedia of Industrial Chemical Analysis*, Vol. 18, *Silicon to Thiophene*, New York, Interscience, pp. 360–440

Sorsa, M., Kolmodin-Hedman, B. & Järventaus, H. (1982) No effect of sulphur dioxide exposure, in aluminium industry, on chromosomal aberrations or sister chromatid exchanges. *Hereditas*, **97**, 159–161

Stevenson, D.D. & Simon, R.A. (1984) Sulfites and asthma. *J. Allergy clin. Immunol.*, **74**, 469–472

Stjernberg, N., Beckman, G., Beckman, L., Nyström, L. & Rosenhall, L. (1984) Alpha-1-antitrypsin types and pulmonary disease among employees at a sulphite pulp factory in northern Sweden. *Hum. Hered.*, **34**, 337–342

Stjernberg, N., Rosenhall, L., Eklund, A. & Nyström, L. (1986) Chronic bronchitis in a community in northern Sweden; relation to environmental and occupational exposure to sulphur dioxide. *Eur. J. respir. Dis.*, **69**, 153–159

Takahashi, M., Hasegawa, R., Furukawa, F., Toyoda, K., Sato, H. & Hayashi, Y. (1986) Effects of ethanol, potassium metabisulfite, formaldehyde and hydrogen peroxide on gastric carcinogenesis in rats after initiation with N-methyl-N'-nitro-N-nitrosoguanidine. *Jpn. J. Cancer Res.*, 77, 118–124

Tanaka, T., Fujii, M., Mori, H. & Hirono, I. (1979) Carcinogenicity test of potassium metabisulfite in mice. *Ecotoxicol. environ. Saf.*, 3, 451–453

Taylor, D.G. (1977) *NIOSH Manual of Analytical Methods*, 2nd ed., Vol. 1 (DHEW (NIOSH) Publ. No. 77-157-A), Washington DC, US Government Printing Office, pp. 146-1–146-7, 160-1–160-9, 163-1–163-7, 204-1–204-11

Taylor, D.G. (1978) *NIOSH Manual of Analytical Methods*, 2nd ed., Vol 4 (DHEW (NIOSH) Publ. No. 78-175), Washington DC, US Government Printing Office, pp. S308-1–S308-7

Tejnorová, I. (1978) Sulfite oxidase activity in liver and kidney tissue in five laboratory animal species. *Toxicol. appl. Pharmacol.*, 44, 251–256

Til, H.P., Feron, V.J. & De Groot, A.P. (1972) The toxicity of sulfite. I. Long-term feeding and multigeneration studies in rats. *Food Cosmet. Toxicol.*, 10, 291–310

Tsutsui, T. & Barrett, J.C. (1990) Sodium bisulfite induces morphological transformation of cultured Syrian hamster embryo cells but lacks the ability to induce detectable gene mutations, chromosome mutations or DNA damage. *Carcinogenesis*, 11, 1869–1873

Turner, S. & Liss, P. (1983) The oceans and the global sulphur budget. *Nature*, 305, 277

Uragoda, C.G. (1981) Long term exposure to sulphur dioxide during bleaching of coir. *J. Soc. occup. Med.*, 31, 76–78

US Environmental Protection Agency (1986) *Acid Rain. An EPA Journal Special Supplement* (OPA-86-009), Washington DC, Office of Public Affairs

US Environmental Protection Agency (1989) Protection of environment. *US Code fed. Regul.*, **Title 40**, Parts 60.82, 60.163, 60.173, 60.183

US Food and Drug Administration (1987) Sulfite. In: Fazio, T. & Sherma, J., eds, *Food Additives Analytical Manual*, Vol. II, *A Collection of Analytical Methods for Selected Food Additives*, Arlington, VA, Association of Official Analytical Chemists, pp. 279–307

US Food and Drug Administration (1989) Food and drugs. *US Code fed. Regul.*, **Title 21**, Parts 182.3637, 182.3739, 182.3766, 182.3798, 182.3862

US National Institute for Occupational Safety and Health (1974) *Criteria for a Recommended Standard...Occupational Exposure to Sulfur Dioxide*, Cincinnati, OH, pp. 16, 105, 108–111

US National Institute for Occupational Safety and Health/Occupational Safety and Health Administration (1981) *Occupational Health Guidelines for Chemical Hazards* (DHHS (NIOSH) Publication No. 81.123), Washington DC

US Occupational Safety and Health Administration (1989) Air contaminants—permissible exposure limits. *Code fed. Regul.*, **Title 29**, Part 1910.1000

Verrett, M.J., Scott, W.F., Reynaldo, E.F., Alterman, E.K. & Thomas, C.A. (1980) Toxicity and teratogenicity of food additive chemicals in the developing chicken embryo. *Toxicol. appl. Pharmacol.*, 56, 265–273

Virginia Basic Chemicals Co. (1991) *Data Sheet: Sodium Metabisulfite Anhydrous, Technical Grade*, Norfolk, VA

Volkova, Z.A. & Bagdinov, Z.M. (1969) Problems of labor hygiene in rubber vulcanization. *Hyg. Sanit.*, 34, 326–333

Warner, C.G., Davies, G.M., Jones, J.G. & Lowe, C.R. (1969) Bronchitis in two integrated steelworks. II. Sulphur dioxide and particulate atmospheric pollution in and around the two works. *Ann. occup. Hyg.*, **12**, 151–170

Weast, R.C., ed. (1989) *CRC Handbook of Chemistry and Physics*, 70th ed., Boca Raton, FL, CRC Press, pp. B-121, B-133, B-135

Weil, E.D. (1983) Sulfur compounds. In: Mark, H.F., Othmer, D.F., Overberger, C.G., Seaborg, G.T. & Grayson, N., eds, *Kirk-Othmer Encyclopedia of Chemical Technology*, 3rd ed., Vol. 22, New York, John Wiley & Sons, pp. 107–167

Welch, K., Higgins, I., Oh, M. & Burchfiel, C. (1982) Arsenic exposure, smoking and respiratory cancer in copper smelter workers. *Arch. environ. Health*, **37**, 325–335

WHO (1979) *Sulfur Oxides and Suspended Particulate Matter* (Environmental Health Criteria No. 8), Geneva

WHO (1987) *Air Quality Guidelines for Europe* (WHO Regional Publication, European Series No. 23), Copenhagen, pp. 341–357

Wilson, W.E. (1978) Sulfates in the atmosphere: a progress report on Project MISTT [Midwest Interstate Sulfur Transformation and Transport]. *Atmos. Environ.*, **12**, 537–547

Winchester, J.W. (1983) Sulfur, acidic aerosols, and acid rain in the eastern United States. In: Schwartz, S.E., ed., *Trace Atmospheric Constituents. Properties, Transformations, and Fates*, New York, John Wiley & Son, pp. 269–301

Wirth, P.J., Doniger, J., Thorgeirsson, S.S. & DiPaolo, J.A. (1986) Altered polypeptide expression associated with neoplastic transformation of Syrian hamster cells by bisulfite. *Cancer Res.*, **46**, 390–399

Wolff, G.T., Ruthkosky, M.S., Stoup, D.P., Korsog, P.E., Ferman, M.A., Wendel, G.J. & Stedman, D.H. (1986) Measurements of SOx, NOx and aerosol species on Bermuda. *Atmos. Environ.*, **20**, 1229–1239

Woodford, D.M., Coutu, R.E. & Gaensler, E.A. (1979) Obstructive lung disease from acute sulfur dioxide exposure. *Respiration*, **38**, 238–245

Yokoyama, E., Yoder, R.E. & Frank, N.R. (1971) Distribution of ^{35}S in the blood and its excretion in urine of dogs exposed to $^{35}SO_2$. *Arch. environ. Health*, **22**, 389–395

HYDROCHLORIC ACID

Hydrogen chloride is a gas; its solutions in water are commonly referred to as hydrochloric acid. This monograph covers both forms.

1. Exposure Data

1.1 Chemical and physical data

1.1.1 *Synonyms, structural and molecular data*

Chem. Abstr. Serv. Reg. No.: 7647-01-0
Replaced CAS Reg. Nos.: 51005-19-7; 61674-62-2; 113962-65-5
Chem. Abstr. Name: Hydrochloric acid
IUPAC Systematic Name: Hydrochloric acid
Synonyms: Anhydrous hydrochloric acid; chlorohydric acid; hydrochloric acid gas; hydrogen chloride; muriatic acid

HCl

HCl   Mol. wt: 36.47

1.1.2 *Chemical and physical properties*

(a) *Description*: Colourless or slightly yellow, fuming pungent liquid or colourless gas with characteristic pungent odour (Sax & Lewis, 1987; Budavari, 1989; Weast, 1989)
(b) *Boiling-point*: Gas, −84.9 °C at 760 mm Hg (101 kPa); constant boiling azeotrope with water containing 20.24% HCl, 110 °C at 760 mm Hg (Weast, 1989)
(c) *Melting-point*: anhydrous (gas), −114.8 °C (Weast, 1989); aqueous solutions, −17.1 °C (10.8% solution); −62.25 °C (20.7% solution); −46.2 °C (31.2% solution); −25.4 °C (39.2% solution) (Budavari, 1989)
(d) *Density*: Aqueous solutions, 39.1% solution (15 °C/4 °C), 1.20 (Budavari, 1989); constant boiling HCl (20.24%), 1.097 (Weast, 1989)
(e) *Specific volume*: Gas, 1/47–1/52 g/l (Linde/Union Carbide Corp., 1985; Matheson Gas Products, 1990; Alphagas/Liquid Air Corp., 1991; Scott Specialty Gases, 1991)
(f) *Solubility*: Soluble in water (g/100 g water): 82.3 at 0 °C, 67.3 at 30 °C; methanol (g/100 g solution): 51.3 at 0 °C, 47.0 at 20° C; ethanol (g/100 g solution): 45.4 at 0 °C, 41.0 at 20 °C; diethyl ether (g/100 g solution): 35.6 at 0 °C, 24.9 at 20 °C (Budavari, 1989); and benzene (Weast, 1989)
(g) *Volatility*: Vapour pressure, 40 atm (4 MPa) at 17.8 °C (Weast, 1989)

(h) *Conversion factor*: mg/m^3 = 1.49 × ppm^a

1.1.3 *Technical products and impurities*

Hydrochloric acid as an aqueous solution is available in several grades (technical, food processing, analytical, commercial, photographic, water white) as 20 °Bé (31.45% HCl), 22 °Bé (35.21% HCl) or 23 °Bé (37.1% HCl), with the following specifications (mg/kg): purity, (20 °Bé) 31.45–32.56%, (22 °Bé) 35.21–36.35%, (23 °Bé) 36.5–38.26; sulfites, 1–10 max; sulfates, 1–15 max; iron (as Fe), 0.2–5 max; free chlorine, 1–30 max; arsenic (see IARC, 1987), 0.01–1 max; heavy metals (as Pb), 0.5–5 max; fluoride, 2; benzene (see IARC, 1987), 0.01–0.05 max; vinyl chloride (see IARC, 1987), 0.01–0.05 max; total fluorinated organic compounds, 25.0 max; toluene (see IARC, 1989), 5.0 max; bromide, 50 max; ammonium, 3 (Dow Chemical USA, 1982, 1983; Atochem North America, 1986a,b; American National Standards Institute, 1987; Vista Chemical Co., 1987; BASF Corp., 1988; Du Pont Co., 1988; BASF Corp., 1989; Dow Chemical USA, 1989; BASF Corp., 1990; Occidental Chemical Corp., 1990).

Hydrogen chloride is also available as a liquefied gas in electronics grade with a purity of 99.99% and the following impurity limits (ppm): nitrogen, 75; oxygen, 10; carbon dioxide, 10; and hydrocarbons, 5 (Dow Chemical USA, 1990).

1.1.4 *Analysis*

Methods have been reported for the analysis of hydrochloric acid in air. One method involves drawing the sample through a silica gel tube, desorbing with sodium bicarbonate/-sodium carbonate solution and heat and analysing for chloride ion with ion chromatography. The lower detection limit for this method is 2 μg/sample (Eller, 1984). A similar method entails collecting a sample from the stack and passing it through dilute (0.1 N) sulfuric acid. The chloride ion concentration is analysed by ion chromatography, with a detection limit of 0.1 μg/ml (US Environmental Protection Agency, 1989).

Hydrogen chloride can be detected in exhaust gas (stack emissions) by: the ion-selective electrode method (absorb in dilute potassium nitrate solution and measure potential difference); silver nitrate titration (absorb in sodium hydroxide solution, add silver nitrate and titrate with ammonium thiocyanate); and a mercuric thiocyanate method (absorb in sodium hydroxide solution, add mercuric thiocyanate and ammonium iron[III] sulfate solutions and measure absorbance of ferric thiocyanate) (Japanese Standards Association, 1982).

1.2 Production and use

1.2.1 *Production*

In the fifteenth century, the German alchemist Valentin heated green vitriol (iron[II] sulfate, FeSO$_4$ · 7H$_2$O) with common salt (sodium chloride) to obtain what was then called 'spirit of salt'. In the seventeenth century, Glauber prepared hydrochloric acid from sodium chloride and sulfuric acid. In 1790, Davy established the composition of hydrogen chloride by

---

^{a}Calculated from: mg/m^3 = (molecular weight/24.45) × ppm, assuming normal temperature (25 °C) and pressure (760 mm Hg [101.3 kPa])

synthesizing it from hydrogen and chlorine. In the same year, Leblanc discovered the process named after him for the production of soda (sodium carbonate), the first stage of which is to react sodium choride with sulfuric acid, liberating hydrogen chloride. This was first considered an undesirable by-product and simply released into the atmosphere in large amounts. In 1863, English soda producers were compelled by the Alkali Act to absorb the hydrogen chloride in water, which quickly led to large-scale industrial use of the acid produced. Excess hydrogen chloride that could not be used as hydrochloric acid was oxidized to chlorine (Austin & Glowacki, 1989).

Following the development of the chlor-alkali electrolytic process early in the twentieth century, the industrial synthesis of hydrogen chloride by burning chlorine in hydrogen gas became an important route. This method generates a product of higher purity than that based on the reaction between chloride salts and sulfuric acid or sodium hydrogen sulfate. These processes are being superseded, however, with the availability of large amounts of hydrogen chloride that arise as by-products of chlorination processes, such as the production of vinyl chloride from ethylene (Leddy, 1983; Austin & Glowacki, 1989).

Hydrogen chloride can thus be formed according to the following reactions: (1) synthesis from the elements (hydrogen and chlorine); (2) reaction of chloride salts, particularly sodium chloride, with sulfuric acid or a hydrogen sulfate; (3) as a by-product of chlorination, e.g., in the production of dichloromethane, trichloroethylene, tetrachloroethylene or vinyl chloride; (4) from spent pickle liquor in metal treatment, by thermal decomposition of the hydrated heavy metal chlorides; and (5) from incineration of chlorinated organic waste. By far the greatest proportion of hydrogen chloride is now obtained as a by-product of chlorination. The degree of purification required depends on the end-use. Recovery from waste materials (Methods 4 and 5) is becoming increasingly important, whereas the amount generated by Method 2 is decreasing (Austin & Glowacki, 1989).

Many impurities in hydrogen chloride gas (e.g., sulfur dioxide, arsenic and chlorine) can be removed by adsorption on activated carbon. As use of the chlorination by-product process increases, removal of chlorinated hydrocarbons from hydrogen chloride gas or hydrochloric acid becomes of greater practical relevance. Gaseous hydrogen chloride can be purified by low-temperature scrubbing with a high-boiling solvent, which may be another chlorinated hydrocarbon (e.g., hexachlorobutadiene (see IARC, 1979) or tetrachloroethane), or with special oil fractions. Chlorine may be removed with carbon tetrachloride (see IARC, 1987), in which it is more soluble than is hydrogen chloride gas. Hydrochloric acid, used as such or for generation of hydrogen chloride, contains mainly volatile impurities, including chlorinated hydrocarbons, and these can be removed from the acid by stripping. An inert gas stream, which results in lower energy consumption, can be used for stripping, although heating the gas is preferable for environmental reasons. Inorganic impurities, in particular iron salts, are removed by ion exchange (Austin & Glowacki, 1989).

Worldwide production of hydrochloric acid in 1980–90 is shown in Table 1. The numbers of companies producing hydrochloric acid/hydrogen chloride are shown in Table 2.

Table 1. Trends in production of hydrochloric acid (thousand tonnes) with time, 1980–90

Country or region	1980	1981	1982	1983	1984	1985	1986	1987	1988	1989	1990
Australia	63	59	55	60	57	58	54	62	69	64	NA
Canada	177	186	135	170	161	158	153	164	180	180	187
China	1177	1292	1483	1583	NA	NA	NA	NA	NA	NA	NA
France	674	700	687	673	767	656	626	647	684	692	675
Germany[a]	889	886	846	898	954	943	929	988	980	956	909
Italy	NA	NA	NA	NA	NA	NA	NA	679	1006	635	742
Japan	570	565	551	511	521	549	549	543	565	571	637
Mexico	36	33	47	79	77	63	83	117	118	NA	NA
Taiwan	179	184	191	212	241	228	242	251	255	217	234
United Kingdom	137	117	118	130	156	153	157	174	176	166	162
USA	2620	2335	2223	2239	2478	2546	2189	2718	2928	2882	2124

From Anon. (1984a,b, 1986, 1987, 1988, 1989, 1990, 1991); NA, not available
[a]Figures prior to 1990 are for western Germany only.

Table 2. Numbers of companies in different countries or regions in which hydrochloric acid/hydrogen chloride were produced in 1988

Country or region	No. of companies	Country or region	No. of companies
Japan	32	Portugal	3
USA	27	Thailand	3
Germany (western)	15	Turkey	3
Italy	13	Austria	2
Spain	13	Greece	2
India	12	Pakistan	2
Brazil	11	Romania	2
United Kingdom	11	South Africa	2
Australia	10	Bulgaria	1
Mexico	8	Chile	1
Canada	7	Colombia	1
France	7	Egypt	1
Argentina	6	Indonesia	1
Sweden	5	Republic of Korea	1
Switzerland	5	Kuwait	1
Yugoslavia	5	New Zealand	1
Taiwan	4	Norway	1
Bangladesh	3	Philippines	1
Belgium	3	Saudi Arabia	1
China	3	Singapore	1
Finland	3	USSR	1
Israel	3	Venezuela	1
Peru	3		

From Chemical Information Services (1988)

1.2.2 Use

Hydrochloric acid is one of the most important basic industrial chemicals. A major use is in the continuous pickling of hot rolled sheet steel; it is also used widely in batch pickling to remove mill scale and fluxing, in cleaning the steel prior to galvanizing and other processes. It is widely used in the production of organic and inorganic chemical products: Inorganic chlorides are prepared by reacting hydrochloric acid with metals or their oxides, sulfides or hydroxides. Hydrochloric acid has long been used in the production of sugars and, more recently, of high fructose corn syrup. It is also involved in the production of monosodium glutamate, for acidizing crushed bone for gelatin and in the production of soya sauce, apple sweetener and vegetable juice. It is used to increase production of oil and gas wells by acidizing and formation fracturing and cleaning and by cleaning and descaling equipment. Acidizing reduces resistance to the flow of oil and gas through limestone or dolomite formations. Inhibited hydrochloric acid is used to remove sludge and hard-water scale from industrial equipment, ranging from boilers and heat exchangers to electrical insulators and glass. Hydrochloric acid has been used in the extraction of uranium, titanium, tungsten and other precious metals. It is used in the production of magnesium from seawater, in water chemistry (from pH control to the regeneration of ion-exchange resins in water purification), brine purification and in pulp and paper production (Sax & Lewis, 1987; Dow Chemical USA, 1988; Austin & Glowacki, 1989; Budavari, 1989).

1.3 Occurrence

1.3.1 Natural occurrence

Hydrochloric acid is produced by human gastric mucosa and is present in the digestive systems of most mammals. The adult human gastric mucosa produces about 1.5 l per day of gastric juices with a normal acid concentration of 0.05–0.10 N (Rosenberg, 1980).

Natural sources of hydrogen chloride may make an important contribution to atmospheric hydrogen chloride. Hydrogen chloride is emitted from volcanoes; total world emissions of hydrogen chloride from this source are very uncertain but have been estimated at 0.8–7.6 million tonnes per year. Methyl chloride, produced in the sea by marine plants or microorganisms and on land during the combustion of vegetation, reacts with OH radicals in the atmosphere to generate hydrogen chloride. Worldwide natural sources produce about 5.6 million tonnes of methyl chloride per year, equivalent to about 4 million tonnes hydrogen chloride. Hydrogen chloride is also produced from the reaction of sea-salt aerosols with atmospheric acids (Lightowlers & Cape, 1988).

1.3.2 Occupational exposure

Occupational exposure to hydrochloric acid is described in the monograph on occupational exposure to mists and vapours from sulfuric acid and other strong inorganic acids (pp. 44–47). Hydrochloric acid occurs in work-room air as a gas or mist. During pickling and other acid treatment of metals, the mean air concentration of hydrochloric acid has been reported to range from < 0.1 (Sheehy *et al.*, 1982) to 12 mg/m^3 (Remijn *et al.*, 1982). Mean levels > 1 mg/m^3 have been reported in the manufacture of sodium sulfate, calcium chloride and hydrochloric acid, in offset printing shops, in zirconium and hafnium extraction and during some textile processing and laboratory work (Bond *et al.*, 1991).

1.3.3 Air

In areas influenced by marine air masses, displacement reactions between either sulfuric acid or nitric acid and aerosol chlorides, such as sea salt, can be an appreciable source of hydrochloric acid (Harrison, 1990).

Atmospheric levels of hydrogen chloride in Europe and in Michigan, USA, are summarized in Table 3 (Kamrin, 1992). Ambient concentrations are generally in the range of 0.4–4 µg/m^3.

Table 3. Atmospheric levels of hydrogen chloride

Location	Season	Sampling duration	Concentration range (µg/m^3)
Maritime, background	All	Weekly	0.07–0.3
Europe			
United Kingdom, rural	Summer	2–4 h	1–3
United Kingdom, rural	All	Daily	0.3–2
United Kingdom, urban	All	Weekly	0.6–1.2
Switzerland	April 1982	1 h	0.2–3
Dübendorf, Switzerland, urban	Winter 1985	Daily	0.03–3
Dubendorf, Switzerland, rural	March 1986–87	-	0.3–1.3
	Winter 1986–87	-	0.2–3
Po River, Italy, rural	November 1984	Daily	0.1–0.5
Ljubljana, Yugoslavia, urban	February 1985	Daily	0.1–0.5
Linz, Austria, urban, industrial	Summer 1985	Daily	0.2–1.6
Vienna, Austria, urban	Winter 1983–84	Daily	0.1–1.5
Dortmund, Germany, urban	September–October 1980	Daily	0.3–11
Michigan, USA			
Northern, rural	Winter 1983–84	Weekly	0.1–0.5
South Haven, urban	July 1990	6 h	0.5–2
Ann Arbor, urban	August 1990	Daily	0.1–2

From Kamrin (1992)

The main anthropogenic sources of hydrogen chloride in the troposphere are the burning of coal and the incineration of chlorinated plastics, such as polyvinyl chloride. Under conditions typical of a modern coal-fired combustion plant, approximately 80 ppm (119 mg/m^3) of hydrogen chloride are contributed to the stack gas for each 0.1% chlorine in the coal. Hydrogen chloride may be an important determinant of precipitation acidity close to incinerators and coal-burning plants (Cocks & McElroy, 1984).

Estimated annual emissions of hydrogen chloride in the United Kingdom in 1983 (total, 260 000 tonnes/year) by source were: coal burning, 92%; waste incineration, 6%; and atmospheric degradation of chlorinated hydrocarbons, automobile exhausts, glass making, fuel oil combustion and steel pickling acid regeneration, 1%. Similarly, in western Germany, power stations and industrial furnaces produced 81.4% of hydrogen chloride emissions, waste incineration produced 17.5% and other sources only 1.1% (Lightowlers & Cape, 1988).

In comparison with the emissions of sulfur dioxide (3.7 million tonnes/year) and nitrogen oxides (1.9 million tonnes/year) in the United Kingdom, hydrogen chloride is a minor source of potential atmospheric acidity, contributing only 4% of the total potential acidity compared to 71% from sulfur dioxide and 25% from nitrogen oxides. In western Europe as a whole, hydrogen chloride contributes less than 2% of the total potential acidity, whereas sulfur dioxide contributes 68% and nitrogen oxides 30% (Lightowlers & Cape, 1988).

Estimated emissions of hydrochloric acid from coal burning, waste incineration and total emissions in 12 western European countries in the early 1980s are presented in Table 4 (Lightowlers & Cape, 1988).

Table 4. Estimated emissions of hydrogen chloride from two sources in 12 European countries (thousand tonnes/year)

Country	Source	
	Coal burning	Waste incineration
Austria	0.5	1.3
Belgium	14	5.9
Denmark	4.3	6.2
Ireland	2.1	0
France	50	64
Germany[a]	93	14
Italy	21	15
Netherlands	9.4	10
Norway	0.5	1.4
Spain	45	2.2
Sweden	2.6	4.7
Switzerland	0.7	12
Total	240 (63%)	140 (27%)

From Lightowlers & Cape (1988)
[a]Western part only

In 1989 in the USA, total air emissions of hydrochloric acid/hydrogen chloride were estimated to be approximately 27 552 tonnes from 3250 locations; total ambient water releases were estimated to be 1389 tonnes; total underground injection releases were estimated to be 136 440 tonnes; and total land releases were estimated to be 1926 tonnes (US National Library of Medicine, 1991).

Hydrochloric acid differs from sulfuric acid and nitric acid in that it is emitted into the atmosphere as a primary pollutant and is not formed by atmospheric chemistry. Oxidation of sulfur dioxide and nitrogen oxides typically proceeds at approximately 1 and 10% per hour or less, respectively. Over appreciable distances from a major source of all three pollutants (e.g., a power plant), hydrochloric acid may therefore predominate, even though it comprises only a small percentage of the total potential acidity (Harrison, 1990).

A municipal incinerator in Newport News, VA, was studied over a four-day period in 1976 to evaluate gaseous emissions when wet chemical and electro-optical methods were used. Hydrogen chloride concentrations in the stack gas averaged 25.1 ppm (37.4 mg/m^3; range, 12.5–56.7 ppm [18.6–84.5 mg/m^3]). The authors compared their results with those from studies of similar facilities (ppm [mg/m^3]): New York City, NY, 41–81 [61–121]; Brooklyn, NY, 64.3 [95.8]; Babylon, NY, 217–248 [323–370]; Hamilton Avenue, NY, 45–89 [67–133]; Oceanside, NY, 96–113 [143–168]; Flushing, NY, 38–40 [57–60]; Yokohama, Japan, 280 [417] (large amounts of industrial plastic wastes incinerated at this source) and Salford, United Kingdom, 227 [338]. The authors noted that use of a water scrubber appeared to provide an effective means of removing hydrochloric acid (Jahnke et al., 1977).

Emissions from a municipal waste incinerator fired by water wall mass and by fuel derived from refuse contained hydrochloric acid at concentrations of 22–336 ppm (33–501 mg/m^3); emission rates were 0.8–27.0 kg/h (0.2–3.3 g hydrochloric acid/kg of refuse burned) (Nunn, 1986).

The exhaust from a space shuttle launch in which a solid rocket fuel was used contained approximately 60 tonnes of hydrochloric acid (Pellett et al., 1983). Partitioning of hydrochloric acid between hydrochloric acid aerosol and gaseous hydrogen chloride in the lower atmosphere was investigated in the exhaust cloud from a solid fuel rocket in humid ambient air. Hydrochloric acid was present at 0.6–16 ppm (0.9–24 mg/m^3); the partitioning studies indicated that unpolluted tropospheric concentrations of hydrochloric acid (< 1 ppb [< 1.5 μg/m^3]) would be in the gaseous phase except under conditions of very high humidity (Sebacher et al., 1980).

Thermal degradation products of polyvinyl chloride food-wrap film were studied under simulated supermarket conditions, using a commercial wrapping machine with either a hot-wire or a cool-rod cutting device. At 240–310 °C, hydrogen chloride is the major volatile thermal degradation production: mean emissions were 3–59 μg/cut (total range, 1–81 μg/cut) when the hot-wire cutting device was used; hydrogen chloride was not detected when the cool-rod cutting device was used. Other compounds found were the plasticizer [di(2-ethylhexyl)adipate, di(2-ethylhexyl)phthalate, acetyl tributyl citrate], benzene, toluene, acrolein and carbon monoxide (Boettner & Ball, 1980).

1.4 Regulations and guidelines

Occupational exposure limits for hydrochloric acid or hydrogen chloride in some countries and regions are presented in Table 5.

Table 5. Occupational exposure limits and guidelines for hydrochloric acid/hydrogen chloride

Country or region	Year	Concentration (mg/m^3)	Interpretation[a]
Australia	1990	7	TWA
Austria	1982	7	TWA
Belgium	1990	7.5	Ceiling
Brazil	1978	5.5	Ceiling
Bulgaria	1977	5	TWA
Chile	1983	5.6	Ceiling
China	1979	15	TWA

Table 5 (contd)

Country or region	Year	Concentration (mg/m^3)	Interpretation[a]
Czechoslovakia	1990	5	TWA
		10	STEL
Denmark	1990	7	Ceiling
Egypt	1967	15	TWA
Germany	1990	7[b]	TWA
Finland	1990	7[b]	STEL (15 min)
France	1990	7.5	STEL
Hungary	1990	5[b]	Ceiling
India	1983	7	Ceiling
Indonesia	1978	7	Ceiling
Italy	1978	4	TWA
Japan	1990	7.5	Ceiling
Mexico	1983	7	TWA
Netherlands	1986	7	Ceiling
Norway	1990	7	Ceiling
Poland	1990	5	TWA
Romania	1975	10	STEL
Sweden	1990	8	Ceiling
Switzerland	1990	7.5	Ceiling
		15	STEL
Taiwan	1981	7[b]	Ceiling
United Kingdom	1990	7	TWA
		7	STEL (10 min)
USA			
ACGIH	1990	7.5	Ceiling
NIOSH	1990	7	Ceiling
OSHA	1989	7	Ceiling
USSR	1990	5	STEL
Venezuela	1978	7	TWA
Yugoslavia	1971	7	Ceiling
		7	TWA

From Cook (1987); US Occupational Safety and Health Administration (OSHA) (1989); American Conference of Governmental Industrial Hygienists (ACGIH) (1990); Direktoratet for Arbeidstilsynet (1990); US National Institute for Occupational Safety and Health (NIOSH) (1990); International Labour Office (1991)
[a]TWA, 8-h time-weighted average; STEL, short-term exposure limit
[b]Skin irritant notation

In 1961, the US Food and Drug Administration listed hydrogen chloride as Generally Recognized as Safe when used as a miscellaneous or a general-purpose food ingredient, with the limitation that it be used as a buffer and neutralizing agent. In 1977, it was reclassified as a multiple-purpose food substance with the same limitation. In 1984, it was also regulated as a food additive to be used to modify food starch and in the manufacture of modified hop extract. It was listed as an optional ingredient in the following food standards: acidified milk, acidified low-fat milk, acidified skim milk, dry curd cottage cheese, tomato paste, tomato purée and catsup (US Food and Drug Administration, 1984). Hydrochloric acid is currently approved by the US Food and Drug Administration (1984, 1989, 1990) for the same uses, except for tomato concentrates (paste, pulp, purée).

The US Environmental Protection Agency has established a limit for emissions of hydrogen chloride from hazardous waste incinerators at a mass rate of 4 pounds (1.8 kg) per hour or 1% of the hydrogen chloride entering the pollution control equipment (Shanklin et al., 1990).

2. Studies of Cancer in Humans

2.1 Cohort studies

In a follow-up study of workers with potential exposure to acrylamide in four US chemical plants, Collins et al. (1989) reported an excess of lung cancer at one of the facilities studied. The excess was due partly to an increased number of lung cancer deaths (11) observed among men who had worked in a muriatic acid (hydrochloric acid) department. [The Working Group noted that the expected numbers were not reported.]

In the study of Beaumont et al. (1987) of 1165 male workers employed in 1940–64 in three US steel-pickling operations for at least six months (described in detail on p. 83), a subset of 189 workers had been exposed to mists of acids other than sulfuric, which were primarily of hydrochloric acid. An excess risk for lung cancer was seen (standardized mortality ratio [SMR], 2.24 [95% confidence interval (CI), 1.02–4.25]; 9 deaths). The excess persisted for workers who had been employed in 1950–54 when other steelworkers were used as a control for socioeconomic and life-style factors such as smoking (SMR, 2.00; 95% CI, 1.06–3.78).

In the study by Steenland et al. (1988) of the same cohort (described on pp. 83–84), an excess of incident cases of laryngeal cancer was observed in steel picklers ([relative risk, 2.6; 95% CI, 1.2–5.0]; 9 cases). Two of the cases had been exposed only to acids other than sulfuric, and three had been exposed to a mixture of acids. [The Working Group noted that confounding by exposure to sulfuric acid could not be ruled out.]

2.2 Case–control studies

A case–control study of primary intracranial neoplasms conducted at a US chemical plant (Bond et al., 1983), described in detail on p. 161, found no association with any exposure to hydrogen chloride (odds ratio, 1.40; 90% CI, 0.70–2.80, using the first control group; odds ratio, 1.02; 90% CI, 0.81–1.29, using the second control group). The odds ratio for exposure to hydrogen chloride for people who had been employed for 1–4 years was 2.02 (90% CI, 0.5–8.1); no association was seen for individuals who had been employed for > 20 years.

In a case–control study of renal cancer (Bond et al., 1985, see pp. 161–162), the odds ratios for exposure to hydrogen chloride were 0.90 (90% CI, 0.44–1.83) in comparison with the first control group and 0.86 (90% CI, 0.40–1.86) in comparison with the second (12 cases).

A case–control study of lung cancer, nested in a cohort of 19 608 men employed at a Dow chemical plant (Bond et al., 1986), is described in detail in the monograph on sulfur dioxide (p. 162). The risk associated with exposure to hydrogen chloride was 1.02 (95% CI, 0.77–1.35; 129 cases); the risk was essentially the same when exposures that had occurred within 15 years of the date of death of the cases were ignored (0.92; 95% CI, 0.68–1.24; 108 cases). The work histories of the 308 cases of lung cancer and 616 controls in this study were augmented with 8-h time-weighted average exposures to hydrochloric acid for each job (0, 0.2–0.3 ppm [0.3–0.5 mg/m^3], 0.9–2.0 ppm [1.3–3.0 mg/m^3] and 2.2–5.1 ppm [3.3–7.6 mg/m^3]) (Bond et al., 1991), and several exposure measures were developed: duration of exposure, a cumulative exposure score, highest average exposure category achieved during a career. In addition, a latency analysis was done excluding all exposures that had occurred within 15 years of the death of the worker. Smoking histories were available for about 71% of the cases and 76% of the controls, based on telephone interviews conducted with the subjects themselves or with a proxy. Calculation of Mantel–Haenszel adjusted relative risks revealed no association between any of the measures of exposure used and lung cancer. [The Working Group noted that the methods used may not have been optimal.]

In the population-based case–control study of Siemiatycki (1991), described in detail on p. 95, no association was found between all cancers of the lung and exposure to hydrogen chloride (7% life-time prevalence of exposure for the population). The odds ratio for oat-cell carcinoma of the lung in exposed workers was 1.6 (19 cases; 90% CI, 1.0–2.6); for workers exposed at the substantial level, the odds ratio was 2.1 (8 cases; 90% CI, 1.0–4.5). In an analysis restricted to the French-Canadian subset of the study population and population controls, the odds ratio for non-Hodgkin's lymphoma was 1.6 (90% CI, 1.0–2.5; 18 cases), and that for rectal cancer was 1.9 (90% CI, 1.1–3.4; 18 cases).

3. Studies of Cancer in Experimental Animals

3.1 Inhalation exposure

Rat: Three groups of 100 male Sprague–Dawley rats, nine weeks old, were unexposed (colony controls), exposed by inhalation to air (air controls) or exposed to 10.0 ± 1.7 (standard deviation) ppm [14.9 ± 2.5 mg/m^3] hydrogen chloride (purity, 99.0%) for 6 h per day on five days per week for life (maximum, 128 weeks). Mortality did not differ significantly between the treated and the air control groups (*t* test). No preoplastic or neoplastic nasal lesion was observed in any group, but hyperplasia of the larynx and trachea was observed in treated animals (22/99 and 26/99, respectively). Tumour responses were similar in the treated and control groups, the total incidences of tumours at various sites being 19/99, 25/99 and 24/99 in treated, air control and colony control animals, respectively (Sellakumar et al., 1985). [The Working Group noted that the experiment was not designed to test the carcinogenicity of hydrogen chloride and that higher doses might have been tolerated.]

3.2 Administration with a known carcinogen

Rat: Five groups of 100 male Sprague-Dawley rats, nine weeks old, were exposed by inhalation for 6 h per day on five days per week for life (128 weeks) to: (i) a mixture of 15.2

ppm [18.7 mg/m^3] formaldehyde [purity unspecified] and 9.9 ppm [14.8 mg/m^3] hydrogen chloride (purity, 99.0%), premixed before entry into the inhalation chamber (average concentration of bis(chloromethyl)ether, which can form from hydrogen chloride and formaldehyde in moist air (see IARC, 1987), < 1 ppb [4.7 µg/m^3]) (Group 1); (ii) a combination of 14.9 ppm [18.3 mg/m^3] formaldehyde and 9.7 ppm [14.5 mg/m^3] hydrogen chloride, mixed after entry into the inlet of the inhalation chamber (Group 2); (iii) 14.8 ppm [18.2 mg/m^3] formaldehyde (Group 3); (iv) 10.0 ppm [14.9 mg/m^3] hydrogen chloride (Group 4); or (v) air (sham-exposed controls; Group 5). A comparable group of rats (Group 6) served as unexposed colony controls. From week 32, mortality in Group 1 was significantly higher ($p < 0.05$; t test) than that in groups 2–4. Tumours of the nasal mucosa occurred only in groups exposed to formaldehyde (groups 1–3), the numbers of tumour-bearing rats being 56/100 (13 papillomas/polyps, 45 squamous-cell carcinomas, one adenocarcinoma and one fibrosarcoma) in Group 1, 39/100 (11 papillomas or polyps, 27 squamous-cell carcinomas and two adenocarcinomas) in Group 2 and 48/100 (10 papillomas or polyps, 38 squamous-cell carcinomas, one fibrosarcoma and one mixed carcinoma) in Group 3. The average latency to tumour appearance was 603–645 days, and there was no remarkable difference among the groups. Statistical analysis of the tumour response (Peto's log rank test) revealed a significantly increased response in Group 1 as compared to Group 2 ($p < 0.001$) and as compared to Group 3 ($p < 0.025$). The authors suggested that formation of alkylating agents by the reaction between hydrogen chloride and formaldehyde was a possible explanation for the higher incidence in Group 1. Tumour response in organs other than the nose did not differ significantly between treated and control groups: the total incidences of tumours at other sites in groups 1–6 were 22/100, 12/100, 10/100, 19/99, 25/99 and 24/99, respectively [statistical method unspecified] (Sellakumar et al., 1985).

4. Other Relevant Data

4.1 Absorption, distribution, metabolism and excretion

4.1.1 *Humans*

Because it is highly soluble in water, hydrogen chloride is normally deposited in the nose and other regions of the upper respiratory tract. By analogy to sulfur dioxide (see p. 96), deeper penetration into the respiratory tract can be expected at high ventilation rates. As with aerosols in general, air flow velocity and the aerodynamic diameter of the particles are important determinants of the deposition of hydrogen chloride aerosols. The acidity within the mucous lining of the respiratory tract may be neutralized, as with sulfuric acid.

Hydrochloric acid is a normal constituent of human gastric juice, in which it plays an important physiological role. The healthy stomach is adapted to deal with the potentially damaging effects of exposure to the acid. The toxicity of hydrochloric acid after inhalation or ingestion is due to local effects on the mucous membranes at the site of absorption. Absorption, distribution, metabolism and excretion of acids and chloride ions have not been studied in relation to toxicology, but these processes are well known from human physiology.

Ingestion by healthy volunteers of hydrochloric acid at 50 mM/day for four days resulted in a fall in blood and urinary urea, with a concomitant rise in urinary excretion of ammonia (Fine et al., 1977).

4.1.2 *Experimental systems*

The absorption, distribution and excretion of hydrochloric acid are similar in humans and other mammals. Following intravenous infusion of 0.15 M hydrochloric acid into rats [50 ml/kg bw per hour] and dogs (20 ml/kg bw per hour), urinary excretion of the chloride ion was increased in both species (Kotchen *et al.*, 1980).

4.2 Toxic effects

4.2.1 *Humans*

Effects of industrial exposures were summarized by Fernandez-Conradi (1983). Exposure to hydrochloric acid can produce burns on the skin and mucous membranes, the severity of which is related to the concentration of the solution. Subsequently, ulceration may occur, followed by keloid and retractile scarring. Contact with the eyes may produce reduced vision or blindness. Frequent contact with aqueous solutions of hydrochloric acid may lead to dermatitis. Vapours of hydrogen chloride are irritating to the respiratory tract, causing laryngitis, glottic oedema, bronchitis, pulmonary oedema and death. Dental decay, with changes in tooth structure, yellowing, softening and breaking of teeth, and related digestive diseases are frequent after exposures to hydrochloric acid.

Kamrin (1991) estimated that the no-effect level for respiratory effects in humans would be 0.2–10 ppm [0.3–14.9 mg/m^3]. Respiratory symptoms were reported in 170 fire fighters who were exposed to hydrogen chloride produced during thermal degradation of polyvinyl chloride. [The Working Group noted that other chemicals were present.] The symptoms included chest discomfort and dyspnoea. One fatal case was reported, and post-mortem examination demonstrated severe pulmonary haemorrhage, oedema and pneumonitis (Dyer & Esch, 1976).

In one of eight asthmatic volunteers exposed to an aerosol of unbuffered hydrochloric acid at pH 2 for 3 min during tidal breathing, airway resistance was increased by 50%. Bronchoconstriction was increased in all eight subjects after inhalation of a mixture of hydrochloric acid and glycine at pH 2 (Fine *et al.*, 1987).

Dental erosion of the incisors was observed in 90% of picklers in a zinc galvanizing plant in the Netherlands, who spent 27% of their time in air containing concentrations of hydrogen chloride above the exposure limit (7 mg/m^3) (Remijn *et al.*, 1982).

Dysphagia and transient ulceration of the oesophagus with luminal narrowing are usually observed following ingestion of hydrochloric acid (Marion *et al.*, 1978; Zamir *et al.*, 1985; Subbarao *et al.*, 1988).

4.2.2 *Experimental systems*

Application of 10 µl hydrochloric acid to the cornea of rabbits caused desquamation of the surface epithelial cells at concentrations of ≥ 0.001 N (Brewitt & Honegger, 1979).

A decreased respiratory rate was observed in Swiss Webster mice exposed to hydrogen chloride at concentrations above 99 ppm [148 mg/m^3] in a study of exposure to 40–943 ppm (60–1405 mg/m^3). The return to control values was slow after exposure to 245 ppm [365 mg/m^3] and above (Barrow *et al.*, 1977).

The 30-min LC$_{50}$s for gaseous hydrogen chloride were estimated to be about 4700 ppm [7000 mg/m^3] for rats and 2600 ppm [3870 mg/m^3] for mice and those for aerosols of hydrogen chloride to be about 5700 ppm [8500 mg/m^3] for rats and 2100 ppm [3130 mg/m^3] for mice. Moderate to severe alveolar emphysema, atelectasia and oedema of the lung were observed (Darmer et al., 1974). All of a group of Swiss Webster mice died or were found moribund after exposure to hydrogen chloride at 304 ppm [453 mg/m^3], which is near the concentration that reduces the respiratory rate by 50% (309 ppm [460 mg/m^3]), for 6 h per day for three days. Respiratory epithelial exfoliation, erosion, ulceration, necrosis and less pronounced lesions in the olfactory epithelium were observed (Buckley et al., 1984).

No pathological change or change in respiratory parameters was seen in guinea-pigs exposed to hydrogen chloride at 15 mg/m^3 for 2 h per day on five days per week for seven weeks, compared to control animals (Oddoy et al., 1982). In guinea-pigs exposed by inhalation to hydrogen chloride at 1309–5708 ppm [1950–8505 mg/m^3], the LC_{50} for a 30-min exposure was about 2500 ppm [3800 mg/m^3] (Kirsch & Drabke, 1982).

In rabbits and guinea-pigs exposed to 0.05–20.5 mg/l [50–20 500 mg/m^3] hydrogen chloride for periods of 5 min to 120 h, the lethal dose after 30 min of exposure was 6.5 mg/l [6500 mg/m^3]; that after 2–6 h of exposure was 1 mg/l [1000 mg/m^3]. The highest non-lethal dose for 5 min was 5.5 mg/l [5500 mg/m^3], and that for five daily 6-h exposures was 0.1 mg/l [100 mg/m^3] (Machle et al., 1942).

Three weeks after intratracheal instillation of 0.5 ml of 0.08 N hydrochloric acid into hamsters, a significant increase in secretory-cell metaplasia was observed in the bronchi, evaluated by estimating the amount of secretory product in the airway epithelium on histological slides (Christensen et al., 1988).

Intratracheal instillation of a single dose of 0.1 N hydrochloric acid (1–3 ml/kg bw) into dogs increased mortality, lung weight and related histological changes; instillation of 2–3 ml/kg bw usually caused a fall in arterial pO_2 and lethality (Greenfield et al., 1969). Similar histological findings were reported in rabbits 4 h after instillation of hydrochloric acid (pH 1.5, 2 ml/kg bw) (Dodd et al., 1976). Instillation of hydrochloric acid (pH 1.6) at 25 meq/l into the oesophagus of sodium phenobarbital-anaesthetized dogs induced tritiated thymidine uptake and mitosis in the oesophageal mucosa within 24 h. This concentration was not sufficient to provoke erosion, ulceration or leukocytic infiltration (De Backer et al., 1985).

In male adult baboons exposed for 15 min to 0, 500, 5000 or 10 000 ppm [745, 7450 or 14 900 mg/m^3] hydrogen chloride, no persistent alteration was observed in pulmonary function three days or three months after exposure (Kaplan et al., 1988).

Studies in experimental animals *in vivo* and *in vitro* have been performed to elucidate the role of hydrochloric acid in the mammalian stomach in inducing peptic ulcers and oesophagitis. Severe damage and increased permeability to H^+ ions were observed in the oesophagus of rabbits after perfusion *in vivo* with solutions of hydrochloric acid (40–80 mM/l) (Chung et al., 1975; Orlando et al., 1981; Kiroff et al., 1987). Oesophagitis was also observed in cats treated with hydrochloric acid (pH 1–1.3) for 1 h (Goldberg et al., 1969). Isolated rat stomach and duodenum treated with 20–50 mM hydrochloric acid for 10 min showed extensive damage of the basal lamina (Black et al., 1985). Oral administration of 0.35 N hydrochloric acid protected the gastric mucosa of rats against 0.6 N HCl-induced gastric lesions for 2 h. The pretreatment significantly increased prostaglandin concentrations in the gastric fundic mucosa (Orihata et al., 1989).

4.3 Reproductive and developmental effects

4.3.1 *Humans*

No data were available to the Working Group.

4.3.2 *Experimental systems*

Groups of 8–15 female Wistar rats were exposed to hydrogen chloride at 450 mg/m^3 for 1 h either 12 days prior to mating or on day 9 of gestation (Pavlova, 1976). Offspring were examined for growth and viability after birth and also underwent pulmonary, hepatic and renal tests at two to three months of age. The authors reported that the exposure was lethal to one-third of the females, and disturbed pulmonary function (decreased oxygen saturation and increased vital dye absorption), renal function (increased chloride and protein excretion) were seen in the survivors. Hepatic function was affected only in exposed animals. Postnatal mortality was increased in the litters of dams exposed during pregnancy (31.9% *versus* 5.6%), and the weight of offspring of dams treated before pregnancy was reduced at four weeks after birth. Renal function was disturbed (increased diuresis and decreased proteinuria in males) in the group exposed during gestation at two but not at three months of age. Increased pulmonary sensitivity was reported in male offspring of females exposed either prior to or during gestation.

4.4 Genetic and related effects (see also Table 6 and Appendices 1 and 2)

4.4.1 *Humans*

No data were available to the Working Group.

4.4.2 *Experimental systems*

Hydrochloric acid did not induce reverse mutations in *Escherichia coli* but caused mutations in L5178Y mouse lymphoma cells at the *tk* locus.

Hydrochloric acid induced chromosomal aberrations in *Vicia faba*, in grasshopper (*Spathosternum prasiniferum*) spermatocytes (by injection), in sea urchin spermatozoa and in cultured Chinese hamster ovary (CHO) cells. There was a threshold in the aberration response to increasing hydrochloric acid concentration. The effect in CHO cells was observed in the absence of rat liver S9 preparations at a nominal hydrochloric acid concentration of 14 mM (pH 5.5) but was greater in the presence of S9, when a nominal hydrochloric acid concentration of 10 mM (pH 5.8) was required (Morita *et al.*, 1989). The greater effect of pH in the presence of S9 was due to generation of substances from S9 at low pH, as demonstrated in experiments in which the pH of medium containing S9 was lowered to 0.9 and readjusted to 7.2 before the cells were exposed. A similar effect was observed in the absence of S9 in medium submitted to this cycle of pH changes with hydrochloric acid [suggesting that clastogens may be generated in serum-containing culture medium at low pH] (A.K. Thilager, reported by Brusick, 1986).

Although only results with hydrochloric acid are reported here, similar results were obtained with other inorganic acids and with acetic acid (A.K. Thilager, personal communication reported by Brusick, 1986) and lactic acid (Ingalls & Shimada, 1974), indicating that the hydrogen ion concentration is the most important factor in experiments with acids, although specific effects of cations cannot be ruled out.

Table 6. Genetic and related effects of hydrochloric acid

Test system	Result[a]		Dose[b] or pH	Reference
	Without exogenous metabolic system	With exogenous metabolic system		
ECR, *Escherichia coli*, (B/Sd-4/1,3,4,5) reverse mutation streptomycin[R]	–	0	15.0000	Demerec et al. (1951)
ECR, *Escherichia coli*, (B/Sd-4/3,4) reverse mutation streptomycin[R]	–	0	15.0000	Demerec et al. (1951)
VFC, Chromosomal aberrations, *Vicia faba* root tips	+	0	pH 4.3	Bradley et al. (1968)
*Chromosomal aberrations, *Sphaerechinus granularis* spermatozoa	+	0	pH 6.0	Cipollaro et al. (1986)
*Chromosomal aberrations, *Spathosternum prasiniferum* spermatocytes *in vivo*	+	0	pH 4	Manna & Mukherjee (1966)
CIC, Chromosomal aberrations, Chinese hamster CHO cells *in vitro*	+	+	380.0000	Morita et al. (1989)
G5T, Gene mutations, mouse lymphoma L5178Y cells, *tk* locus	(+)	+	0.0000	Cifone et al. (1987)

[a]+, positive; (+), weakly positive; –, negative; 0, not tested; ?, inconclusive (variable response in several experiments within an adequate study)
[b]In-vitro tests, µg/ml; in-vivo tests, mg/kg bw
*Not displayed on profile

5. Summary of Data Reported and Evaluation

5.1 Exposure data

Hydrochloric acid is one of the most widely used industrial chemicals. It is used in pickling and cleaning steel and other metals, in the production of many inorganic and organic chemicals, in food processing, in cleaning industrial equipment, in extraction of metals and for numerous other purposes.

Hydrochloric acid may occur in workroom air as a gas or mist. The mean concentration of hydrochloric acid during pickling, electroplating and other acid treatment of metals has been reported to range from < 0.1 to 12 mg/m^3. Mean levels exceeding 1 mg/m^3 may also occur in the manufacture of sodium sulfite, calcium chloride and hydrochloric acid, in offset printing shops, in zirconium and hafnium extraction, and during some textile processing and laboratory work.

Hydrochloric acid levels in ambient air usually do not exceed 0.01 mg/m^3.

5.2 Human carcinogenicity data

One US study of steel-pickling workers showed an excess risk for cancer of the lung in workers exposed primarily to hydrochloric acid. An increased risk for laryngeal cancer was observed in the same cohort; however, no analysis was performed of workers exposed to hydrochloric acid. None of three US industry-based case–control studies suggested an association between exposure to hydrogen chloride and cancers of the lung, brain or kidney. In one Canadian population-based case–control study, an increased risk for oat-cell carcinoma was suggested in workers exposed to hydrochloric acid; however, no excess risk was observed for other histological types of lung cancer.

5.3 Animal carcinogenicity data

In one lifetime study in male rats exposed by inhalation at one dose level, hydrogen chloride did not produce a treatment-related increase in the incidence of tumours. Hydrogen chloride was tested at one dose level in combination with formaldehyde by inhalation exposure in the same long-term experiment in male rats. Hydrogen chloride did not influence the nasal carcinogenicity of formaldehyde when mixed with it upon entry into the inhalation chamber. When the two compounds were premixed before entry into the inhalation chamber, an increased incidence of nasal tumours was observed over that seen in animals treated with the combination mixed on entry or with formaldehyde alone.

5.4 Other relevant data

In single studies, hydrochloric acid induced mutation and chromosomal aberrations in mammalian cells; it also induced chromosomal aberrations in insects and in plants. Hydrochloric acid did not induce mutation in bacteria.

5.5 Evaluation[1]

There is *inadequate evidence* for the carcinogenicity in humans of hydrochloric acid.

There is *inadequate evidence* for the carcinogenicity in experimental animals of hydrochloric acid.

Overall evaluation

Hydrochloric acid *is not classifiable as to its carcinogenicity to humans (Group 3)*.

6. References

Alphagas/Liquid Air Corp. (1991) *Specialty Gas Products Catalog*, Walnut Creek, CA, pp. 14, 129

American Conference of Governmental Industrial Hygienists (1990) *1990-1991 Threshold Limit Values for Chemical Substances and Physical Agents and Biological Exposure Indices*, Cincinnati, OH, p. 23

American National Standards Institute (1987) *Specification for Photographic Grade Hydrochloric Acid. HCl* (ANSI PH4.104), New York City

Anon. (1984a) Facts & figures for the chemical industry. *Chem. Eng. News*, **62**, 32–74

Anon. (1984b) Chemical industry statistics. 1. Statistical data of China chemical industry. In: Guangqi, Y., ed., *China Chemical Industry* (World Chemical Industry Yearbook), English ed., Beijing, Scientific & Technical Information, Research Institute of the Ministry of Chemical Industry of China, p. 497

Anon. (1986) Facts & figures for the chemical industry. *Chem. Eng. News*, **64**, 32–86

Anon. (1987) Facts & figures for the chemical industry. *Chem. Eng. News*, **65**, 24–76

Anon. (1988) Facts & figures for the chemical industry. *Chem. Eng. News*, **66**, 34–82

Anon. (1989) Facts & figures for the chemical industry. *Chem. Eng. News*, **67**, 86

Anon. (1990) Facts & figures for the chemical industry. *Chem. Eng. News*, **68**, 34–83

Anon. (1991) Facts & figures for the chemical industry. *Chem. Eng. News*, **69**, 28–69

Atochem North America (1986a) *Technical Data Sheet: Hydrochloric Acid, 20 °Baumé*, Philadelphia, PA

Atochem North America (1986b) *Technical Data Sheet: Hydrochloric Acid, 22 °Baumé*, Philadelphia, PA

Austin, S. & Glowacki, A. (1989) Hydrochloric acid. In: Elvers, B., Hawkins, S., Ravenscroft, M. & Schulz, G., eds, *Ullmann's Encyclopedia of Industrial Chemistry*, 5th rev. ed., Vol. A-13, New York, VCH Publishers, pp. 283–296

Barrow, C.S., Alarie, Y., Warrick, J.C. & Stock, M.F. (1977) Comparison of the sensory irritation response in mice to chlorine and hydrogen chloride. *Arch. environ. Health*, **32**, 68–76

BASF Corp. (1988) *Technical Bulletin: Hydrochloric Acid—Food Grade* (Food Chemical Codex III), Geismar, LA

BASF Corp. (1989) *Technical Bulletin: Muriatic Acid—20 °Be and 22 °Be Technical Grade*, Geismar, LA

---

[1]For definition of the italicized terms, see Preamble, pp. 26–29.

BASF Corp. (1990) *Technical Bulletin: Hydrochloric Acid—ACS Grade (Meets ACS and NF Specifications)*, Geismar, LA

Beaumont, J.J., Leveton, J., Knox, K., Bloom, T., McQuiston, T., Young, M., Goldsmith, R., Steenland, N.K., Brown, D.P. & Halperin, W.E. (1987) Lung cancer mortality in workers exposed to sulfuric acid mist and other acid mists. *J. natl Cancer Inst.*, **79**, 911–921

Black, B.A., Morris, G.P. & Wallace, J.L. (1985) Effects of acid on the basal lamina of the rat stomach and duodenum. *Virchows Arch.*, **50**, 109–118

Boettner, E.A. & Ball, G.L. (1980) Thermal degradation products from PVC film in food-wrapping operations. *Am. ind. Hyg. Assoc. J.*, **41**, 513–522

Bond, G.G., Cook, R.R., Wight, P.C. & Flores, G.H. (1983) A case–control study of brain tumor mortality at a Texas chemical plant. *J. occup. Med.*, **25**, 377–386

Bond, G.G., Shellenberger, R.J., Flores, G.H., Cook, R.R. & Fishbeck, W.A. (1985) A case–control study of renal cancer mortality at a Texas chemical plant. *Am. J. ind. Med.*, **7**, 123–139

Bond, G.G., Flores, G.H., Shellenberger, R.J., Cartmill, J.B., Fishbeck, W.A. & Cook, R.R. (1986) Nested case–control study of lung cancer among chemical workers. *Am. J. Epidemiol.*, **124**, 53–66

Bond, G.G., Flores, G.H., Stafford, B.A. & Olsen, G.W. (1991) Lung cancer and hydrogen chloride exposure: results from a nested case–control study of chemical workers. *J. occup. Med.*, **33**, 958–961

Bradley, M.V., Hall, L.L. & Trebilcock, S.J. (1968) Low pH of irradiated sucrose in induction of chromosome aberrations. *Nature*, **217**, 1182–1183

Brewitt, H. & Honegger, H. (1979) Early morphological changes of the corneal epithelium after burning with hydrochloric acid. A scanning electron microscope study. *Ophthalmologica*, **178**, 327–336

Brusick, D. (1986) Genotoxic effects in cultured mammalian cells produced by low pH treatment conditions and increased ion concentrations. *Environ. Mutag.*, **8**, 879–886

Buckley, L.A., Jiang, X.Z., James, R.A., Morgan, K.T. & Barrow, C.S. (1984) Respiratory tract lesions induced by sensory irritants at the RD_{50} concentration. *Toxicol. appl. Pharmacol.*, **74**, 417–429

Budavari, S., ed. (1989) *The Merck Index*, 11th ed., Rahway, NJ, Merck & Co., pp. 756, 759–760

Chemical Information Services (1988) *Directory of World Chemical Producers 1989/90 Edition*, Oceanside, NY, pp. 322–323

Christensen, T.G., Lucey, E.C., Breuer, R. & Snider, G.L. (1988) Acid-induced secretory cell metaplasia in hamster bronchi. *Environ. Res.*, **45**, 78–90

Chung, R.S.K., Magri, J. & DenBesten, L. (1975) Hydrogen ion transport in the rabbit esophagus. *Am. J. Physiol.*, **229**, 496–500

Cifone, M.A., Myhr, B., Eiche, A. & Bolcsfoldi, G. (1987) Effect of pH shifts on the mutant frequency at the thymidine kinase locus in mouse lymphoma L5178Y $TK^{+/-}$ cells. *Mutat. Res.*, **189**, 39–46

Cipollaro, M., Corsale, G., Esposito, A., Ragucci, E., Staiano, N., Giordano, G.G. & Pagano, G. (1986) Sublethal pH decrease may cause genetic damage to eukaryotic cells: a study on sea urchins and *Salmonella typhimurium*. *Teratog. Carcinog. Mutag.*, **6**, 275–287

Cocks, A.T. & McElroy, W.J. (1984) The absorption of hydrogen chloride by aqueous aerosols. *Atmos. Environ.*, **18**, 1471–1483

Collins, J.J., Swaen, G.M.H., Marsh, G.M., Utidjian, H.M.D., Caporossi, J.C. & Lucas, L.J. (1989) Mortality patterns among workers exposed to acrylamide. *J. occup. Med.*, **31**, 614–617

Cook, W.A. (1987) *Occupational Exposure Limits—Worldwide*, Akron, OH, American Industrial Hygiene Association, pp. 122, 142, 192

Darmer, K.I., Jr, Kinkead, E.R. & DiPasquale, L.C. (1974) Acute toxicity in rats and mice exposed to hydrogen chloride gas and aerosols. *Am. ind. Hyg. Assoc. J.*, **35**, 623–631

De Backer, A., Haentjes, P. & Willems, G. (1985) Hydrochloric acid. A trigger of cell proliferation in the oesophagus of dogs. *Digest. Dis. Sci.*, **30**, 884–890

Demerec, M., Bertani, G. & Flint, J. (1951) A survey of chemicals for mutagenic action on *E. coli. Am. Nat.*, **85**, 119–136

Direktoratet for Arbeidstilsynet (Directorate of Labour Inspection) (1990) *Administrative Normer for Forurensning i Arbeidsatmosfaere 1990* [Administrative Norms for Pollution in Work Atmosphere 1990], Oslo, p. 12

Dodd, D.C., Marshall, B.E., Soma, L.R. & Leatherman, J. (1976) Experimental acid-aspiration pneumonia in the rabbit. A pathologic and morphometric study. *Vet. Pathol.*, **13**, 436–448

Dow Chemical USA (1982) *Specification: Hydrochloric Acid, Technical Grade Low Colour, 22 °Baumé*, Midland, MI

Dow Chemical USA (1983) *Specification: Hydrochloric Acid, Technical Grade Low Colour, 23 °Baumé*, Midland, MI

Dow Chemical USA (1988) *Hydrochloric Acid Handbook*, Midland, MI

Dow Chemical USA (1989) *Specification: Hydrochloric Acid, Technical Grade Low Colour, 20 °Baumé*, Midland, MI

Dow Chemical USA (1990) *Specification: Anhydrous Hydrogen Chloride, Electronics Grade*, Midland, MI

Du Pont Co. (1988) *Data Sheet: Hydrochloric Acid—Technical and Food Processing*, Wilmington, DE

Dyer, R.F. & Esch, V.H. (1976) Polyvinyl chloride toxicity in fires. Hydrogen chloride toxicity in fire fighters. *J. Am. med. Assoc.*, **235**, 393–397

Eller, P.M., ed. (1984) *NIOSH Manual of Analytical Methods*, 3rd ed., Vol. 1, (DHHS (NIOSH) Publ. No. 84-100), Washington DC, US Government Printing Office, pp. 7903-1–7903-6

Fernandez-Conradi, L. (1983) Hydrochloric acid. In: Parmeggiani, L., ed., *Encyclopedia of Occupational Health and Safety*, Vol. 1, Geneva, International Labour Office, pp. 1084–1085

Fine, A., Carlyle, J.E. & Bourke, E. (1977) The effects of administrations of HCl, NH_4Cl and NH_4HCO_3 on the excretion of urea and ammonium in man. *Eur. J. clin. Invest.*, **7**, 587–589

Fine, J.M., Gordon, T., Thompson, J.E. & Sheppard, D. (1987) The role of titratable acidity in acid aerosol-induced bronchoconstriction. *Am. Rev. respir. Dis.*, **135**, 826–830

Goldberg, H.I., Dodds, W.J., Gee, S., Montgomery, C. & Zboralske, F.F. (1969) Role of acid and pepsin in acute experimental esophagitis. *Gastroenterology*, **56**, 223–230

Greenfield, L.J., Singleton, R.P., McCaffree, D.R. & Coalson, J.J. (1969) Pulmonary effects of experimental graded aspiration of hydrochloric acid. *Ann. Surg.*, **170**, 74–86

Harrison, R.M. (1990) Chemistry of the troposphere. In: Harrison, R.M., ed., *Pollution: Causes, Effects, and Control*, 2nd ed., Boca Raton, FL, CRC Press, pp. 157–180

IARC (1979) *IARC Monographs on the Evaluation of the Carcinogenic Risk of Chemicals to Humans*, Vol. 20, *Some Halogenated Hydrocarbons*, Lyon, pp. 179–193

IARC (1987) *IARC Monographs on the Evaluation of Carcinogenic Risks to Humans*, Suppl. 7, *Overall Evaluations of Carcinogenicity. An Updating of IARC Monographs Volumes 1 to 42*, Lyon, pp. 100–106, 120–122, 131–133, 143–144, 373–376

IARC (1989) *IARC Monographs on the Evaluation of Carcinogenic Risks to Humans*, Vol. 47, *Some Organic Solvents, Resin Monomers and Related Compounds, Pigments and Occupational Exposures in Paint Manufacture and Painting*, Lyon, pp. 79–123

Ingalls, T.H. & Shimada, T. (1974) pH Disturbances and chromosomal anomalies. *Lancet*, **i**, 872–873

International Labour Office (1991) *Occupational Exposure Limits for Airborne Toxic Substances*, 3rd ed. (Occupational Safety and Health Series No. 37), Geneva, pp. 222–223

Jahnke, J.A., Cheney, J.L., Rollins, R. & Fortune, C.R. (1977) A research study of gaseous emissions from a municipal incinerator. *J. Air Pollut. Control Assoc.*, **27**, 747–753

Japanese Standards Association (1982) *Japanese Industrial Standard. Methods for Determination of Hydrogen Chloride in Exhaust Gas* (Doc. No. K-0107), Tokyo

Kamrin, M.A. (1992) Workshop on the health effects of hydrochloric acid in ambient air. *Regul. Toxicol. Pharmacol.*, **15**, 73–82

Kaplan, H.L., Anzueto, A., Switzer, W.G. & Hinderer, R.K. (1988) Effects of hydrogen chloride on respiratory response and pulmonary function of the baboon. *J. Toxicol. environ. Health*, **23**, 473–493

Kiroff, G.K., Mukerjhee, T.M., Dixon, B., Devitt, P.G. & Jamieson, G.G. (1987) Morphological changes caused by exposure of rabbit oesophageal mucosa to hydrochloric acid and sodium taurocholate. *Aust. N.Z. J. Surg.*, **57**, 119–126

Kirsch, H. & Drabke, P. (1982) Assessment of the biological effects of hydrogen chloride (Ger.). *Z. ges. Hyg.*, **28**, 107–109

Kotchen, T.A., Krzyzaniak, K.E., Anderson, J.E., Ernst, C.B., Galla, J.H. & Luke, R.G. (1980) Inhibition of renin secretion by HCl is related to chloride in both dog and rat. *Am. J. Physiol.*, **239**, F44–F49

Leddy, J.J. (1983) Salt, chlor-alkali and related heavy chemicals. In: Kent, J.A., ed., *Riegel's Handbook of Industrial Chemistry*, 8th ed., New York, Van Nostrand Reinhold, pp. 231–232

Lightowlers, P.J. & Cape, J.N. (1988) Sources and fate of atmospheric HCl in the UK and western Europe. *Atmos. Environ.*, **22**, 7–15

Linde/Union Carbide Corp. (1985) *Specialty Gases Catalog*, Somerset, NJ, pp. 1–22

Machle, W., Kitzmiller, K.V., Scott, E.W. & Treon, J.F. (1942) The effect of the inhalation of hydrogen chloride. *J. ind. Hyg. Toxicol.*, **24**, 222–225

Manna, G.K. & Mukherjee, P.K. (1966) Spermatocyte chromosome aberrations in two species of grasshoppers at two different ionic activities. *Nucleus*, **9**, 119–131

Marion, L., Sanders, B., Nayfield, S. & Zfass, A.M. (1978) Gastric and esophageal dysfunction after ingestion of acid. *Gastroenterology*, **75**, 502–503

Matheson Gas Products (1990) *Specialty Gases and Equipment Catalog*, East Rutherford, NJ, pp. 28, 89–90

Morita, T., Watanabe, Y., Takeda, K. & Okumura, K. (1989) Effects of pH in the in vitro chromosomal aberration test. *Mutat. Res.*, **225**, 55–60

Nunn, A.B., III (1986) *Gaseous HCl and Chlorinated Organic Compound Emissions from Refuse Fired Waste-to-energy Systems (Final report)* (EPA Report No. EPA-600/3-84-094; US NTIS PB86-145661), Research Triangle Park, NC, Office of Research and Development

Occidental Chemical Corp. (1990) *Product Data Sheet: Muriatic Acid (Hydrochloric Acid)*, Dallas, TX

Oddoy, A., Drabke, P., Felgner, U., Kirsch, H., Lachmann, B., Merker, G., Robertson, B. & Vogel, J. (1982) Intermittent hydrogen chloride gas exposure and lung function in guinea pigs (Ger.). *Z. Erkrank. Atm.-Org.*, **158**, 285–290

Orihata, M., Watanabe, Y., Tanaka, M., Okubo, T. & Sakakibara, N. (1989) The relationship between adaptive cytoprotection and prostaglandin contents in the rat stomachs after oral administration of 0.35 N HCl. *Scand. J. Gastroenterol.*, **24** (Suppl. 162), 79–82

Orlando, R.C., Powell, D.W. & Carney, C.N. (1981) Pathophysiology of acute acid injury in rabbit esophageal epithelium. *J. clin. Invest.*, **68**, 286-293

Pavlova, T.E. (1976) Disturbance of development of the progeny of rats exposed to hydrogen chloride. *Bull. exp. Biol. Med.*, **82**, 1078-1081

Pellett, G.L., Sebacher, D.I., Bendura, R.J. & Wornom, D.E. (1983) HCl in rocket exhaust clouds: atmospheric dispersion, acid aerosol characteristics, and acid rain deposition. *J. Air Pollut. Control Assoc.*, **33**, 304-311

Remijn, B., Koster, P., Houthuijs, D., Boleij, J., Willems, H., Brunekreef, B., Biersteker, K. & van Loveren, C. (1982) Zinc chloride, zinc oxide, hydrochloric acid exposure and dental erosion in a zinc galvanizing plant in the Netherlands. *Ann. occup. Hyg.*, **25**, 299-307

Rosenberg, D.S. (1980) Hydrogen chloride. In: Mark, H.F., Othmer, D.F., Overberger, C.G., Seaborg, G.T. & Grayson, N., eds, *Kirk-Othmer Encyclopedia of Chemical Technology*, 3rd ed., Vol. 12, New York, John Wiley & Sons, pp. 983-1015

Sax, N.I. & Lewis, R.J., Sr (1987) *Hawley's Condensed Chemical Dictionary*, 11th ed., New York, Van Nostrand Reinhold, pp. 614, 617

Scott Specialty Gases (1991) *Electronic Group Catalog*, Plumsteadville, PA, pp. 36-37

Sebacher, D.I., Bendura, R.J. & Wornom, D.E. (1980) Hydrochloric acid aerosol and gaseous hydrogen chloride partitioning in a cloud contaminated by solid rocket exhaust. *Atmos. Environ.*, **14**, 543-547

Sellakumar, A.R., Snyder, C.A., Solomon, J.J. & Albert, R.E. (1985) Carcinogenicity of formaldehyde and hydrogen chloride in rats. *Toxicol. appl. Pharmacol.*, **81**, 401-406

Shanklin, S.A., Steinsberger, S.C., Logan, T.J. & Rollins, R. (1990) *Evaluation of HCl Measurement Techniques at Municipal and Hazardous Waste Incinerators* (EPA Report No. EPA-600/D-90-031; US NTIS PB90-221896), Research Triangle Park, NC, Office of Research and Development

Sheehy, J.W., Spottswood, S., Hurley, D.E., Amendola, A.A. & Cassinelli, M.E. (1982) *In-depth Survey Report, Honeywell, Incorporated, Minneapolis, MN* (Report No. ECTB 106-11a), Cincinnati, OH, National Institute for Occupational Safety and Health

Siemiatycki, J., ed. (1991) *Risk Factors for Cancer in the Workplace*, Boca Raton, FL, CRC Press

Steenland, K., Schnorr, T., Beaumont, J., Halperin, W. & Bloom, T. (1988) Incidence of laryngeal cancer and exposure to acid mists. *Br. J. ind. Med.*, **45**, 766-776

Subbarao, K.S.V.K., Kakar, A.K., Chandrasekhar, V., Ananthakrishnan, N. & Banerjee, A. (1988) Cicatrical gastric stenosis caused by corrosive ingestion. *Aust. N.Z. J. Surg.*, **58**, 143-146

US Environmental Protection Agency (1989) Method 26—Determination of hydrogen chloride emissions from stationary sources. *Fed. Regist.*, **54**, 52201-52207

US Food and Drug Administration (1984) Hydrochloric acid; proposed affirmation of GRAS status as a direct human food ingredient. *Fed. Regist.*, **49**, 17966-17968

US Food and Drug Administration (1989) Food and drugs. *US Code fed. Regul.*, **Title 21**, Parts 172.560, 172.892, 182.1057

US Food and Drug Administration (1990) Food and drugs. *US Code fed. Regul.*, **Title 21**, Parts 131.111, 131.136, 131.144, 133.129, 155.194

US National Institute for Occupational Safety and Health (1990) *NIOSH Pocket Guide to Chemical Hazards* (DHHS (NIOSH) Publ. No. 90-117), Washington DC, US Department of Health and Human Services, p. 126

US National Library of Medicine (1991) *Toxic Chemical Release Inventory (TRI) Data Bank*, Bethesda, MD

US Occupational Safety and Health Administration (1989) Air contaminants—permissible exposure limits. *Fed. Regul.*, **Title 29**, Part 1910.1000

Vista Chemical Co. (1987) *Specification Sheet: Muriatic Acid*, Houston, TX

Weast, R.C., ed. (1989) *CRC Handbook of Chemistry and Physics*, 70th ed., Boca Raton, FL, CRC Press, pp. B-94, D-198

Zamir, O., Hod, G., Lernau, O.Z., Mogle, P. & Nissan, S. (1985) Corrosive injury to the stomach due to acid ingestion. *Am. Surg.*, **51**, 170–172

DIETHYL SULFATE

Diethyl sulfate was considered by previous IARC Working Groups, in 1973 and 1987 (IARC, 1974, 1987). Since then, new data have become available, and these are included in the present monograph and have been taken into consideration in the evaluation.

1. Exposure Data

1.1 Chemical and physical data

1.1.1 *Synonyms, structural and molecular data*

Chem. Abstr. Serv. Reg. No.: 64-67-5
Replaced CAS Reg. No.: 98503-29-8
Chem. Abstr. Name: Sulfuric acid, diethyl ester
IUPAC Systematic Name: Diethyl sulfate
Synonyms: Diethyl sulphate; diethyl tetraoxosulfate; DS; ethyl sulfate

$$CH_3CH_2-O-\underset{\underset{O}{\|}}{\overset{\overset{O}{\|}}{S}}-O-CH_2CH_3$$

$C_4H_{10}O_4S$ Mol. wt: 154.19

1.1.2 *Chemical and physical properties*

(a) *Description*: Colourless, oily liquid with faint peppermint odour (Sax & Lewis, 1987; Budavari, 1989)
(b) *Boiling-point*: 208–209.5 °C (decomposes) (Sax & Lewis, 1987; Budavari, 1989; Union Carbide Chemicals and Plastics Co., 1990)
(c) *Melting-point*: −25 °C (Budavari, 1989)
(d) *Density*: 1.1803 at 20 °C/20 °C (McCormack & Lawes, 1983; Sax & Lewis, 1987)
(e) *Spectroscopy data*: Infrared and nuclear magnetic resonance spectroscopy data have been reported (Aldrich Chemical Co., 1990).
(f) *Solubility*: Practically insoluble in water, 0.7 g/100 ml at 20 °C; miscible with ethanol and diethyl ether (McCormack & Lawes, 1983; Sax & Lewis, 1987; Budavari, 1989; Union Carbide Chemicals and Plastics Co., 1990)
(g) *Volatility*: Vapour pressure, 0.19 mm Hg [25 Pa] at 20 °C (Sax & Lewis, 1987); relative vapour density (air = 1), 5.31 (Budavari, 1989)
(h) *Stability*: Decomposes to diethyl ether, ethylene and sulfur oxides at temperatures above 100 °C (Union Carbide Chemicals and Plastics Co., 1990)

(i) *Reactivity*: Hydrolyses slowly in water (about 0.05%/h) at 25 °C to monoethyl sulfate and ethanol; reacts rapidly with water or aqueous alkali at temperatures above 50 °C; forms ethyl ether by reaction with ethanol. Diethyl sulfate is a strong alkylating agent (Budavari, 1989; Union Carbide Chemicals and Plastics Co., 1990).

(j) *Conversion factor*: mg/m^3 = 6.31 × ppm^a

1.1.3 Technical products and impurities

Diethyl sulfate is available as a technical-grade product with a minimal purity of 99.5% and a maximal acidity of 0.03% (calculated as sulfuric acid) (Union Carbide Chemicals and Plastics Co., 1989). It is also available as a laboratory chemical at a purity of ≥ 98% (American Tokyo Kasei, 1988; Aldrich Chemical Co., 1990; Janssen Chimica, 1990; Riedel-deHaen, 1990) or 95% (Eastman Fine Chemicals, 1990).

1.1.4 Analysis

An analytical method for the determination of diethyl sulfate in air involves adsorption of samples on silica gel, desorbtion with acetone and determination by gas chromatography using a flame photometric detector. The minimal concentration of diethyl sulfate detectable was 0.1 ppm [0.6 mg/m^3] (Gilland & Bright, 1980). A method for the analysis of diisopropyl sulfate in air (Kingsley *et al.*, 1984) can also be used for diethyl sulfate.

In a method for the analysis of diethyl sulfate in the work place, samples are adsorbed on a porous polymer such as Tenax TA, thermally desorbed and determined by gas chromatography using either flame ionization detection or flame photometric detection. The minimal quantities detectable were 0.1 ng with flame ionization detection and approximately 1 ng with flame photometry (Düblin & Thöne, 1988).

1.2 Production and use

1.2.1 Production

Commercial manufacture of diethyl sulfate starts with ethylene and 96 wt% sulfuric acid heated at 60 °C. The resulting mixture of 43 wt% diethyl sulfate, 45 wt% ethyl hydrogen sulfate and 12 wt% sulfuric acid is heated with anhydrous sodium sulfate under vacuum, and diethyl sulfate is obtained in 86% yield; the commercial product is > 99% pure. Dilution of the ethylene–sulfuric acid concentrate with water and extraction gives a 35% yield. In the reaction of ethylene with sulfuric acid, losses can occur due to several side reactions, including oxidation, hydrolysis–dehydration and polymerization, especially at sulfuric acid concentrations > 98 wt% (McCormack & Lawes, 1983).

Diethyl sulfate is believed to be produced commercially by two companies, one in the USA and one in Japan. Annual US production is estimated at 5000 tonnes.

Diethyl sulfate is an intermediate in the indirect hydration (strong acid) process for the production of ethanol involving ethylene and sulfuric acid. The reaction of ethylene with sulfuric acid is complex, and water plays a major role in determining the concentrations of the intermediate alkyl sulfates.

---

^{a}Calculated from: mg/m^3 = (molecular weight/24.45) × ppm, assuming normal temperature (25 °C) and pressure (760 mm Hg [101.3 kPa])

$$CH_2=CH_2 + H_2SO_4 \rightarrow CH_3\text{-}CH_2\text{-}O\text{-}SO_3H$$
$$CH_3\text{-}CH_2\text{-}O\text{-}SO_3H + CH_2=CH_2 \rightarrow (CH_3\text{-}CH_2)_2SO_4$$
$$(CH_3\text{-}CH_2)_2SO_4 + H_2SO_4 \rightleftharpoons 2CH_3\text{-}CH_2\text{-}O\text{-}SO_3H$$
$$(CH_3\text{-}CH_2)_2SO_4 + H_2O \rightarrow CH_3\text{-}CH_2\text{-}O\text{-}SO_3H + CH_3\text{-}CH_2OH$$
$$CH_3\text{-}CH_2\text{-}O\text{-}SO_3H + H_2O \rightarrow CH_3\text{-}CH_2OH + H_2SO_4$$

In ethanol production, the more water present in the extracting acid, the less ethylene is absorbed to produce the initial monoethyl sulfate. In addition, the more water that is present, the more monoethyl sulfate, once formed, is converted to ethanol. Diethyl sulfate can also be removed by rapid hydrolysis with acidic water. Therefore, increasing the water content in the sulfuric acid decreases the concentration of diethyl sulfate in the acid extract. Efficient ethanol production requires use of at least 90% sulfuric acid in the absorber. For example, in the Exxon Baton Rouge ethanol plant, 98.5% sulfuric acid is used (Lynch *et al.*, 1979). Details of this industrial process are given in the monograph on occupational exposure to mists and vapours from sulfuric acid and other strong inorganic acids (pp. 43–44).

1.2.2 *Use*

Diethyl sulfate is used chiefly as an ethylating agent in organic synthesis. The principal uses are as an intermediate in dye manufacture, as an ethylating agent in pigment production, as a finishing agent in textile manufacture and as a dye-set agent in carbonless paper. Smaller applications are in agricultural chemicals, in household products, in the pharmaceutical and cosmetic industries, as a laboratory reagent, as an accelerator in the sulfation of ethylene and in some sulfonation processes (McCormack & Lawes, 1983; Sax & Lewis, 1987; Budavari, 1989).

1.3 Occurrence

1.3.1 *Natural occurrence*

Diethyl sulfate is not known to occur as a natural product.

1.3.2 *Occupational exposure*

No data on occupational levels of exposure to diethyl sulfate were available to the Working Group.

On the basis of the US National Occupational Exposure Survey, the US National Institute for Occupational Safety and Health (1990) estimated that 2260 workers were potentially exposed to diethyl sulfate in the USA in 1981–83, in textile mills and the lumber and wood industries. Exposure to diethyl sulfate could also occur during its production or its use in the synthesis of a variety of intermediates and products (Center for Chemical Hazard Assessment, 1985). Exposure to diethyl sulfate in ethanol manufacturing plants has been inferred from its presence at concentrations ~30% in acid extracts. The maximal vapour concentration over a spill was calculated as 2000 ppm [12 620 mg/m^3]. Actual exposure of workers from spills or leaks would probably be much less, because of dilution in the surrounding air.

An analysis of historical records and interviews with unit supervisors in a US ethanol production plant indicated that there was frequent opportunity for exposure to diethyl sulfate, since the equipment had to be opened often to clean sticky deposits in absorbers and extract soakers and since there was almost continual leakage from extract pump seals (Lynch *et al.*, 1979). Diethyl sulfate might be inhaled as aerosol during the opening of reaction vessels (Teta *et al.*, 1992).

Other potential exposures encountered in these processes are described in the monograph on occupational exposure to mists and vapours from sulfuric acid and other inorganic acids.

1.3.3 *Environmental occurrence*

In 1989, total air emissions of diethyl sulfate in the USA were estimated at approximately 4 tonnes from 28 locations; total land releases were estimated at 114 kg (US National Library of Medicine, 1991).

Diethyl sulfate has not been identified in the atmosphere. A study of the atmospheric chemistry of gaseous diethyl sulfate found no evidence for the formation of diethyl sulfate during the ozonolysis of olefins in the presence of sulfur dioxide and ethanol (Japar *et al.*, 1990).

1.4 Regulations and guidelines

The technical guiding concentration (TRK) of 0.2 mg/m^3 for diethyl sulfate, valid in Germany in 1985, was cancelled in 1989, and this compound was classified as III A2, compounds that 'have proven so far to be unmistakably carcinogenic in animal experimentation only; namely under conditions which are comparable to those for possible exposure of a human being at the workplace, or from which such comparability can be deduced' (Cook, 1987; Deutsche Forschungsgemeinschaft, 1989). No threshold limit value is applicable to diethyl sulfate, because it is considered to be carcinogenic in several countries (e.g., Finland, France, Sweden) (International Labour Office, 1991).

2. Studies of Cancer in Humans

2.1 Cohort studies

A historical cohort study was conducted of 335 US workers in ethanol and isopropanol units (Lynch *et al.*, 1979), described in detail on p. 81. The relative risk for developing laryngeal cancer was 5.04 [95% confidence interval (CI), 1.36–12.90], based on four cases. When the cohort was expanded to include mechanical craftsmen and supervisors, for a total of 740 men, the relative risk was 3.2 [95% CI, 1.3–6.6] based on seven cases. The ethanol process involved strong concentrations of sulfuric acid (98.5% wt), while the isopropanol process involved sulfuric acid at 'weak' concentrations (65–75 wt%). Dialkyl sulfates are generated as intermediates in these processes, but the ethanol process generated some 30 times more than the weak-acid process, owing to the use of more concentrated acid. The excess risk was determined for the two process units combined and was tentatively attributed to the dialkyl (diethyl and diisopropyl) sulfates. [The Working Group noted that the excess risk was determined over two units in which sulfuric acid was used at different concentrations.]

The mortality experience of 1031 ethanol and isopropanol process workers in two plants in the USA (Teta *et al.*, 1992) was determined as an extension to the study by Weil *et al.* (1952) (described on pp. 80–82). The mortality patterns of the combined cohort of strong-acid workers were markedly different from those of weak-acid workers, among whom no cancer death was seen. In the strong-acid group, two laryngeal cancers and three buccal cavity and pharyngeal cancers were observed, giving elevated but nonsignificant standardized mortality ratios; mortality from lung cancer was not increased. The authors recognized the lack of power in their study to detect significant effects.

2.2 Case–control studies

A nested case-control study comprising 17 glioma deaths and six controls each was conducted among workers in a US petrochemical plant in 1950–77 (Leffingwell *et al.*, 1983). Controls without cancer were individually matched on race, sex and year of birth (within three years); the year of first employment for each control was not earlier than three years before that of the case; the date of last employment was later for controls than for the case. Possible associations between gliomas of the brain and job title, employment history by department, history of chemical exposure, location within the plant, dates of employment and residence were examined. Estimated exposure to diethyl sulfate gave an odds ratio of 2.10 (90% CI, 0.57–7.73); duration of exposure was not related to disease status. In a parallel analysis of 21 brain tumours [including the 17 gliomas studied by Leffingwell *et al.* (1983)], which used a different series of controls, the proportion of cases exposed was similar to that of controls (Austin & Schnatter, 1983).

Soskolne *et al.* (1984) conducted a case–control study (described in detail on p. 89) to examine the role of exposure to sulfuric acid in laryngeal cancer at the same plant studied by Lynch *et al.* (1979). They found a high correlation with exposure to sulfuric acid in any of three processes (strong-, intermediate- or weak-acid). Exposure–response relationships were seen. Similar results were obtained even after exclusion of those cases studied by Lynch *et al.* (1979) that were associated with the ethanol and isopropanol units. [The Working Group noted that this finding supports the role of sulfuric acid independent of dialkyl sulfates; however, it does not preclude a role for dialkyl sulfates.]

3. Studies of Cancer in Experimental Animals

3.1 Oral administration

Rat: Two groups of 12 BD rats [sex unspecified], about 100 days old, received 25 or 50 mg/kg bw diethyl sulfate [purity unspecified] in arachis oil once weekly by gavage for 81 weeks (total dose, 1.9 or 3.7 g/kg bw) and were observed until death [time of death unspecified]. One squamous-cell carcinoma of the forestomach was found in each group, and 6/24 rats [distribution of tumours by group unspecified] had a number of benign papillomas of the forestomach (Druckrey *et al.*, 1970). [The Working Group noted the small number of animals used and the absence of a concurrent control group.]

3.2 Subcutaneous administration

Rat: Two groups of 12 BD rats [sex unspecified], about 100 days old, received subcutaneous injections of 25 or 50 mg/kg bw diethyl sulfate [purity unspecified] in arachis oil (concentrations, 1.25 or 2.50%) once weekly for 49 weeks (total dose, 0.8 or 1.6 g/kg bw) and were observed until death (295–685 days). Local tumours (three spindle-cell sarcomas, three fibrosarcomas, three myosarcomas, one polymorphocellular sarcoma and one glandular carcinoma of unknown origin) developed at the site of injection in the 11 surviving rats in the high-dose group during a mean survival time of 350 ± 50 (standard deviation) days (one rat in this group died prematurely from pneumonia). Two cases of metastasis to the lungs occurred. Local tumours (three fibrosarcomas, two spindle-cell sarcomas, one myosarcoma) developed at the site of injection in 6/12 rats in the low-dose group, during an average survival period of 415 days [standard deviation unspecified] (Druckrey *et al.*, 1970). [The Working Group noted the absence of a concurrent control group and that historical vehicle controls had no local tumour even when injected subcutaneously with high doses of the vehicle.]

3.3 Other experimental systems

Rat: A single subcutaneous injection of 85 mg/kg bw (25% of LD_{50}) diethyl sulfate [purity unspecified; vehicle most probably arachis oil] was given to three pregnant BD rats [age unspecified] on day 15 of gestation. One of the rats died with multiple mammary gland carcinomas at the age of 742 days. Thirty offspring [sex unspecified] were observed until death; two developed malignant neurinomas, one of the cauda equina (in a rat found dead at the age of 285 days) and one of the lumbal nerve (in a rat dead at day 541). Spontaneous tumours of this type had not been observed in untreated historical control BD rats (Druckrey *et al.*, 1970). [The Working Group noted the small number of pregnant females treated and the absence of a concurrent control group.]

4. Other Relevant Data

4.1 Absorption, distribution, metabolism and excretion

4.1.1 *Humans*

No data were available to the Working Group

4.1.2 *Experimental systems*

After male CFE albino rats were administered 1 ml of a 5% (v/v) solution of diethyl sulfate in arachis oil by gavage or by intraperitoneal or subcutaneous injection, ethylmercapturic acid and a sulfoxide were identified as metabolites (Kaye, 1974).

4.2 Toxic effects

4.2.1 *Humans*

No data were available to the Working Group.

DIETHYL SULFATE

4.2.2 *Experimental systems*

The LD$_{50}$s of diethyl sulfate have been summarized as 150 mg/kg bw by intraperitoneal injection in mice, 350 mg/kg bw by subcutaneous injection in rats, 350–1000 mg/kg bw by oral administration in rats, and 600 mg/kg bw by percutaneous administration in rabbits (Druckrey *et al.*, 1970; Deutsche Forschungsgemeinschaft, 1990).

Diethyl sulfate is a strong skin irritant (Sax & Lewis, 1987; Deutsche Forschungsgemeinschaft, 1990).

4.3 Reproductive and developmental effects

4.3.1 *Humans*

No data were available to the Working Group.

4.3.2 *Experimental systems*

In a mammalian spot test, C57 × T-stock mice were treated intraperitoneally with 0–225 mg/kg bw diethyl sulfate on day 10.25 of gestation. No effect on litter size at birth was noted (Braun *et al.*, 1984).

4.4 Genetic and related effects (see also Table 1 and Appendices 1 and 2)

4.4.1 *Humans*

No data were available to the Working Group.

4.4.2 *Experimental systems*

The genetic effects of diethyl sulfate have been reviewed (Hoffmann, 1980). It reacts with DNA *in vitro* to produce, primarily, ethylation at the *N*7 position of guanine (Lawley, 1966). It induced SOS repair and forward and reverse mutations in bacteria and mitotic recombination and mutation in *Saccharomyces cerevisiae*.

Diethyl sulfate induced unscheduled DNA synthesis in pollen of *Petunia hybrida*. It induced chromosomal aberrations in meiotic cells and chlorophyll mutations in rice, ring chromosomes in *Allium sativum* root tips and anaphase and telophase aberrations in *Papaver somniferum* root meristemic cells.

Sex-linked recessive lethal mutations were induced in *Drosophila melanogaster* after larval feeding and after exposure to diethyl sulfate vapour. Larval feeding of this compound induced crossing-over and autosomal recessive lethal mutations, but it did not induce reciprocal translocations between the second and third chromosomes in male *D. melanogaster*.

Diethyl sulfate induced DNA single-strand breaks in Chinese hamster ovary (CHO) cells and unscheduled DNA synthesis in primary cultures of adult rat hepatocytes. Mutations were induced at the *hprt* and Na$^+$/K$^+$ ATPase loci in CHO cells and Chinese hamster lung (V79) cells. Diethyl sulfate induced sister chromatid exchange in V79 cells. It induced alkali-labile sites, numerical and structural aberrations and micronuclei in cultured human lymphocytes.

Micronucleated erythrocytes were induced in larvae of newts (*Pleurodeles waltl*) treated with diethyl sulfate. In mice, diethyl sulfate alkylated DNA to produce mainly

Table 1. Genetic and related effects of diethyl sulfate

Test system	Result[a] Without exogenous metabolic system	Result[a] With exogenous metabolic system	Dose[b] LED/HID	Reference
PRB, SOS functions, *Escherichia coli*	+	0	40.0000	Barbé et al. (1983)
PRB, SOS functions, *Escherichia coli*	+	0	1170.0000	Vericat et al. (1986)
PRB, SOS functions, *Escherichia coli*	+	0	30.0000[c]	de Oliveira et al. (1986)
PRB, *umu* test, *Salmonella typhimurium* TA1535/pSK1002	0	+	0.2000	Nakamura et al. (1987)
SAF, *Salmonella typhimurium* SV50 (Ara[r]), forward mutation	+	0	75.0000	Xu et al. (1984)
SAF, *Salmonella typhimurium* BA13 (Ara[r]), forward mutation	+	0	154.0000	Roldán-Arjona et al. (1990)
SAF, *Salmonella typhimurium* TM677, forward mutation	+	0	65.0000	Skopek & Thilly (1983)
ECK, *Escherichia coli* K12–343/113, forward mutation	+	0	308.0000	Mohn & van Zeeland (1985)
SA0, *Salmonella typhimurium* TA100, reverse mutation	+	0	0.0000	McCann et al. (1975)
SA0, *Salmonella typhimurium* TA100, reverse mutation	+	+	2500.0000[c]	Waskell (1978)
SA0, *Salmonella typhimurium* TA100, reverse mutation	+	0[d]	0.0000	Probst et al. (1981)
SA5, *Salmonella typhimurium* TA1535, reverse mutation	+	0	0.0000	McCann et al. (1975)
SA9, *Salmonella typhimurium* TA98, reverse mutation	–	–	2500.0000[c]	Waskell (1978)
SAS, *Salmonella typhimurium* TA97, reverse mutation	+	0	5000.0000[c]	Levin et al. (1982)
SAS, *Salmonella typhimurium* TS1121, reverse mutation	+	0	600.0000	Hoffmann et al. (1988)
SAS, *Salmonella typhimurium* TS1157, reverse mutation	+	0	600.0000	Hoffmann et al. (1988)
SAS, *Salmonella typhimurium* TA90, reverse mutation	+	0	5000.0000	Levin et al. (1982)
SAS, *Salmonella typhimurium* TA2637, reverse mutation	–	0	5000.0000	Levin et al. (1982)
SA7, *Salmonella typhimurium* TA1537, reverse mutation	+	0	2500.0000	Levin et al. (1982)
SA8, *Salmonella typhimurium* TA1538, reverse mutation	–	0	2500.0000	Levin et al. (1982)
SAS, *Salmonella typhimurium* TA88, reverse mutation	+	0	2500.0000	Levin et al. (1982)
SAS, *Salmonella typhimurium* TR3243 (*his* D6610), reverse mutation	+	0	5000.0000	Levin et al. (1982)
SAS, *Salmonella typhimurium hisC3076*, reverse mutation	+	0	2500.0000	Levin et al. (1982)
SAS, *Salmonella typhimurium hisD3052*, reverse mutation	–	0	2500.0000	Levin et al. (1982)
ECW, *Escherichia coli* WP2 *uvrA*⁻, mutation	+	0[d]	0.0000	Probst et al. (1981)
EC2, *Escherichia coli* WP2, mutation	+	0[d]	0.0000	Probst et al. (1981)
SCH, *Saccharomyces cerevisiae* D1, mitotic recombination	+	0	4500.0000[c]	Zimmermann et al. (1966)

Table 1 (contd)

Test system	Result[a]		Dose[b] LED/HID	Reference
	Without exogenous metabolic system	With exogenous metabolic system		
SCR, *Saccharomyces cerevisiae* D1, reverse mutation	+	0	4500.0000[c]	Zimmermann et al. (1966)
PLU, *Petunia hybrida*, Mature pollen, unscheduled DNA synthesis	+	0	15400.0000	Jackson & Linskens (1980)
ACC, *Allium cepa* root-tip cells, chromosomal aberrations	−	0	4600.0000	Gohil & Kaul (1983)
PLC, *Papaver somniferum*, chromosomal aberrations	+	0	1200.0000	Floria & Ghiorghita (1980)
PLC, *Allium sativum* root-tip cells, chromosomal aberrations	+	0	3850.0000	Gohil & Kaul (1983)
PLM, *Oryza sativa* (rice) chlorophyll mutations	+	0	600.0000	Reddy et al. (1974)
PLC, *Oryza sativa* (rice), chromosomal aberrations	+	0	350.0000	Seetharami Reddi & Reddi (1985)
DMG, *Drosophila melanogaster*, genetic crossing-over	+	0	6000.0000[c]	Pelecanos (1966)
DMM, *Drosophila melanogaster*, autosomal recessive lethal mutation	+	0	6000.0000[c]	Pelecanos (1966)
DMX, *Drosophila melanogaster*, sex-linked recessive lethal mutation	+	0	0.0000	Abraham et al (1979)
DMX, *Drosophila melanogaster mei-9¹*, sex-linked recessive lethal mutation	+	0	1500.0000[c]	Vogel (1989)
DMX, *Drosophila melanogaster, exr*⁺, sex-linked recessive lethal mutation	+	0	1500.0000[c]	Vogel (1989)
Drosophila melanogaster, sex chromosome loss	−	0	0.0000 (vapour, 5-15 min)	Abraham et al. (1979)
DMC, *Drosophila melanogaster*, reciprocal translocation 2nd–3rd chromosome	−	0	6000.0000	Pelecanos (1966)
DIA, DNA single-strand breaks, Chinese hamster ovary cells *in vitro*	+	0	154.0000	Abbondandolo et al. (1982)
DIA, DNA single-strand breaks, Chinese hamster ovary cells *in vitro*	+	0	385.0000[c]	Dogliotti et al. (1984)
URP, Unscheduled DNA synthesis, rat primary hepatocyte cells	+	0	15.4000	Probst et al. (1981)
GCO, Gene mutation (6TG^r), Chinese hamster ovary K1-BH4 cells	+	0	46.0000	Couch et al. (1978)
GCO, Gene mutation (6TG^r), Chinese hamster ovary K1 cells	+	0	154.0000	Bignami et al. (1988)
GCO, Gene mutation (Oua^r), Chinese hamster ovary K1 cells	+	0	154.0000	Bignami et al. (1988)
G9H, Gene mutation (6TG^r), Chinese hamster V79 cells *in vitro*	+	0	100.0000	Nishi et al. (1984)
G9H, Gene mutation (6TG^r), Chinese hamster V79 cells *in vitro*	+	0	308.0000	Mohn & van Zeeland (1985)
SIC, Sister chromatid exchange, Chinese hamster V79 cells *in vitro*	+	0	100.0000	Nishi et al. (1984)

Table 1 (contd)

Test system	Result[a]		Dose[b] LED/HID	Reference
	Without exogenous metabolic system	With exogenous metabolic system		
MIA, Micronucleus test, Chinese hamster V79 cells *in vitro*	+	0	154.0000	Bonatti et al. (1986)
MIA, Micronucleus test, Chinese hamster V79 cells *in vitro*	+	0	40.0000	De Ferrari et al. (1988)
MIA, Micronucleus test, Chinese hamster V79 cells *in vitro*	+	0	460.0000	Nüsse et al. (1989)
CIC, Chromosomal aberrations, Chinese hamster ovary cells *in vitro*	+	0	100.0000	Asita (1989)
DIH, Alkali-labile site, human leukocytes *in vitro*	+	0	154.0000	Schutte et al. (1988)
MIH, Micronucleus test, human lymphocytes *in vitro*	+	0	154.0000	De Ferrari et al. (1988)
AIH, Chromosomal aberrations (numerical), human lymphocytes *in vitro*	+	0	15.0000	De Ferrari et al. (1988)
CHL, Chromosomal aberrations (structural), human lymphocytes *in vitro*	+	0	154.0000	De Ferrari et al. (1988)
DVA, Alkaline elution, Sprague-Dawley rat brain cells *in vivo*	+		40.0000[c]	Robbiano & Brambilla (1987)
BVD, DNA adduct formation, mouse germ/testis/bone-marrow/liver *in vivo*	+		48.0000	van Zeeland et al. (1990)
MST, Mouse spot test, C57Bl/6 Jena × T stock *in vivo*	?		225.0000	Braun et al. (1984)
SLP, Mouse specific locus test *in vivo*	(+)		200.0000	Ehling & Neuhäuser-Klaus (1988)
MVM, Micronucleus test, ddY mouse peripheral blood cells *in vivo*	+		400.0000	Asita et al. (1992)
*Micronucleus test, *Pleurodeles waltl* larvae erythrocytes	+		6.0000 in water	Jaylet et al. (1986)
COE, Chromosomal aberrations, embryonic NMRI mouse cells *in vivo*	+		150.0000	Braun et al. (1986)
DLM, Dominant lethal test, mice *in vivo*	+		100.0000	Ehling & Neuhäuser-Klaus (1988)

[a] +, positive; (+), weakly positive; −, negative; 0, not tested; ?, inconclusive (variable response in several experiments within an adequate study)
[b] In-vitro tests, µg/ml; in-vivo tests, mg/kg bw
[c] Single dose level tested
[d] Result not clear
[e] Not displayed on profile

*N*7-ethylguanine in germ cells, testis tubuli, bone marrow and liver (van Zeeland *et al.*, 1990). Brain DNA was fragmented in male rats treated intraperitoneally with diethyl sulfate. An inconclusive result was obtained in the mouse somatic coat colour mutation test (spot test). Diethyl sulfate induced specific locus mutations in mouse germ-line cells at 200 mg/kg but not at 300 mg/kg. It induced dominant lethal mutations and chromosomal aberrations, which were mainly chromatid breaks and gaps, in mouse embryonal cells after transplacental treatment. It induced micronuclei in mouse peripheral reticulocytes.

5. Summary of Data Reported and Evaluation

5.1 Exposure data

Diethyl sulfate is manufactured from ethylene and sulfuric acid. It is used principally as an intermediate (ethylating agent) in the manufacture of dyes, pigments and textile chemicals, and as a finishing agent in textile production. It is an obligatory intermediate in the indirect hydration (strong acid) process for the preparation of synthetic ethanol from ethylene.

No data were available on levels of occupational exposure to diethyl sulfate.

5.2 Human carcinogenicity data

One cohort study at a US isopropanol and ethanol manufacturing plant revealed an increased risk for laryngeal cancer. A subsequent case–control study nested in an expanded cohort at this plant indicated that the increased risk was related to exposure to sulfuric acid; the risk persisted even after exclusion of workers in the ethanol and isopropanol units. A cohort study from two US plants producing ethanol and isopropanol suggested an increased risk for cancers of the larynx, buccal cavity and pharynx, but not of the lung, in strong-acid workers. An association between estimated exposure to diethyl sulfate and risk for brain tumour was suggested in a study of workers at a US petrochemical plant.

No measurement of exposure diethyl sulfate was available for the industrial processes investigated in the epidemiological studies. It is therefore difficult to assess the contribution of diethyl sulfate to the increased cancer risks. Furthermore, exposure to mists and vapours from strong inorganic acids, primarily sulfuric acid, may play a role in increasing these risks.

5.3 Animal carcinogenicity data

Diethyl sulfate was tested for carcinogenicity by oral and subcutaneous administration in one strain of rats. After subcutaneous administration, a high incidence of malignant tumours occurred at the injection site. Following oral gavage of diethyl sulfate, forestomach tumours were observed. A low incidence of malignant tumours of the nervous system was observed in the same strain of rats after prenatal exposure.

5.4 Other relevant data

Diethyl sulfate induced specific locus mutations in mouse germ-line cells. It was clastogenic in mice and newts, induced DNA damage in mice and rats and ethylated DNA in mice. Diethyl sulfate induced chromosomal aberrations and micronucleus formation in cultured human lymphocytes. It induced alkali-labile sites in cultured human leukocytes in one study. In cultured mammalian cells, diethyl sulfate induced chromosomal aberrations, micronucleus formation, sister chromatid exchange, forward mutation and DNA single-strand breaks; it also induced unscheduled DNA synthesis in primary cultures of rat hepatocytes. In single studies, diethyl sulfate did not induce aneuploidy or reciprocal translocation in *Drosophila melanogaster* but did induce sex-linked recessive lethal mutations and genetic crossing-over. In plant cells, diethyl sulfate induced chromosomal aberrations, mutation and unscheduled DNA synthesis. It induced reverse mutation and mitotic recombination in yeast. Diethyl sulfate induced mutation and DNA damage in bacteria.

5.5 Evaluation[1]

There is *inadequate evidence* for the carcinogenicity in humans of diethyl sulfate.

There is *sufficient evidence* for the carcinogenicity in experimental animals of diethyl sulfate.

Diethyl sulfate is a strong alkylating agents which ethylates DNA. As a result, it is genotoxic in virtually all test systems examined including induction of potent effects in somatic and germ cells of mammals exposed *in vivo*.

Overall evaluation

Diethyl sulfate *is probably carcinogenic to humans (Group 2A)*.

6. References

Abbondandolo, A., Dogliotti, E., Lohman, P.H.M. & Berends, F. (1982) Molecular dosimetry of DNA damage caused by alkylation. I. Single-strand breaks induced by ethylating agents in cultured mammalian cells in relation to survival. *Mutat. Res.*, 92, 361–377

Abraham, S.K., Goswami, V. & Kesavan, P.C. (1979) Mutagenicity of inhaled diethyl sulphate vapour in *Drosophila melanogaster* and its implications for the utility of the system for screening air pollutants. *Mutat. Res.*, 66, 195–198

Aldrich Chemical Co. (1990) *1990–1991 Aldrich Catalog Handbook of Fine Chemicals*, Milwaukee, WI, p. 461

American Tokyo Kasei (1988) *Organic Chemicals 88/89 Catalog*, Portland, OR, p. 434

Asita, A. (1989) A comparative study of the clastogenic activity of ethylating agents. *Mutagenesis*, 4, 432–436

Asita, A.O., Hayashi, M., Kodama, Y., Matsuoka, A., Suzuki, T. & Sofuni, T. (1992) Micronucleated reticulocyte induction by ethylating agents in mice. *Mutat. Res.*, 271, 29–37

Austin, S.G. & Schnatter, A.R. (1983) A case–control study of chemical exposures and brain tumors in petrochemical workers. *J. occup. Med.*, 25, 313–320

Barbé, J., Vericat, J.A. & Guerrero, R. (1983) Discriminated induction of SOS functions in *Escherichia coli* by alkylating agents. *J. gen. Microbiol.*, 129, 2079–2089

---

[1]For definition of the italicized terms, see Preamble, pp. 26–29.

Bignami, M., Vitelli, A., Di Muccio, A., Terlizzese, M., Calcagnile, A., Zapponi, G.A., Lohman, P.H.M., den Engelse, L. & Dogliotti, E. (1988) Relationship between specific alkylated bases and mutations at two gene loci induced by ethylnitrosourea and diethyl sulfate in CHO cells. *Mutat. Res.*, **193**, 43-51

Bonatti, S., De Ferrari, M., Pisano, V. & Abbondandolo, A. (1986) Cytogenetic effects induced by alkylated guanine in mammalian cells. *Mutagenesis*, **1**, 99-105

Braun, R., Hüttner, E. & Schöneich, J. (1984) Transplacental genetic and cytogenetic effects of alkylating agents in the mouse. I: Induction of somatic coat color mutations. *Teratog. Carcinog. Mutag.*, **4**, 449-457

Braun, R., Hüttner, E. & Schöneich, J. (1986) Transplacental genetic and cytogenetic effects of alkylating agents in the mouse. II. Induction of chromosomal aberrations. *Teratog. Carcinog. Mutag.*, **6**, 69-80

Budavari, S., ed. (1989) *The Merck Index*, 11th ed., Rahway, NJ, Merck & Co., pp. 493-494

Center for Chemical Hazard Assessment (1985) *Monograph on Human Exposure to Chemicals in the Work Place: Diethyl Sulfate*, Syracuse, NY, Syracuse Research Corporation

Cook, W.A. (1987) *Occupational Exposure Limits—Worldwide*, Akron, OH, American Industrial Hygiene Association, p. 256

Couch, D.B., Forbes, N.L. & Hsie, A.W. (1978) Comparative mutagenicity of alkylsulfate and alkanesulfonate derivatives in Chinese hamster ovary cells. *Mutat. Res.*, **57**, 217-224

De Ferrari, M., Bonatti, S., Pisano, V., Viaggi, S. & Abbondandolo, A. (1988) The induction of numerical chromosome aberrations in human lymphocyte cultures and V79 Chinese hamster cells by diethyl sulfate. *Mutat. Res.*, **205**, 409-414

Deutsche Forschungsgemeinschaft [German Research Association] (1989) *Maximum Concentrations at the Workplace and Biological Tolerance Values for Working Materials, 1989* (Report No. 25), Weinheim, VCH Verlagsgesellschaft, pp. 33, 68

Deutsche Forschungsgemeinschaft [German Research Association] (1990) Diethylsulfate. In: Henschler, D., ed., *Gesundheitsschädliche Arbeitstoffe, Toxikologisch-arbeitsmedizinische Begründung von MAK-Werten* [Industrial Substances Harmful to Health. Toxicological and Occupational Medical Basis for TLV Values] (Ger.), Weinheim, VCH Verlagsgesellschaft, pp. 1-8

Dogliotti, E., Lakhanisky, T., van der Schans, G.P. & Lohman, P.H.M. (1984) Molecular dosimetry of DNA damage caused by alkylation. II. The induction and repair of different classes of single-strand breaks in cultured mammalian cells treated with ethylating agents. *Mutat. Res.*, **132**, 41-49

Druckrey, H., Kruse, H., Preussmann, R., Ivankovic, S. & Landschütz, C. (1970) Carcinogenic alkylating substances. III. Alkyl-halogenides, -sulfates, -sulfonates and strained heterocyclic compounds (Ger.). *Z. Krebsforsch.*, **74**, 241-270

Düblin, T. & Thöne, H.J. (1988) Thermal desorption-capillary gas chromatography for the quantitative analysis of dimethyl sulphate, diethyl sulphate and ethylene oxide in the workplace. *J. Chromatogr.*, **456**, 233-239

Eastman Fine Chemical (1990) *Kodak Laboratory Chemicals* (Catalog No. 54), Rochester, NY, p. 268

Ehling, U.H. & Neuhäuser-Klaus, A. (1988) Induction of specific-locus and dominant-lethal mutations in male mice by diethyl sulfate (DES). *Mutat. Res.*, **199**, 191-198

Floria, F.G. & Ghiorghita, G.I. (1980) The influence of the treatment with alkylating agents on *Papaver somniferum* L., in M_1. *Rev. Roum. Biol.*, **25** 151-155

Gilland, J.C., Jr & Bright, A.P. (1980) Determination of dimethyl and diethyl sulfate in air by gas chromatography. *Am. ind. Hyg. Assoc. J.*, **41**, 459-461

Gohil, R.N. & Kaul, A. (1983) Formation of ring chromosomes by diethyl sulphate and gamma-rays. *Experientia*, **39**, 1152–1155

Hoffmann, G.R. (1980) Genetic effects of dimethyl sulfate, diethyl sulfate, and related compounds. *Mutat. Res.*, **75**, 63–129

Hoffmann, G.R., Boyle, J.F. & Freemer, C.S. (1988) Induction of genetic duplications in *Salmonella typhimurium* by dialkyl sulfates. *Environ. mol. Mutag.*, **11**, 545–551

IARC (1974) *IARC Monographs on the Evaluation of Carcinogenic Risk of Chemicals to Man*, Vol. 4, *Some Aromatic Amines, Hydrazine and Related Substances, N-Nitroso Compounds and Miscellaneous Alkylating Agents*, Lyon, pp. 277–281

IARC (1987) *IARC Monographs on the Evaluation of Carcinogenic Risks to Humans*, Suppl. 7, *Overall Evaluations of Carcinogenicity: An Updating of* IARC Monographs Volumes 1 to 42, Lyon, pp. 198, 229

International Labour Office (1991) *Occupational Exposure Limits for Airborne Toxic Substances*, 3rd ed. (Occupational Safety and Health Series 37), Geneva, pp. 158–159

Jackson, J.F. & Linskens, H.F. (1980) DNA repair in pollen: range of mutagens inducing repair, effect of replication inhibitors and changes in thymidine nucleotide metabolism during repair. *Mol. gen. Genet.*, **180**, 517–522

Janssen Chimica (1990) *1991 Catalog Handbook of Fine Chemicals*, Beerse, p. 436

Japar, S.M., Wallington, T.J., Andino, J.M. & Ball, J.C. (1990) Atmospheric chemistry of gaseous diethyl sulfate. *Environ. Sci. Technol.*, **24**, 894–897

Jaylet, A., Deparis, P., Ferrier, V., Grinfeld, S. & Siboulet, R. (1986) A new micronucleus test using peripheral blood erythrocytes of the newt *Pleurodeles waltl* to detect mutagens in fresh-water pollution. *Mutat. Res.*, **164**, 245–257

Kaye, C.M. (1974) The synthesis of mercapturic acids from diethyl sulphate and di-*n*-propyl sulphate in the rat. *Xenobiotica*, **4**, 329–336

Kingsley, B.A., Gunderson, E.C. & Coulson, D.M. (1984) Sampling and analysis of diisopropyl sulfate in air. In: Keith, L., ed., *Identification and Analysis of Organic Pollutants in Air*, Boston, MA, Butterworth, pp. 127–137

Lawley, P.D. (1966) Effects of some chemical mutagens and carcinogens on nucleic acids. *Prog. nucleic Acids Res. mol. Biol.*, **5**, 89–131

Leffingwell, S.S., Waxweiler, R., Alexander, V., Ludwig, H.R. & Halperin, W. (1983) Case–control study of gliomas of the brain among workers employed by a Texas City, Texas chemical plant. *Neuroepidemiology*, **2**, 179–195

Levin, D.E., Yamasaki, E. & Ames, B.N. (1982) A new *Salmonella* tester strain, TA97, for the detection of frameshift mutagens. A run of cytosines as a mutational hot-spot. *Mutat. Res.*, **94**, 315–330

Lynch, J., Hanis, N.M., Bird, M.G., Murray, K.J. & Walsh, J.P. (1979) An association of upper respiratory cancer with exposure to diethyl sulfate. *J. occup. Med.*, **21**, 333–341

McCann, J., Choi, E., Yamasaki, E. & Ames, B.N. (1975) Detection of carcinogens as mutagens in the *Salmonella*/microsome test: assay of 300 chemicals. *Proc. natl Acad. Sci. USA*, **72**, 5135–5139

McCormack, W.B. & Lawes, B.C. (1983) Sulfuric and sulfurous esters. In: Mark, H.F., Othmer, D.F., Overberger, C.G., Seaborg, G.T. & Grayson, N., eds, *Kirk–Othmer Encyclopedia of Chemical Technology*, 3rd ed., Vol. 22, New York, John Wiley & Sons, pp. 233–254

Mohn, G.R. & van Zeeland, A.A. (1985) Quantitative comparative mutagenesis in bacteria, mammalian cells, and animal-mediated assays. A convenient way of estimating genotoxic activiy in vivo? *Mutat. Res.*, **150**, 159–175

Nakamura, S.-I., Oda, Y., Shimada, T., Oki, I. & Sugimoto, K. (1987) SOS-inducing activity of chemical carcinogens and mutagens in *Salmonella typhimurium* TA1535/pSK1002: examination with 151 chemicals. *Mutat. Res.*, **192**, 239–246

Nishi, Y., Hasegawa, M.M., Taketomi, M., Ohkawa, Y. & Inui, N. (1984) Comparison of 6-thioguanine-resistant mutation and sister chromatid exchanges in Chinese hamster V79 cells with forty chemical and physical agents. *Cancer Res.*, **44**, 3270–3279

Nüsse, M., Viaggi, S. & Bonatti, S. (1989) Induction of kinetochore positive and negative micronuclei in V79 cells by the alkylating agent diethylsulphate. *Mutagenesis*, **4**, 174–178

de Oliveira, R.C., Laval, J. & Boiteux, S. (1986) Induction of SOS and adaptive responses by alkylating agents in *Escherichia coli* mutants deficient in 3-methyladenine-DNA glycosylase activities. *Mutat. Res.*, **183**, 11–20

Pelecanos, M. (1966) Induction of cross-overs, autosomal recessive lethal mutations, and reciprocal translocations in *Drosophila* after treatment with diethyl sulphate. *Nature*, **210**, 1294–1295

Probst, G.S., McMahon, R.E., Hill, L.E., Thompson, C.Z., Epp, J.K. & Neal, S.B. (1981) Chemically-induced unscheduled DNA synthesis in primary rat hepatocyte cultures: a comparison with bacterial mutagenicity using 218 compounds. *Environ. Mutag.*, **3**, 11–32

Reddy, T.P., Reddy, C.S. & Reddy, G.M. (1974) Interaction of certain base-specific chemicals and diethylsulphate in the induction of chlorophyll mutations in *Oryza sativa* L. *Mutat. Res.*, **22**, 127–132

Riedel-deHaen (1990) *Laboratory Chemicals 1990*, Hanover, p. 471

Robbiano, L. & Brambilla, M. (1987) DNA damage in the central nervous system of rats after in vivo exposure to chemical carcinogens: correlation with the induction of brain tumors. *Teratog. Carcinog. Mutag.*, **7**, 175–181

Roldán-Arjona, T., Luque-Romero, F.L., Ruiz-Rubio, M. & Pueyo, C. (1990) Quantitative relationship between mutagenic potency in the Ara test of *Salmonella typhimurium* and carcinogenic potency in rodents. A study of 11 direct-acting monofunctional alkylating agents. *Carcinogenesis*, **11**, 975–980

Sax, N.I. & Lewis, R.J., Sr (1987) *Hawley's Condensed Chemical Dictionary*, 11th ed., New York, Van Nostrand Reinhold, p. 395

Schutte, H.H., van der Schans, G.P. & Lohman, P.H.M. (1988) Comparison of induction and repair of adducts and of alkali-labile sites in human lymphocytes and granulocytes after exposure to ethylating agents. *Mutat. Res.*, **194**, 23–37

Seetharami Reddi, T.V.V. & Reddi, V.R. (1985) Cytogenetical effects of chemical mutagens in rice. *Cytologia*, **50**, 499–505

Skopek, T.R. & Thilly, W.G. (1983) Rate of induced forward mutation at 3 genetic loci in *Salmonella typhimurium*. *Mutat. Res.*, **108**, 45–56

Soskolne, C.L., Zeighami, E.A., Hanis, N.M., Kupper, L.L., Herrmann, N., Amsel, J., Mausner, J.S. & Stellman, J.M. (1984) Laryngeal cancer and occupational exposure to sulfuric acid. *Am. J. Epidemiol.*, **120**, 358–369

Teta, J., Perlman, G.D. & Ott, M.G. (1992) Mortality study of ethanol and isopropanol production workers at two facilities. *Scand. J. Work Environ. Health* (in press)

Union Carbide Chemicals and Plastics Co. (1989) *Product Specification Sheet: Diethyl Sulfate*, South Charleston, WV

Union Carbide Chemicals and Plastics Co. (1990) *Material Safety Data Sheet: Diethyl Sulfate*, Danbury, CT

US National Institute for Occupational Safety and Health (1990) *National Occupational Exposure Survey 1981–83*, Cincinnati, OH

US National Library of Medicine (1991) *Toxic Chemical Release Inventory (TRI) Data Bank*, Bethesda, MD

Vericat, J.-A., Guerrero, R. & Barbé, J. (1986) Effect of alkylating agents on the expression of inducible genes of *Escherichia coli*. *J. gen. Microbiol.*, **132**, 2677–2684

Vogel, E.W. (1989) Nucleophilic selectivity of carcinogens as a determinant of enhanced mutational response in excision repair-defective strains in *Drosophila*: effects of 30 carcinogens. *Carcinogenesis*, **10**, 2093–2106

Waskell, L. (1978) A study of the mutagenicity of anesthetics and their metabolites. *Mutat. Res.*, **57**, 141–153

Weil, C.S., Smyth, H.F., Jr & Nale, T.W. (1952) Quest for a suspected industrial carcinogen. *Arch. ind. Hyg.*, **5**, 535–547

Xu, J., Whong, W.-Z. & Ong, T.-M. (1984) Validation of the *Salmonella* (SV50)/arabinose-resistant forward mutation assay system with 26 compounds. *Mutat. Res.*, **130**, 79–86

van Zeeland, A.A., de Groot, A. & Neuhäuser-Klaus, A. (1990) DNA adduct formation in mouse testis by ethylating agent: a comparison with germ-cell mutagenesis. *Mutat. Res.*, **231**, 55–62

Zimmermann, F.K., Schwaier, R. & von Laer, U. (1966) Mitotic recombination induced in *Saccharomyces cerevisiae* with nitrous acid, diethyl sulfate and carcinogenic, alkylating nitrosamides. *Z. Vererbungsl.*, **98**, 230–246

DIISOPROPYL SULFATE

The strong-acid process for producing isopropanol, in which diisopropyl sulfate occurs, was evaluated previously (IARC, 1987).

1. Exposure Data

1.1 Chemical and physical data

1.1.1 *Synonyms, structural and molecular data*

Chem. Abstr. Serv. Reg. No.: 2973-10-6
Chem. Abstr. Name: Sulfuric acid, bis(1-methylethyl) ester
IUPAC Systematic Name: Sulfuric acid, diisopropyl ester
Synonyms: Di-isopropylsulphate; diisopropylsulfate; diisopropyl tetraoxosulfate; DIPS; isopropyl sulfate

$$\begin{array}{c} H_3C \\ \diagdown \\ CH-O- \end{array} \overset{\overset{O}{\|}}{\underset{\underset{O}{\|}}{S}} \begin{array}{c} \\ -O-CH \diagup \\ \diagdown CH_3 \end{array}$$

$C_6H_{14}O_4S$ Mol. wt: 182.24

1.1.2 *Chemical and physical properties*

(a) *Description*: Colourless, oily liquid (Druckrey *et al.*, 1973)
(b) *Boiling-point*: 94 °C at 7 mm Hg [933 Pa]; 106 °C at 18 mm Hg [2400 Pa] (decomposes) (STN International, 1991)
(c) *Melting-point*: –19 °C (STN International, 1991)
(d) *Density*: 1.0941 at 20 °C/4 °C (STN International, 1991)
(e) *Solubility*: 0.5% in water (Druckrey *et al.*, 1973)
(f) *Stability*: Highly reactive; degrades rapidly at room temperature, forming coloured species, followed by phase separation resulting in the formation of oligomers (Kingsley *et al.*, 1984); hydrolysed when heated to the monoisopropyl sulfate (Druckrey *et al.*, 1973). Diisopropyl sulfate is an alkylating agent (Wright, 1979).
(g) *Conversion factor*: mg/m^3 = 7.45 × ppm[a]

---

[a]Calculated from: mg/m^3 = (molecular weight/24.45) × ppm, assuming normal temperature (25 °C) and pressure (760 mm Hg [101.3 kPa]).

1.1.3 Technical products and impurities

Diisopropyl sulfate is not available as a commercial product (Kingsley *et al.*, 1984).

1.1.4 Analysis

Sampling and analysis of airborne (personal exposure) diisopropyl sulfate produced in the propylene/sulfuric acid process of isopropanol manufacture have been described (Kingsley *et al.*, 1984). The sample was collected on a solid sorbent (Chromosorb 102), with a filter to prevent the collection of sulfuric acid, and extracted with carbon tetrachloride. The sample was analysed by gas chromatography with sulfur-specific flame photometric detection. The method was shown to be applicable over a range of 0.1–10 ppm [0.75–75 mg/m^3].

1.2 Production and use

1.2.1 Production

There is no commercial production of diisopropyl sulfate as such; however, it occurs as an intermediate in the production of isopropanol.

The reaction of olefins with sulfuric acid and water *via* intermediate alkylsulfates to produce alcohols has been known since the middle of the nineteenth century. It was not until the 1920s, however, that the reaction was used commercially to produce isopropanol from propylene. In manufacturing plants, a mixture of propylene and propane is contacted in the absorber with concentrated sulfuric acid. Initially, a sulfuric acid strength of > 90% was required for the reaction to occur (strong-acid process). With time, however, it was found that the acid strength could be reduced to 65–75%, for the propylene reaction ('weak'-acid process) (Lynch *et al.*, 1979).

The reaction of propylene with sulfuric acid is complex, and water plays a major role in determining the concentrations of the intermediate alkyl sulfates.

$$CH_3-CH=CH_2 + H_2SO_4 \rightarrow (CH_3)_2-CH-O-SO_3H$$
$$(CH_3)_2-CH-O-SO_3H + CH_3-CH=CH_2 \rightarrow ((CH_3)_2-CH)_2SO_4$$
$$((CH_3)_2-CH)_2SO_4 + H_2SO_4 \rightleftharpoons 2(CH_3)_2-CH-O-SO_3H$$
$$((CH_3)_2-CH)_2SO_4 + H_2O \rightarrow (CH_3)_2-CH-O-SO_3H + (CH_3)_2-CHOH$$
$$(CH_3)_2-CH-O-SO_3H + H_2O \rightarrow (CH_3)_2-CHOH + H_2SO_4$$

The more water present in the extracting acid, the less propylene is absorbed to produce the initial monoisopropyl sulfate. In addition, the more water that is present, the more monoisopropyl sulfate, once formed, is converted to isopropanol. Diisopropyl sulfate can also be removed by rapid hydrolysis with acidic water. Therefore, increasing the water content in the sulfuric acid decreases the concentration of diisopropyl sulfate in the acid extract. The concentration of diisopropyl sulfate is reduced by approximately 85% when the sulfuric acid concentration is reduced from 97 to 84 wt%. The diisopropyl sulfate concentration of a 75 wt% propylene–sulfuric acid system is about 1% (Lynch *et al.*, 1979).

Details of the commercial process are presented in the monograph on occupational exposure to mists and vapours from sulfuric acid and other strong inorganic acids (pp. 42–43).

1.2.2 *Use*

Diisopropyl sulfate has no known industrial use; however, it occurs as an intermediate in the production of isopropanol.

1.3 Occurrence

1.3.1 *Natural occurrence*

Diisopropyl sulfate is not known to occur as a natural product.

1.3.2 *Occupational exposure*

No data were available to the Working Group on levels of occupational exposure to diisopropyl sulfate.

Exposure to diisopropyl sulfate in isopropanol manufacturing plants has been inferred from its presence at a concentration of about 20% in acid extracts obtained in the strong-acid processes and about 0.3% in the weak-acid process. The maximal vapour concentration over a spill was calculated to be 520 ppm [3874 mg/m^3] in the strong-acid process and 13 ppm [93 mg/m^3] in the weak-acid process. Actual exposures of workers from spills or leaks would probably be much less, because of dilution in the surrounding air (Lynch *et al.*, 1979). Diisopropyl sulfate might be inhaled as aerosol or vapours during periodic opening of reaction vessels and clean-out operations in these types of plants (Weil *et al.*, 1952; Teta *et al.*, 1992).

Other potential exposures encountered in these processes are described in the monograph on occupational exposure to mists and vapours from sulfuric acid and other strong inorganic acids.

1.4 Regulations and guidelines

No information on the regulatory status of diisopropyl sulfate was found by the Working Group.

2. Studies of Cancer in Humans

Fuller descriptions of the studies summarized below are given in the monograph on occupational exposures to mists and vapours of sulfuric acid and other strong inorganic acids.

2.1 Cohort studies

Weil *et al.* (1952) first raised concern by describing an excess cancer risk associated with work in a US isopropanol unit using a strong-acid process. Cancers at three sites were noted, but significance could be attached only to the few sinonasal cancers and not to the one case of lung and one of laryngeal cancer. Hueper (1966) reviewed the data of Weil *et al.* (1952) and calculated a significant, age-specific excess incidence in men aged 45–54 years, with a relative risk of 21 for cancers of the nasal sinuses and larynx combined.

A cohort study of men at an isopropanol plant in the United Kingdom was reported by Alderson and Rattan (1980). Deaths from cancer gave a nonsignificant standardized mortality ratio (SMR) of 1.45; one death from nasal cancer was seen, with 0.02 expected, and two each from lung cancer (SMR, 0.78), kidney cancer (SMR, 6.45) and brain tumour (SMR, 16.67). Only the latter was significant.

Enterline (1982), reporting on a US cohort of isopropanol workers, found an SMR for cancer of 0.99, based on 16 deaths; two of these were cancers of the buccal cavity and pharynx (0.50 expected) and seven were of the lung, to give an SMR of 1.18 (not significant). Neither of the subjects with cancers of buccal cavity and pharynx had worked with epichlorohydrin, and their high risk was attributed to employment in the isopropanol unit.

Two cohort studies (Lynch et al., 1979; Teta et al., 1992) have been described not only in the monograph on occupational exposures to mists and vapours from sulfuric acid and other strong inorganic acids but also in the monograph on diethyl sulfate. Lynch et al. (1979) demonstrated an excess risk for laryngeal cancer among workers employed in an isopropanol plant (strong- and weak-acid processes) and in an ethanol plant (strong-acid process) in a petrochemical complex. Teta et al. (1992) found no effect with the weak-acid process but found an association with work in strong-acid processes, including isopropanol manufacture (one death due to laryngeal cancer and two due to cancer of the buccal cavity and pharynx in men with fewer than five years of employment). The authors noted the inadequate power of their study.

2.2 Case–control studies

The nested case–control study of Soskolne et al. (1984), expanded from the study of Lynch et al. (1979), found an increased risk for laryngeal cancer in association with exposure to sulfuric acid and demonstrated that there was no confounding of the relationship between exposure to sulfuric acid and laryngeal cancer by employment in either an ethanol or an isopropanol unit: Similar risks were seen after exclusion of workers in these units.

3. Studies of Cancer in Experimental Animals

3.1 Subcutaneous administration

3.1.1 *Mouse*

In a screening assay for lung adenoma induction, groups of 40 A/J or C3H/HeJ mice [sex and age unspecified] received weekly subcutaneous injections of 0.025 ml undiluted diisopropyl sulfate [purity unspecified] or two parts diisopropyl sulfate plus one part diisopropyl oil [purity unspecified] for eight (A/J mice) or 13 (C3H/HeJ mice) weeks. Groups of 40 untreated mice of each strain served as controls. Survival was shorter in the treated groups than in controls. The study was terminated after 24 weeks, and lungs were examined grossly. The incidences of lung adenomas in surviving A/J mice were 9/39 controls, 11/18 ($p < 0.05$) diisopropyl sulfate-treated animals and 10/11 ($p < 0.001$) animals given diisopropyl sulfate plus diisopropyl oil; the incidences in surviving C3H/HeJ mice were 5/40 controls, 14/28 ($p < 0.01$) diisopropyl sulfate-treated animals and 10/37 given diisopropyl sulfate plus diisopropyl oil (Mellon Institute, 1985). [The Working Group noted the limited reporting of the study and the lack of data on animals that died before the end of the study.]

3.1.2 *Rat*

A group of 15 male and female BD-II rats, 100 days old, received weekly subcutaneous injections of 100 mg/kg bw diisopropyl sulfate [purity unspecified] in arachis oil for 15 weeks. Local sarcomas occurred in 14/15 treated rats, which had a mean survival time of 314 ± 24 (standard deviation) days. In a separate experiment, 15 rats received a single subcutaneous injection of 300 mg/kg bw diisopropyl sulfate in arachis oil. Sarcomas developed at the site of injection in 8/15 rats, which had a mean survival time of 476 ± 42 days. In another experiment, 5/18 rats injected subcutaneously with a single dose of 1000 mg/kg bw diisopropyl sulfate in arachis oil developed sarcomas at the site of injection, with a mean induction time of 325 days. No local tumour was found in historical control groups treated with arachis oil (Druckrey *et al.*, 1973). [The Working Group noted that concurrent control groups were not included.]

3.2 Skin application

Mouse: Groups of 28 C3H/HeJ mice [sex and age unspecified] received skin applications [dose unspecified] of a 40% solution of diisopropyl sulfate [purity unspecified] in acetone or a 40% solution of two parts diisopropyl sulfate plus one part diisopropyl oil [purity unspecified] in acetone three times a week for 14 months. A control group of 40 mice received applications of acetone only. Skin papillomas developed in 19/28 mice given diisopropyl sulfate and in 26/28 given diisopropyl sulfate plus diisopropyl oil. Skin carcinomas developed in 12/28 mice given diisopropyl sulfate alone and in 21/28 given the combination. No skin tumour was observed in controls (Mellon Institute, 1985). [The Working Group noted the limited reporting of the study.]

4. Other Relevant Data

No data were available to the Working Group.

5. Summary of Data Reported and Evaluation

5.1 Exposure data

Diisopropyl sulfate is an intermediate in the indirect hydration (strong- or weak-acid) process for the preparation of isopropanol from propylene. It has no other known industrial use.

No data were available on levels of occupational exposure to diisopropyl sulfate.

5.2 Human carcinogenicity data

An early US cohort study of isopropanol manufacture using the strong-acid process in a petrochemical plant demonstrated an excess risk for nasal sinus cancer. An increased risk for cancer of the buccal cavity and pharynx was suggested in a cohort of workers at an isopropanol unit in the USA. A cohort study at an isopropanol plant in the United Kingdom indicated an increased risk for nasal cancer (based on one case only) and for brain tumours.

One cohort study at a US isopropanol and ethanol manufacturing plant revealed an increased risk for laryngeal cancer. A subsequent case–control study nested in an expanded cohort at this plant indicated that the increased risk was related to exposure to sulfuric acid; the risk persisted even after exclusion of workers in the ethanol and isopropanol units. A cohort study from a US plant producing ethanol and isopropanol suggested an increased risk for cancers of the larynx, buccal cavity and pharynx, but not of the lung, in strong-acid workers.

No measurement of exposure to diisopropyl sulfate was available for the industrial processes investigated in the epidemiological studies. It is therefore difficult to assess the contribution of diisopropyl sulfate to the increased cancer risks. Furthermore, exposure to mists and vapours from strong inorganic acids, primarily sulfuric acid, probably plays a role.

5.3 Animal carcinogenicity data

Diisopropyl sulfate was tested for carcinogenicity by subcutaneous injection in one strain of rats and by skin application in one strain of mice. It produced local sarcomas in rats and skin papillomas and carcinomas in mice. In a screening study in two strains of mice, an increased incidence of lung adenomas was observed following subcutaneous injection.

5.4 Other relevant data

No data were available to the Working Group.

5.5 Evaluation[1]

There is *inadequate evidence* for the carcinogenicity in humans of diisopropyl sulfate.

There is *sufficient evidence* for the carcinogenicity in experimental animals of diisopropyl sulfate.

Overall evaluation

Diisopropyl sulfate *is possibly carcinogenic to humans (Group 2B)*.

6. References

Alderson, M.R. & Rattan, N.S. (1980) Mortality of workers on an isopropyl alcohol plant and two MEK dewaxing plants. *Br. J. ind. Med.*, **37**, 85–89

Druckrey, H., Gimmy, J. & Landschütz, C. (1973) Carcinogenicity of diisopropyl sulfate (DIPS) and noncarcinogenicity of monomethylsulfate in BD rats (Ger.). *Z. Krebsforsch.*, **79**, 135–140

Enterline, P.E. (1982) Importance of sequential exposure in the production of epichlorohydrin and isopropanol. *Ann. N.Y. Acad. Sci.*, **381**, 344–349

Hueper, W.C. (1966) Occupational and environmental cancers of the respiratory system. *Recent Results Cancer Res.*, **3**, 105–107, 183

---

[1]For definition of the italicized terms, see Preamble, pp. 26–29.

IARC (1987) *IARC Monographs on the Evaluation of Carcinogenic Risks to Humans*, Suppl. 7, *Overall Evaluation of Carcinogenicity: An Updating of* IARC Monographs *Volumes 1 to 42*, Lyon, p. 229

Kingsley, B.A., Gunderson, E.C. & Coulson, D.M. (1984) Sampling and analysis of diisopropyl sulfate in air. In: Keith, L., ed., *Identification and Analysis of Organic Pollutants in Air*, Boston, MA, Butterworth, pp. 127–137

Lynch, J., Hanis, N.M., Bird, M.G., Murray, K.J. & Walsh, J.P. (1979) An association of upper respiratory cancer with exposure to diethyl sulfate. *J. occup. Med.*, 21, 333–341

Mellon Institute (1985) *Results of Long-term Mouse Skin Painting and Subcutaneous Injection Tests for Carcinogenicity of Diisopropyl Sulfate and of the Sulfate in Diisopropyl Oil* (EPA/OTS; FYI-OTS-1285-0466), Washington DC, National Technical Information Service

Soskolne, C.L., Zeighami, E.A., Hanis, N.M., Kupper, L.L., Herrmann, N., Amsel, J., Mausner, J.S. & Stellman, J.M. (1984) Laryngeal cancer and occupational exposure to sulfuric acid. *Am. J. Epidemiol.*, 120, 358–369

STN International (1991) *Beilstein Database*, Columbus, OH

Teta, M.J., Perlman, G.D. & Ott, M.G. (1992) Mortality study of ethanol and isopropanol production workers at two facilities. *Scand. J. Work Environ. Health* (in press)

Weil, C.S., Smyth, H.F., Jr & Nale, T.W. (1952) Quest for a suspected industrial carcinogen. *Arch. ind. Hyg.*, 5, 535–547

Wright, U. (1979) The hidden carcinogen in the manufacture of isopropyl alcohol. In: Deichmann, W.B., ed., *Developments in Toxicology and Environmental Science*, Vol. 4, *Toxicology and Occupational Medicine*, New York, Elsevier North Holland, pp. 93–98

1,3-BUTADIENE

This substance was considered by previous working groups in June 1985 (IARC, 1986a; see also correction, IARC, 1987a) and March 1987 (IARC, 1987b). Since that time, new data have become available, and these have been incorporated into the monograph and taken into consideration in the present evaluation.

1. Exposure data

1.1 Chemical and physical data

1.1.1 *Synonyms, structural and molecular data*

Chem. Abstr. Serv. Reg. No.: 106-99-0
Chem. Abstr. Name: 1,3-Butadiene
IUPAC Systematic Name: 1,3-Butadiene
Synonyms: Biethylene; bivinyl; butadiene; buta-1,3-diene; α,γ-butadiene; *trans*-butadiene; divinyl; erythrene; pyrrolylene; vinylethylene

$$CH_2 = CH - CH = CH_2$$

C_4H_6 Mol. wt: 54.09

1.1.2 *Chemical and physical properties*

(a) *Description*: Colourless gas with mildly aromatic odour; easily liquefied (Sax & Lewis, 1987)
(b) *Boiling-point*: −4.4 °C (Weast, 1989)
(c) *Melting-point*: −108.9 °C (Weast, 1989)
(d) *Density*: 0.6211 g/ml at 20 °C/liquefied (Kirshenbaum, 1978; Verschueren, 1983)
(e) *Spectroscopy data*: Ultraviolet (Grasselli & Ritchey, 1975), infrared (Sadtler Research Laboratories, 1980; prism [893[a]], grating [36758]), nuclear magnetic resonance and mass spectral data (US National Institutes of Health/Environmental Protection Agency Chemical Information System, 1983) have been reported.
(f) *Solubility*: Very slightly soluble in water (735 mg/l at 20 °C); soluble in ethanol, diethyl ether and organic solvents (Verschueren, 1983; Sax & Lewis, 1987; Budavari, 1989)
(g) *Volatility*: Vapour pressure, 1790 mm Hg (239 kPa) at 20 °C (Santodonato, 1985); relative vapour density (air = 1), 1.87 (Verschueren, 1983)

---

[a]Spectrum number in Sadtler compilation

(h) *Stability*: Flash-point, −76 °C (Sax & Lewis, 1987); slowly dimerizes to 4-vinyl-1-cyclohexene (US Occupational Safety and Health Administration, 1990); may form peroxides upon exposure to air (Kirshenbaum, 1978)

(i) *Reactivity*: Polymerizes readily, particularly if oxygen is present (Sax & Lewis, 1987)

(j) *Conversion factor*[b]: mg/m^3 = 2.21 × ppm

1.1.3 Technical products and impurities

1,3-Butadiene is available commercially as a liquefied gas under pressure in several grades of purity, including a special purity or instrument grade of 99.4–99.5 mol% purity, a research grade of 99.86 mol% purity, a technical–commercial grade of 98 mol% purity and a rubber grade (Santodonato, 1985). Analytical, polymer, rubber and liquid grades (Aldrich Chemical Co., 1990; Kuney, 1990) range in minimal purity from 99.0 to 99.5%, with the following typical impurities: 1,2-butadiene, acetaldehyde (see IARC, 1987b), acetylenes (alpha, vinyl), propadiene, butadiene dimer (4-vinylcyclohexene, see IARC, 1986b), peroxides, sulfur and C$_5$ hydrocarbons. Oxidation/polymerization of 1,3-butadiene is inhibited by addition of hydroquinone, di-*n*-butylamine, *tert*-butylcatechol, aliphatic mercaptans or *ortho*-dihydroxybenzene (Exxon Chemical Co., 1973; Kirshenbaum, 1978; Lyondell Petrochemical Co., 1988; Budavari, 1989).

Crude 1,3-butadiene is also available from many producers for use as a feedstock. Such grades contain a minimum of 36–65% 1,3-butadiene, with specifications typically given for acetylenes, C$_3$ compounds and lighter hydrocarbons, C$_5$ compounds and heavier, peroxides, carbonyl compounds, sulfur and organic chlorides. Inhibitors (e.g., *tert*-butylcatechol, 50–200 ppm) are also added (Vista Chemical Co., 1985; Union Carbide Corp., 1987).

1.1.4 Analysis

Selected methods for the analysis of 1,3-butadiene in various matrices are listed in Table 1 (methods used previously are given in section 1.3.2).

The specificity and the detection limit of methods for determining simple, small molecules present in packaging materials which migrate into packaged goods have been discussed (Vogt, 1988). 1,3-Butadiene can be determined in plastic polymers, foods and food simulants by chromatographic methods.

Several gas detector tubes are used in conjunction with common colorimetric reactions to detect 1,3-butadiene. The reactions include the reduction of chromate or dichromate to chromous ion and the reduction of ammonium molybdate and palladium sulfate to molybdenum blue (Saltzman & Harman, 1989).

1.2 Production and use

1.2.1 Production

1,3-Butadiene was first produced in 1886 by the pyrolysis of petroleum hydrocarbons (Kirshenbaum, 1978). Commercial production started in the 1930s (Kosaric *et al.*, 1987).

---

[b]Calculated from: mg/m^3 = (molecular weight/24.45) × ppm, assuming normal temperature (25°C) and pressure (760 mm Hg [101.3 kPa])

Table 1. Methods for the analysis of 1,3-butadiene

Sample matrix	Sample preparation	Assay procedure	Limit of detection	Reference
Air	Collect on solid sorbent tube; desorb with dichloromethane; chill in ice	GC/FID	0.044 mg/m^3	Eller (1987)
	Collect on solid sorbent tube of charcoal coated with *tert*-butylcatechol; desorb with carbon disulfide	GC/FID	0.35 mg/m^3	Hendricks & Schultz (1986)
	Inject sample into GC using a temperature-programmed, fused-silica, porous layer, open tubular Al$_2$O$_3$/KCl column	GC/FID	0.01 ppm by volume (0.01 μl/l)	Locke *et al.* (1987)
	Assay directly	FT-IR	5 ppm (10 mg/m^3)	Harman (1987)
Plastics, liquid foods	Dissolve in *ortho*-dichlorobenzene; inject headspace sample	GC/FID	2–20 μg/kg	US Food and Drug Administration (1987)
Solid foods	Cut or mash sample; inject headspace sample	GC/FID	2–20 μg/kg	US Food and Drug Administration (1987)

Abbreviations: FT-IR, Fourier transform–infrared absorption spectroscopy; GC, gas chromatograph; GC/FID, gas chromatography/flame ionization detection

1,3-Butadiene has been produced commercially by three processes: catalytic dehydrogenation of *n*-butane and *n*-butene (the Houdry process), oxidative dehydrogenation of *n*-butene (the Oxo-D or O-X-D process) and recovery from the C$_4$ co-product (by-product) stream from the steam cracking process used to manufacture ethylene (the ethylene co-product process). All three processes involve the production of 1,3-butadiene from a C$_4$ hydrocarbon stream, and solvent extraction and extractive distillation are used in all three to further concentrate the 1,3-butadiene. There has recently been a shift to the use of cheaper, heavier feedstocks for ethylene production, with a concomitant increase in the volume of co-product containing 1,3-butadiene (Krishnan & Corwin, 1987). The ethylene co-product process accounts for approximately 95% of US and 85% of worldwide production (Morrow, 1990).

The production of 1,3-butadiene is thus a two-stage process: (i) production of a C$_4$ co-product during ethylene manufacture and (ii) recovery of 1,3-butadiene from the co-product. The first stage consists of cracking a hydrocarbon such as naphtha to produce ethylene as the primary product and a co-product stream composed of C$_4$ hydrocarbons. The amount of 1,3-butadiene in the co-product depends on the feedstock used and the severity of the cracking process: the heavier the feedstock and the more severe the cracking, the more 1,3-butadiene is produced. The 1,3-butadiene content of the co-product C$_4$ stream is 20–70%; the C$_4$ feed streams are usually blended with a feed stream containing 40–50% 1,3-butadiene for processing. In the extraction plants, solvents such as dimethylformamide, acetonitrile, furfural, dimethylacetamide and methylpyrrolidone are used (US Occupational Safety and Health Administration, 1990) to alter the volatility of components in a fractional distillation selectively and to produce a high purity (> 99.0%) 1,3-butadiene monomer (Krishnan & Corwin, 1987).

In 1987, worldwide production of 1,3-butadiene was approximately 5.5 million tonnes (Morrow, 1990). A more detailed accounting of the production of 1,3-butadiene in several countries in 1980–90 is presented in Table 2. Global 1,3-butadiene consumption in 1987 was estimated at 5.5 million tonnes, 1.5 million tonnes of which were used in the USA. As in most years, the US demand exceeded its supply, so approximately 227 thousand tonnes of 1,3-butadiene monomer were imported in 1987 (Morrow, 1990).

Table 2. Trends in production of 1,3-butadiene in several countries (thousand tonnes)

Country	1980	1981	1982	1983	1984	1985	1986	1987	1988	1989	1990
Canada	NA	126	118	133	127	132	146	167	182	175	192
France	259	266	258	281	303	288	291	307	335	329	281
Germany[a]	NA	NA	579	717	754	840	683	701	761	717	771
Italy	183	166	159	195	181	NA	NA	NA	NA	NA	NA
Japan	574	518	522	556	627	639	656	707	780	827	827
Mexico	17	12	15	19	20	18	18	21	12	NA	NA
United Kingdom	192	207	228	237	259	297	192	231	239	226	195
USA[b]	1270	1356	869	1068	1113	1062	1156	1329	1437	1417	1435

From Anon. (1984, 1986, 1988, 1991b); NA, not available
[a]Figures prior to 1990 are for western Germany only
[b]Rubber grade

Information available in 1988 indicated that 1,3-butadiene was produced by nine companies in Germany, eight in Japan, four in the United Kingdom and in Brazil, three in France, two in Australia, Belgium, Canada, the Netherlands and Spain, and one each in Argentina, Austria, Bulgaria, China, Czechoslovakia, Finland, India, Italy, Mexico, Poland, Saudi Arabia, Singapore, Taiwan and Yugoslavia (Chemical Information Services, 1988). It was produced by eight companies in the USA in 1991 (Anon., 1991a).

1.2.2 *Use*

1,3-Butadiene is used principally as a monomer in the manufacture of a wide range of polymers and copolymers. Polymerization of styrene and 1,3-butadiene yields styrene–butadiene rubber, the largest single use of butadiene; almost 80% of the styrene–butadiene rubber produced is used in tyres and tyre products. Polymerization of 1,3-butadiene produces polybutadiene, almost all of which used for car and bus tyres. Nitrile rubber is produced by copolymerizing 1,3-butadiene and acrylonitrile; it is used in hoses, gaskets, seals, latexes, adhesives and footwear. Acrylonitrile–butadiene–styrene resins are graft terpolymers of polybutadiene on a styrene-acrylonitrile copolymer; they are used in automotive parts, pipes, appliances, business machines and telephones. Styrene–butadiene latexes are suspensions of particles or globules of the elastomer in water and are used in paper coatings and paints and as carpet backing (Santodonato, 1985; US Occupational Safety and Health Administration, 1990).

1,3-Butadiene is used as a chemical intermediate in the production of a number of important chemicals. Neoprene is made by chlorinating 1,3-butadiene and treating the resultant chloroprene with sodium hydroxide; two-thirds of the neoprene produced is used for industrial and automotive rubber goods. Adiponitrile is produced by chlorinating 1,3-butadiene and cyanating the product to 1,4-dicyanobutene, which is then reduced to adiponitrile; this is converted to hexamethylenediamine for the production of Nylon 66. 1,4-Hexadiene, made by reacting 1,3-butadiene with ethylene, is used as a monomer for ethylene–propylene terpolymer. Sulfolane, produced by reacting sulfur dioxide and 1,3-butadiene and dehydrogenating the product, is a valuable solvent for extraction. 1,5,9-Cyclodecatriene is produced by trimerizing 1,3-butadiene and is used for the production of various nylon fibres and resins. Some other nonpolymer applications include manufacture of agricultural fungicides (captan and captafol) and anthraquinone dyes (Santodonato, 1985; US Occupational Safety and Health Administration, 1990).

In 1990, 1,3-butadiene was used in the USA for: styrene–butadiene rubber (30%), polybutadiene rubber (20%), adiponitrile/hexamethylenediamine (15%), styrene–butadiene latex (10%), neoprene rubber (5%), acrylonitrile–butadiene–styrene resins (5%), exports (4%), nitrile rubber (3%) and other (including specialty polymers) (8%) (Anon., 1991a).

(For more detailed discussions of the production and use of 1,3-butadiene, see Miller, 1978; Leviton, 1983; Greek, 1984.)

1.3 Occurrence

1.3.1 *Natural occurrence*

1,3-Butadiene is not known to occur as a natural product (Santodonato, 1985).

1.3.2 *Occupational exposure*

On the basis of a National Occupational Exposure Survey, the US National Institute for Occupational Safety and Health (1990) estimated that 52 000 workers were potentially exposed to 1,3-butadiene in the USA in 1981–83. Potential exposure to 1,3-butadiene can occur in the following industrial activities: petroleum refining and related operations (production of C_4 fractions containing 1,3-butadiene, production and distribution of gasoline), production of purified 1,3-butadiene monomer, production of various 1,3-butadiene-based rubber and plastics polymers and other derivatives, and the rubber and plastics products manufacturing industry (production of tyres, hoses and a variety of moulded objects).

In the descriptions below, the accuracy of the levels of exposure to 1,3-butadiene may have been affected by inability to distinguish between 1,3-butadiene and other C_4 compounds, low desorption efficiency at low concentrations, possible sample breakthrough in charcoal tubes and possible loss during storage, in methods used until the mid-1980s (Lunsford *et al.*, 1990). No data are available on levels of exposure to 1,3-butadiene before the 1970s, when different processes and working conditions (e.g., during the Second World War) would have resulted in exposure conditions different from those now prevalent in developed countries.

(a) *Petroleum refining and production of crude 1,3-butadiene*

Gasoline contains a small percentage of 1,3-butadiene, and exposures of workers in various job groups in the production and distribution of gasoline are shown in Table 3. Table 4 shows the exposures since 1984 of workers in different areas of petroleum refineries and petrochemical facilities where crude 1,3-butadiene is produced (usually a C_4 stream obtained as a by-product of ethylene production).

Table 3. Personal exposures (mg/m^3) to 1,3-butadiene associated with gasoline during 1984–85 in 13 European countries

Activity	Mean	Range	Exposure duration (TWA)
Production on-site (refining)	0.3	ND–11.4	8 h
Production off-site (refining)	0.1	ND–1.6	8 h
Loading ships (closed system)	6.4	ND–21.0	8 h
Loading ships (open system)	1.1	ND–4.2	8 h
Loading barges	2.6	ND–15.2	8 h
Jettyman	2.6	ND–15.9	8 h
Bulk loading road tankers			
Top loading < 1 h	1.4	ND–32.3	< 1 h
Top loading > 1 h	0.4	ND–4.7	8 h
Bottom loading < 1 h	0.2	ND–3.0	< 1 h
Bottom loading > 1 h	0.4	ND–14.1	8 h
Road tanker delivery (bulk plant to service station)	ND		
Railcar top loading	0.6	ND–6.2	8 h
Drumming	ND		
Service station attendant (dispensing fuel)	0.3	ND–1.1	8 h
Self-service station (filling tank)	1.6	ND–10.6	2 min

From CONCAWE (1987); ND, not detected; TWA, time-weighted average

Table 4. Mean 8-h time-weighted average concentrations of 1,3-butadiene to which workers in different jobs in petroleum refineries and petrochemical facilities have been exposed since 1984

Job area	No. of facilities	Mean[a]		Range	
		ppm	mg/m^3	ppm	mg/m^3
Production	7	0.24	0.53	0.008–2.0	0.02–4.4
Maintenance	6	0.11	0.24	0.02–0.37	0.04–0.82
Distribution	1	2.9	64.1		
Laboratory	4	0.18	0.40	0.07–0.4	0.16–0.88

From Heiden Associates (1987)
[a]Weighted by number of exposed workers

(b) *Monomer production*

Detailed industrial hygiene surveys were conducted by the US National Institute for Occupational Safety and Health in 1985 in four of 10 US facilities where 1,3-butadiene was produced by solvent extraction of C_4 fractions originating as ethylene co-product streams (Krishnan *et al.*, 1987). Levels of 1,3-butadiene to which workers in various job categories were exposed are summarized in Table 5. Jobs that require workers to handle or transport containers, such as voiding sample cylinders or loading and unloading tank trucks or rail cars, present the greatest potential exposure. Geometric means of full-shift exposure levels for other job categories were below 1 ppm [2.2 mg/m^3]. Short-term samples showed that such activities as open-loop sampling and cylinder voiding were associated with peak exposures of 100 ppm [220 mg/m^3]. Full-shift area samples indicated that ambient concentrations of 1,3-butadiene were greatest in the railcar terminals (geometric mean, 1.77 [3.4 mg/m^3]) and in the tank storage farm (2.12 ppm [3.4 and 4.7 mg/m^3]).

Table 5. Full-shift, time-weighted average exposure levels in personal breathing-zone samples at four US 1,3-butadiene monomer production facilities, 1985

Job category	No. of samples	Exposure level (ppm [mg/m^3])		
		Arithmetic mean	Geometric mean	Range
Process technician Control room	10	0.45 [1.0]	0.09 [0.20]	< 0.02–1.87 [< 0.04–4.1]
Process technician Process area	28	2.23 [4.9]	0.64 [1.4]	< 0.08–34.9 [< 0.18–77.1]
Loading area				
Railcar	9	14.64 [32.4]	1.00 [2.2]	0.12–123.57 [0.27–273.1]
Tank truck	3	2.65 [5.9]	1.02 [2.3]	0.08–5.46 [0.18–12.1]
Tank farm	5	0.44 [0.97]	0.20 [0.44]	< 0.04–1.53 [< 0.09–3.4]
Laboratory technician	29	1.06 [2.3]	0.40 [0.88]	0.03–6.31 [0.07–14.0]
Cylinder voiding	3	125.52 [277.4]	7.46 [16.5]	0.42–373.54 [0.93–825.5]

From Krishnan *et al.* (1987)

In 1984, the US Chemical Manufacturers' Association obtained data on personal exposure to 1,3-butadiene before 1984 from 13 monomer-producing companies, categorized broadly by job type (Table 6). These data were collected by an older method and provide a historical perspective on the data reported in Table 5. The highest exposures were in the maintenance and distribution jobs. Out of a total of 1287 samples, 91% were less than or equal to 10 ppm [22.1 mg/m^3] and 68% were less than or equal to 5 ppm [11.1 mg/m^3]. Factors that limit generalization of these data are unspecified sampling and analytical techniques, lack of detailed job descriptions and different or unspecified average times of sampling (JACA Corp., 1987).

Monitoring in a Finnish plant generally indicated ambient air levels of less than 10 ppm [22.1 mg/m^3] at different sites (33 samples; mean sampling time, 5.3 h). In personal samples for 16 process workers, the concentration ranged from < 0.1 to 477 ppm [< 0.22–1054.2

Table 6. Time-weighted average exposure to 1,3-butadiene in 13 US monomer production plants before 1984

Job area	No. of samples	Exposure (ppm [mg/m³])									
		0.00–5.00 [0–11.05]		5.01–10.00 [11.07–22.12]		10.01–25.00 [22.12–55.25]		25.01–50.00 [55.27–110.50]		50.01–100.00 [110.52–221.23]		> 100.00 [> 221.23]
		No.	%	No.	%	No.	%	No.	%	No.	%	No.	%
Production	562	446	79.4	111	19.7	5	0.9						
Maintenance	329	247	75.1			47	14.3	35	10.6				
Supervisory	64	60	93.8	4	6.2								
Distribution	206	60	29.1	121	58.7	16	7.8	5	2.4	2	1.0	2	1.0
Laboratory	126	58	46.0	68	54.0								
Total	1287	871	67.8	304	23.6	68	5.3	40	3.1	2	0.1	2	0.1

From JACA Corp. (1987)

mg/m^3] (mean, 11.5 ppm [25.4 mg/m^3]; median, < 0.1 ppm [< 0.22 mg/m^3]; 46 samples; mean sampling time, 2.5 h). The highest concentrations were measured during sample collection. Protective clothing and respirators were used during this operation (Arbetsmiljöfonden, 1991).

Potential exposure in the monomer industry other than to 1,3-butadiene includes extraction solvents and components of the C$_4$ feedstock. Extraction solvents differ among facilities; some common ones are dimethylformamide, dimethylacetamide, acetonitrile, β-methoxypropylnitrile (Fajen, 1985a), furfural and cuprous ammonium acetate (US Occupational Safety and Health Administration, 1990). Stabilizers are commonly used to prevent formation of peroxides in air and polymerization (see p. 238). No information was available on these other exposures, or on exposures to chemicals other than 1,3-butadiene that are produced in some facilities, such as butylenes, ethylene, propylene, polyethylene and polypropylene resins, methyl-*tert*-butyl ether and aromatic hydrocarbons (Fajen, 1985b,c).

(c) Production of polymers and derivatives

Detailed industrial hygiene surveys were conducted in 1986 in five of 17 US facilities where 1,3-butadiene was used to produce styrene–butadiene rubber, nitrile–butadiene rubber, polybutadiene rubber, neoprene and adiponitrile (Fajen, 1988). Levels of 1,3-butadiene to which workers in various job categories were exposed are summarized in Table 7. Process technicians in unloading, the tank farm, purification, polymerization and reaction, laboratory technicians and maintenance technicians were exposed to the highest levels. Short-term sampling showed that activities such as sampling a barge and laboratory work were associated with peak exposures to more than 100 ppm [221 mg/m^3]. Full-shift area sampling indicated that geometric mean ambient concentrations of 1,3-butadiene were less than 0.5 ppm [1.1 mg/m^3] and usually less than 0.1 ppm [0.22 mg/m^3] in all locations at the five plants.

Eight-hour time-weighted average (TWA) exposures to 1,3-butadiene in the polymer industry were obtained by personal sampling in 11 North American synthetic rubber plants in 1978–84 and reported by the International Institute of Synthetic Rubber Producers in 1984 (JACA Corp., 1987) (Table 8). The highest exposures were found for tank car loaders (15% of exposures, > 10 ppm [> 22.1 mg/m^3]), reactor operators (18% of exposures, > 10 ppm) and laboratory technicians (6% of exposures, > 10 ppm). Sampling and analytical techniques and job descriptions were not available.

Other data on levels of exposure to 1,3-butadiene have been collected during health surveys and epidemiological studies (Table 9). In a US styrene–butadiene rubber manufacturing plant in 1979, the only two departments in which levels were greater than 10 ppm [22.1 mg/m^3] were tank farm (53.4 ppm [118 mg/m^3]) and maintenance (20.7 ppm [45.8 mg/m^3]) (Checkoway & Williams, 1982). In samples taken at one of two US styrene–butadiene rubber plants in 1976, levels above 100 ppm [221 mg/m^3] were encountered by technical services personnel (114.6 ppm [253.3 mg/m^3]) and an instrument man (174.1 ppm [384.78 mg/m^3]) (Meinhardt *et al.*, 1978). Overall mean 8-h TWA exposure levels differed considerably between the two plants, however: 1.24 ppm [2.74 mg/m^3] in one plant and 13.5 ppm [29.84 mg/m^3] in the other (Meinhardt *et al.*, 1982).

Table 7. Full-shift time-weighted average exposure levels in personal breathing-zone samples at five US plants producing 1,3-butadiene-based polymers and derivatives, 1986

Job category	No. of samples	Exposure level (ppm [mg/m^3])		
		Arithmetic mean	Geometric mean	Range
Process technician				
Unloading area	2	14.6 [32.27]	4.69 [10.37]	0.770–28.5 [1.7–63.0]
Tank farm	31	2.08 [4.60]	0.270 [0.60]	< 0.006–23.7 [< 0.01–52.4]
Purification	18	7.80 [17.24]	6.10 [13.48]	1.33–24.1 [3.0–53.3]
Polymerization or reaction	81	0.414 [0.92]	0.062 [0.14]	< 0.006–11.3 [< 0.01–25.0]
Solutions and coagulation	33	0.048 [0.11]	0.029 [0.06]	< 0.005–0.169 [< 0.01–0.4]
Crumbing and drying	35	0.033 [0.07]	0.023 [0.05]	< 0.005–0.116 [< 0.01–0.26]
Packaging	79	0.036 [0.08]	0.022 [0.05]	< 0.005–0.154 [< 0.01–0.34]
Warehouse	20	0.020 [0.04]	0.010 [0.02]	< 0.005–0.068 [< 0.01–0.15]
Control room	6	0.030 [0.07]	0.019 [0.04]	< 0.012–0.070 [< 0.03–0.16]
Laboratory technician	54	2.27 [5.02]	0.213 [0.47]	< 0.006–37.4 [< 0.01–82.65]
Maintenance technician	72	1.37 [3.02]	0.122 [0.27]	< 0.006–43.2 [< 0.01–95.47]
Utilities operator	6	0.118 [0.26]	0.054 [0.12]	< 0.006–0.304 [< 0.01–0.67]

From Fajen (1988)

The manufacture of butadiene-based polymers and butadiene derivatives implies potential occupational exposure to a number of other chemical agents, which varies according to product and process. These include other monomers (styrene (see IARC, 1987b), acrylonitrile (see IARC, 1987b), chloroprene (see IARC, 1979)), solvents, additives (e.g., activators, antioxidants, modifiers), catalysts, mineral oils (see IARC, 1987b), carbon black (see IARC, 1987b), chlorine, inorganic acids and caustic solution (Fajen, 1986a,b; Roberts, 1986). Styrene, benzene (see IARC, 1987b) and toluene (see IARC, 1989) were measured in various departments of a US styrene–butadiene rubber manufacturing plant in 1979: mean 8-h TWA levels of styrene were below 2 ppm [8.4 mg/m^3], except for tank farm workers (13.7 ppm [57.5 mg/m^3], 8 samples); mean benzene levels did not exceed 0.1 ppm [0.3 mg/m^3], and those of toluene did not exceed 0.9 ppm [3.4 mg/m^3] (Checkoway & Williams, 1982). Meinhardt et al. (1982) reported that the mean 8-h TWA levels of styrene were 0.94 ppm [3.9 mg/m^3] (55 samples) and 1.99 ppm [8.4 mg/m^3] (35 samples) in two styrene–butadiene rubber manufacturing plants in 1977; the average benzene level measured in one of the plants was 0.1 ppm [0.3 mg/m^3] (3 samples). Average levels of styrene, toluene, benzene, vinyl cyclohexene and cyclooctadiene were reported to be lower than 1 ppm in another styrene–butadiene rubber plant in 1977 (Burroughs, 1977).

(d) Rubber and plastics products manufacturing industries

Unreacted 1,3-butadiene was detected as only a trace (0.04–0.2 ng/mg) in 15 of 37 bulk samples of polymers and other chemicals synthesized from 1,3-butadiene and analysed in 1985–86. Only two samples contained measurable amounts of 1,3-butadiene: tetrahydrophthalic anhydride (53 ng/mg) and vinyl pyridine latex (16.5 ng/mg) (JACA Corp., 1987).

Table 8. Time-weighted average exposures to 1,3-butadiene in 11 North American plants producing synthetic rubber, 1978-84

Occupational group	No. of samples	Exposure (ppm [mg/m³])													
		0.00-5.00 [0-11.05]		5.01-10.00 [11.07-22.12]		10.01-25.00 [22.12-55.25]		25.01-50.00 [55.27-110.50]		50.01-100.00 [110.52-221.23]		100.01-200.00 [221.23-420.00]		200.01-500.00 [442.02-1105.00]		500.01-1000.00 [1105.02-2210.00]	
		No.	%	No.	%	No.	%	No.	%	No.	%	No.	%	No.	%	No.	%
Tank car loader	102	78	76.5	9	8.8	9	8.8	4	3.9	2	2.0						
Vessel cleaner	214	199	93	9	4.2	4	1.9	2	0.9								
Charge solution make-up	89	83	93.2	3	3.4			2	2.3	1	1.1						
Reactor operator	190	133	70	22	11.6	14	7.4	7	3.7	7	3.7	5	2.6	1	0.5	1	0.5
Recovery operator	108	100	92.6	5	4.6	2	1.9	1	0.9								
Coagulation operator	185	173	93.5	9	4.9	2	1.1	1	0.5								
Dryer operator	85	84	98.8	1	1.2												
Baler and packager	167	164	98.2	2	1.2	1	0.6										
Warehouseman	22	22	100														
Laboratory technician	116	103	88.8	6	5.2	6	5.2	1	0.9								
Maintenance technician	262	241	92.0	12	4.6	4	1.5	2	0.8	3	1.1						
Supervisor	123	111	90.2	6	4.9	6	4.9										
Waste treatment operator	9	9	100														
Total	1672	1500	89.7	84	5.0	48	2.9	20	1.2	13	0.78	5	0.30	1	0.06	1	0.06

From JACA Corp. (1987)

Table 9. Mean 8-h time-weighted average concentrations of 1,3-butadiene measured in two US styrene–butadiene rubber manufacturing plants

Job classification or department	No. of samples	Concentration		Year of sampling	Reference
		ppm	mg/m³		
Instrument man	3	58.62	129.55	1976	Meinhardt et al. (1978)
Technical services personnel	12	19.85	43.87		
Head production operator	5	15.50	34.26		
Carpenter	4	7.80	17.24		
Production operator	24	3.30	7.29		
Maintenance mechanic	17	3.15	6.96		
Common labourer	17	1.52	3.36		
Production foreman	1	1.16	2.56		
Operator helper	3	0.79	1.75		
Pipefitter	8	0.74	1.64		
Electrician	5	0.22	0.49		
Tank farm	8	20.03	44.3	1979	Checkoway & Williams (1982)
Maintenance	52	0.97	2.14		
Reactor and recovery	28	0.77	1.7		
Solution	12	0.59	1.3		
Factory service	56	0.37	0.82		
Shipping and receiving	2	0.08	0.18		
Storeroom	1	0.08	0.18		

Detailed industrial hygiene surveys were conducted in 1984–87 in a US rubber tyre plant and a US industrial hose plant where styrene–butadiene rubber, polybutadiene and acrylonitrile–butadiene rubber were processed. No 1,3-butadiene was detected in any of a total of 124 personal full-shift samples from workers in the following job categories, which were identified as involving potential exposure to 1,3-butadiene: Banbury operators, mill operators, extruder operators, curing operators, conveyer operators, calendering operators, wire winders, tube machine operators, tyre builders and tyre repair and buffer workers (Fajen et al., 1990).

Measurements taken in 1978 and 1979 in personal 8-h samples in companies where acrylonitrile–butadiene–styrene moulding operations were conducted showed levels of < 0.05–1.9 mg/m³ (Burroughs, 1979; Belanger & Elesh, 1980; Ruhe & Jannerfeldt, 1980). In a polybutadiene rubber warehouse, levels of 0.003 ppm [0.007 mg/m³] were found in area samples; area and personal samples taken in tyre plants contained 0.007–0.05 ppm [0.016–0.11 mg/m³] (Rubber Manufacturers' Association, 1984). In a US tyre and tube manufacturing plant in 1975, a cutter man/Banbury operator was reported to have been exposed to 1,3-butadiene at 2.1 ppm [4.6 mg/m³] (personal 6-h sample) (Ropert, 1976).

Occupational exposures to many other agents in the rubber goods manufacturing industry were reviewed in a previous monograph (IARC, 1982).

1.3.3 Air

In 1989, total emissions of 1,3-butadiene to the air in the USA were estimated at approximately 2512 tonnes from 158 locations; total land releases were estimated at 6.7 tonnes (US National Library of Medicine, 1991).

Data on annual emissions of 1,3-butadiene from US facilities producing 1,3-butadiene, polybutadiene, neoprene/chloroprene and styrene–butadiene rubber and from miscellaneous facilities where 1,3-butadiene was used were collected in 1984 by the US Environmental Protection Agency. Data on episodic emissions were collected from most of the same facilities in 1985–86 (US Environmental Protection Agency, 1987; Mullins, 1990). Average annual emissions, the average rates and durations of episodic emissions and the highest rates for specific types of emissions are presented in Table 10.

Table 10. 1,3-Butadiene emissions from US manufacturing facilities in 1984–86

Activity of facility	No. of facilities	Total emissions (tonnes/year)		Episodic emissions (1986)		
		Average	Range	Average rate (kg/min)	Highest average rate (kg/min)	Average duration (min)
1,3-Butadiene production	10[a]	135.9	6.8–752	355	1600[b] 1100[c]	2170
Polybutadiene production	7	57.4	22.1–176	24	81.4[c] 24.0[d]	7.5
Chloroprene/neoprene production	2	10, 32.2		2.9	181[b]	38.8
Styrene–butadiene rubber production	17	49.3	0.9–145	3.9	9.9[e] 9.2[c]	49.6
Using 1,3-butadiene	11[f]	63.5	2.2–350	NR	NR	NR

From US Environmental Protection Agency (1987); NR, not reported
[a]Episodic emissions reported for eight facilities
[b]Pressure relief discharges
[c]Accidental liquid releases
[d]Equipment openings
[e]Accidental gas releases
[f]Episodic emissions reported for five facilities

Few data are available on levels of 1,3-butadiene in ambient air; reported concentrations in urban air generally range from less than 1 to 10 ppb [2–22 µg/m^3] (Neligan, 1962; Cote & Bayard, 1990). In the USA, combined levels of 1,3-butadiene and 2-butene were 5.9–24.4 ppb (0.01–0.05 mg/m^3) in 1978 in Tulsa, OK (Arnts & Meeks, 1981), and 0–0.019 ppm (0–0.042 mg/m^3) in 1973–74 in Houston, TX (Siddiqi & Worley, 1977). Levels of 1,3-butadiene were 0.004 mg/m^3 in Denver, CO, and < 0.001–0.028 mg/m^3 in various cities in Texas (Hunt et al., 1984); urban air in Los Angeles and Riverside, CA, contained levels as high as 9 ppb [0.02 mg/m^3] (Parsons & Wilkins, 1976).

1,3-Butadiene was found in 32% of 24-h ambient air samples taken in 19 US cities in 1987–88, at a mean concentration of 1.39 µg/m³ (range, 0.11–6.94) (US Environmental Protection Agency, 1989).

1.3.4 *Water*

1,3-Butadiene has been detected in drinking-water in the USA (US Environmental Protection Agency, 1978; Kraybill, 1980). Total releases to ambient water in 1989 were estimated to be 65 tonnes (US National Library of Medicine, 1991).

1.3.5 *Food*

Levels of < 0.2 µg/kg 1,3-butadiene were found in retail soft margarine; the plastic tubs containing the margarine contained < 5–310 µg/kg (Startin & Gilbert, 1984).

1.3.6 *Miscellaneous*

The US Environmental Protection Agency (1990) estimated that 1,3-butadiene is emitted in automobile exhaust at 8.9–9.8 mg/mile [5.6–6.1 mg/km] and comprises about 0.35% of total hydrocarbon in exhaust emissions. It has been detected in smoke generated during house fires at up to 15 ppm [33 mg/m³] (Berg *et al.*, 1978).

Sidestream cigarette smoke contains 1,3-butadiene at approximately 0.4 mg/cigarette, and levels of 1,3-butadiene in smoky indoor environments are typically 10–20 µg/m³ (Löfroth *et al.*, 1989).

1.4 Regulations and guidelines

Occupational exposure limits and guidelines for 1,3-butadiene in some countries and regions are presented in Table 11. Exposure limits were lowered in many countries in the late 1980s.

1,3-Butadiene is regulated by the US Food and Drug Administration (1989) for use in resinous and polymeric coatings in can-end cements; for use only as a coating or coating component and limited to a level not to exceed 1% by weight of paper or paperboard in contact with foods; for use in semi-rigid and rigid acrylic and modified acrylic plastics in repeat-use articles; for use in acrylonitrile–butadiene–styrene copolymers used in closures with sealing gaskets for food containers; and for use in textiles and textile fibres that come in contact with food.

2. Studies of Cancer in Humans

2.1 Cohort studies

The rubber industry, i.e., the manufacture of finished rubber goods, in which there is potential exposure to 1,3-butadiene, among other chemicals, has been evaluated previously; it was concluded that exposure in the rubber industry is carcinogenic to humans (IARC, 1982, 1987b). The epidemiological studies that were evaluated did not, however, include specific information on styrene–butadiene rubber manufacture, and it is these that are summarized below. In these descriptions, the histological descriptions of observed tumours given by the authors are used, with ICD codes when available.

Table 11. Occupational exposure limits and guidelines for 1,3–butadiene

Country or region	Year	Concentration (mg/m^3)	Interpretation[a]
Australia	1990	22 (carcinogen)	
Austria	1982	2200	TWA
Belgium	1990	22 (carcinogen)	TWA
Brazil	1978	1720	TWA
Bulgaria	1984	100	TWA
Czechoslovakia	1990	20	TWA
		40	STEL
Denmark	1990	22 (carcinogen)	TWA
Finland	1987	73 (carcinogen)	TWA
Germany	1989	0 (carcinogen in animals; III A2)	
Hungary	1990	10 (carcinogen)	STEL
Indonesia	1978	2200	TWA
Italy	1978	1000	TWA
Mexico	1983	2200	TWA
Netherlands	1989	110	TWA
Norway	1990	2.2 (carcinogen)	TWA
Poland	1984	100	TWA
Romania	1975	1500[b]	TWA
		2000[b]	Ceiling
Sweden	1990	20 (carcinogen)	TWA
		40	STEL (15-min)
Switzerland	1990	11 (carcinogen)	TWA
Taiwan	1981	2200	TWA
United Kingdom	1991	22	TWA
USA			
ACGIH	1991	22 (suspected human carcinogen; A2)	TWA
OSHA	1989	2200[c]	TWA
USSR	1984	100	MAC
Venezuela	1978	2200	TWA
		2750	Ceiling
Yugoslavia	1971	500	TWA

From Cook (1987); US Occupational Safety and Health Administration (OSHA) (1989); Direktoratet for Arbeidstilsynet (1990); Dutch Expert Committee for Occupational Standards (1990); American Conference of Governmental Industrial Hygienists (ACGIH) (1991); Health and Safety Executive (1991); International Labour Office (1991)

[a]TWA, 8-h time-weighted average; STEL, short-term exposure limit; MAC, maximum allowable concentration

[b]Skin notation

[c]The US OSHA has proposed to reduce the permissible exposure limits to 4.4 mg/m^3 for an 8-h TWA, 22 mg/m^3 for a 15-min STEL and 2.2 mg/m^3 for an 8-h TWA 'action level'; for a detailed discussion of this proposal, see US Occupational Safety and Health Administration (1990).

Follow-up of mortality in a cohort of workers who manufactured 1,3-butadiene monomer in Texas (USA) (Downs *et al.*, 1987) was extended through 1985 (Divine, 1990). The cohort comprised men who had been employed for six months or more between the opening of the plant in 1943 and 31 December 1979. Vital status was ascertained through the Social Security Administration or from state health departments. Of 2582 male employees, 1.9% were lost to follow-up and 32.0% were dead, 6% of these with no death certificate. Using US white men as the comparison population, the standardized mortality ratio (SMR) for mortality from all causes was 0.84 (826 deaths; 95% confidence interval [CI], 0.79–0.90) and that for all cancers was 0.80 (163 deaths; 95% CI, 0.69–0.94). The only significantly elevated SMR was for lymphosarcoma and reticulosarcoma (ICD8, 200) (2.29; 9 deaths; 95% CI, 1.04–4.35), thus confirming the earlier report (Downs *et al.*, 1987). Seven of the nine subjects had first been employed before 1946. When analysis was carried out by years of employment, there was no trend in SMR with increasing length of employment for lymphosarcoma or reticulosarcoma, and the only excess was seen for men with fewer than 10 years of employment. On the basis of the department listed on workers' personnel records, exposure to 1,3-butadiene was classified as low (not normally exposed to 1,3-butadiene), routine (exposed to 1,3-butadiene on a daily basis), non-routine (exposed intermittently to 1,3-butadiene, with possible exposure to peak concentrations higher than those with routine exposure) or unknown. Workers ever employed with routine exposure had a significant excess of lympho- and reticulosarcoma (5 deaths; SMR, 5.61; 95% CI, 1.81–13.10); all five deaths were seen in workers who had been employed fewer than 10 years. The rates for cancers of the kidney and large intestine were nonsignificantly increased among men who had worked for more than 10 years. Men who had had non-routine exposure had nonsignificantly increased risks for leukaemia (ICD8, 204–207) (SMR, 1.85; 6 deaths; 95% CI, 0.68–4.03) and lymphosarcoma and reticulosarcoma (SMR, 1.26; 2 deaths; 95% CI, 0.14–4.54).

Results were available from a study on the mortality of white male workers who had been employed for at least six months in two US styrene–butadiene rubber plants (Meinhardt *et al.*, 1982). A total of 1662 workers employed in plant A between 1943 and 1976 and 1094 workers employed in plant B between 1950 and 1976 were followed-up through 31 March 1976. Nine deaths from cancer of the lymphatic and haematopoietic tissues (ICD7, 200–205) were seen in workers in plant A (SMR, 1.55 [95% CI, 0.71–2.95]); all these deaths occurred among men who had first been employed between January 1943 and December 1945 (SMR, 2.12; [95% CI, 0.97–4.02]), after which the process changed from batch to continuous feed operation. No information was available, however, on the work histories of the subjects. The SMR for leukaemia (ICD7, 204) in plant A among workers employed between 1943 and 1945 was 2.78 (5 deaths [95% CI, 0.65–4.72]); two of the deaths had occurred within three years of first employment. In plant B, the numbers were very small: one death from leukaemia was observed (0.99 expected), which occurred within four years of first employment; the SMR for lymphatic and haematopoietic neoplasms was 0.78 (2 deaths [95% CI, 0.10–2.83]). Time-weighted average exposure to 1,3-butadiene was estimated after 1976 to be about 10 times higher in plant B (mean, 13.5 ppm; SD, 29.9; range, 0.34–174) than in plant A (mean, 1.24 ppm; SD, 1.20; range, 0.11–4.17). Concomitant exposure to styrene had occurred in plants A and B, and to traces of benzene at least in plant A.

Matanoski *et al.* (1990a) investigated mortality patterns from 1943 (synthetic rubber production began in 1942) through 1982 of employees from eight styrene–butadiene rubber plants in Canada and the USA, previously followed up through 1979 by Matanoski and Schwartz (1987). The study included all men who had been employed for at least one year between 1943 — or when their plant records were complete — and 1976. Canadian workers were included in the more recent study only if they had worked 10 or more years or had reached age 45 while still employed, since this enabled more complete ascertainment of their vital status through the company's insurance records. Of 12 113 employees, 2441 (20.2%) were deceased, 416 (3.4%) had unknown vital status and 9256 (76.4%) were still living at the end of follow-up. Death certificates were obtained for 97.2% of deceased individuals. On the basis of US death rates for black and white men (since Ontario rates were similar to US rates), the SMRs for the entire cohort were as follows: 0.81 for all causes (2441 deaths; 95% CI, 0.78–0.85); 0.85 for all cancers (518 deaths; 95% CI, 0.78–0.93), 0.61 for lymphosarcoma (ICD8, 200) (seven deaths; 95% CI, 0.25–1.26), 1.20 for Hodgkin's disease (ICD8, 201) (eight deaths; 95% CI, 0.52–2.37), 0.96 for leukaemia (ICD8, 204–207) (22 deaths; 95% CI, 0.60–1.46) and 1.11 for 'other lymphatic' system cancers (ICD8, 202, 203, 208) (17 deaths; 95% CI, 0.64–1.77). The SMR for lymphatic or haematopoietic cancers showed no clear trend of increasing with increasing number of years worked or years since first exposure. When employees were classified according to the job held longest, production workers (presumed by the authors to be those with highest exposures to 1,3-butadiene) had an SMR for deaths from all causes of 0.88 (594 deaths; 95% CI, 0.81–0.95) and a significant excess of other lymphatic cancer (SMR, 2.60; nine deaths; 95% CI, 1.19–4.94). When mortality among production workers was examined by race, the only significant excess was seen for leukaemia in blacks (three deaths; SMR, 6.56; 95% CI, 1.35–19.06). Of 92 deaths among black production workers, six were due to all lymphopoietic cancers (5.07; 1.87–11.07), and three of these were leukaemias (6.56; 1.35–19.06). The rates for haematopoietic cancers among maintenance workers were lower than those of the production workers. Maintenance workers showed increased risk for some digestive cancers, which were not evident in production workers. Workers in the two other job classification categories ('utility' and 'other') showed no significant increase in SMR for any type of cancer. A limitation of this study, pointed out by the authors, was that missing information on 2391 employees meant that they were excluded from the analysis of job department. Since many of these men were active in 1976 and are thus more likely to be alive than dead, the analysis by job is biased toward including more dead workers. The SMRs in this analysis may therefore be higher than those in the total cohort and are thus not directly comparable.

2.2 Case–control studies

In a case–control study nested within a cohort of 6678 US male rubber workers, deaths from cancers at the following sites were compared to those in a sample of the whole cohort: stomach (ICD8, 151) (41 deaths), colorectal (ICD8, 153–154) (63), respiratory tract (ICD8, 160–163) (119), prostate (ICD8, 185) (52), urinary bladder (ICD8, 188) (13), lymphatic and haematopoietic (ICD8, 200–209) (51) and lymphatic leukaemia (ICD8, 204) (14) (McMichael *et al.*, 1976). A 6.2-fold increase in risk for lymphatic and haematopoietic cancers (99.9% CI, 4.1–12.5) and a 3.9-fold increase for lymphatic leukaemia (99.9% CI,

2.6–8.0) were found in association with more than five years' work in manufacturing units producing mainly styrene–butadiene rubber during 1940-60. Of the five other cancer sites investigated, only cancer of the stomach was associated with a significant (two-fold) increase in risk. [The Working Group noted that, although the confidence limits were calculated by a method not used commonly, the results are significant at the 5% level.]

A case–control study nested within the US and Canadian cohort study described above (Matanoski *et al.*, 1990a) involved 59 workers with lymphopoietic cancers, identified using both underlying and contributing causes listed on death certificates. Controls were 193 workers without cancer, matched to the cases for plant, age, sex, date of hire, duration of work and survival up to date of death of the case (Santos-Burgoa, 1988; Matanoski *et al.*, 1990b). Since the exposures to 1,3-butadiene and to styrene were highly correlated, an attempt was made to discern to what extent each exposure contributed to the risk for leukaemia. Four industrial engineers who had no knowledge of the case or control status of the subjects estimated the intensity of exposure in each job, and duration of work was determined from job histories. The sum of the product of intensity and duration for each job resulted in a cumulative ranked exposure index for 1,3-butadiene and styrene separately. When the log of the ranked exposure indexes was dichotomized above and below the mean score for each exposure, 1,3-butadiene alone was associated with a risk for leukaemia (26 deaths) of 7.61 (95% CI, 1.62-35.64), and styrene alone gave a risk of 2.92 (95% CI, 0.83–10.27), each without adjustment for the other chemical. The relative risk for exposure to styrene, adjusted for 1,3-butadiene, was 1.06 (95% CI, 0.23-4.96), while the risk for 1,3-butadiene, adjusted for styrene, was 7.39 (95% CI, 1.32-41.33). The same type of analysis for other lymphatic cancers (18 deaths), including non-Hodgkin's lymphoma (ICD8, 202) and multiple myeloma (ICD8, 203), gave a risk of 0.81 (95% CI, 0.28-2.38) for styrene adjusted for 1,3-butadiene and a risk of 1.68 (95% CI, 0.55-5.15) for 1,3-butadiene adjusted for styrene.

In the population-based case–control study of cancers at multiple sites (excluding leukaemia) carried out in Montréal, Canada (Siemiatycki, 1991), described in detail on p. 95, 4% of the entire study population had been exposed at some time to styrene–butadiene rubber. Elevated odds ratios were seen for cancer of the kidney: 2.0 (90% CI, 1.2-3.4) for 12 cases with 'any' exposure and 2.9 (1.0-8.3) for three cases with 'substantial' exposure. For non-Hodgkin's lymphoma, the odds ratios were 0.9 (0.5-1.7) for seven cases with 'any' exposure and 1.5 (0.4-5.1) for two cases with 'substantial' exposure.

3. Studies of Cancer in Experimental Animals

3.1 Inhalation

3.1.1 *Mouse*

Groups of 50 male and 50 female B6C3F$_1$ mice, eight to nine weeks of age, were exposed to 625 or 1250 ppm (1380 or 2760 mg/m^3) 1,3-butadiene (minimum purity, > 98.9%) for 6 h per day on five days per week for 60 weeks (males) or 61 weeks (females). An equal number of animals sham-exposed in chambers served as controls. The study was terminated after 61 weeks because of a high incidence of lethal neoplasms in the exposed animals. The numbers of survivors were: males—49/50 controls, 11/50 low-dose and 7/50 high-dose; females—46/50 controls, 14/50 low-dose and 30/50 high-dose. Haemangiosarcomas originating in the heart with metastases to various organs were found in: males—0/50 controls, 16/49 ($p < 0.001$) low-dose and 7/49 ($p = 0.006$) high-dose—and females—0/50 controls, 11/48 ($p < 0.001$) low-dose and 18/49 ($p < 0.001$) high-dose (Fisher exact test). [The Working Group noted that the incidence of haemangiosarcomas of the heart in historical controls was 1/2372 in males and 1/2443 in females.] Other types of neoplasm for which the incidences were increased (Fisher exact test) in animals of each sex were malignant lymphomas: males—0/50 controls, 23/50 ($p < 0.001$) low-dose and 29/50 ($p < 0.001$) high-dose; females—1/50 controls, 10/49 ($p = 0.003$) low-dose and 10/49 ($p = 0.003$) high-dose; alveolar bronchiolar adenomas or carcinomas of the lung: males—2/50 controls, 14/49 ($p < 0.001$) low-dose and 15/49 ($p < 0.001$) high-dose; females—3/49 controls, 12/48 ($p = 0.01$) low-dose and 23/49 ($p < 0.001$) high-dose; papillomas or carcinomas of the forestomach: males—0/49 controls, 7/40 ($p = 0.003$) low-dose and 1/44 ($p = 0.473$) high-dose; females—0/49 controls, 5/42 ($p = 0.018$) low-dose and 10/49 ($p < 0.001$) high-dose. Tumours that occurred with statistically significantly increased incidence in females only included hepatocellular adenoma or carcinoma of the liver: 0/50 controls, 2/47 ($p = 0.232$) low-dose and 5/49 ($p = 0.027$) high-dose; acinar-cell carcinoma of the mammary gland: 0/50 controls, 2/49 low-dose and 6/49 ($p = 0.012$) high-dose; and granulosa-cell tumours of the ovary: 0/49 controls, 6/45 ($p = 0.01$) low-dose and 12/48 ($p < 0.001$) high-dose (US National Toxicology Program, 1984; Huff et al., 1985).

Groups of 60 male $B6C3F_1$ and 60 male NIH Swiss mice, four to six weeks of age, were exposed to 0 or 1250 ppm (2760 mg/m^3) 1,3-butadiene (> 99.5% pure) for 6 h per day on five days per week for 52 weeks. A group of 50 male $B6C3F_1$ mice was exposed similarly to 1,3-butadiene for 12 weeks and held until termination of the experiment at 52 weeks. The incidence of thymic lymphomas was 1/60 control $B6C3F_1$ mice, 10/48 $B6C3F_1$ mice exposed for 12 weeks, 34/60 $B6C3F_1$ mice exposed for 52 weeks and 8/57 NIH Swiss mice exposed for 52 weeks. Haemangiosarcomas of the heart were observed in 5/60 $B6C3F_1$ mice and 1/57 NIH Swiss mice (Irons et al., 1989). [The Working Group noted the absence of reporting on NIH Swiss control mice.]

In studies designed to characterize exposure–response relationships further, groups of 70–90 male and 70–90 female $B6C3F_1$ mice, 6.5 weeks of age, were exposed to 0, 6.25, 20, 62.5, 200 or 625 ppm (0.14, 44, 138, 440 or 1380 mg/m^3) 1,3-butadiene (purity, > 99%) for 6 h per day on five days per week for up to two years. Ten animals per group were killed and evaluated after 40 and 65 weeks of exposure. Survival was significantly reduced ($p < 0.05$) in all groups of mice exposed to 1,3-butadiene at 20 ppm or higher; terminal survivors were: males, 35/70 controls, 39/70 at 6.25 ppm, 24/70 at 20 ppm, 22/70 at 62.5 ppm, 3/70 at 200 ppm and 0/90 at 625 ppm; females, 37/70 controls, 33/70 at 6.25 ppm, 24/70 at 20 ppm; 11/70 at 62.5 ppm; 0/70 at 200 ppm and 0/90 at 625 ppm. Tumours for which the rates were significantly increased by exposure to 1,3-butadiene are shown in Table 12 (Melnick et al., 1990).

Groups of 50 male $B6C3F_1$ mice, 6.5 weeks of age, were exposed to 1,3-butadiene (purity, > 99%) for 6 h per day on five days per week at 200 ppm (442 mg/m^3) for 40 weeks, 625 ppm (1380 mg/m^3) for 13 weeks, 312 ppm (690 mg/m^3) for 52 weeks or 625 ppm

Table 12. Tumour incidences (I) and percentage mortality-adjusted tumour rates (R) in mice exposed to 1,3-butadiene for up to two years

Tumour	Sex	Exposure concentration (ppm)											
		0		6.25		20		62.5		200		625	
		I	R	I	R	I	R	I	R	I	R	I	R
Lymphoma	M	4/70	8	3/70	6	8/70	19	11/70	25[a]	9/70	27[a]	69/90	97[a]
	F	10/70	20	14/70	30	18/70	41[a]	10/70	26	19/70	58[a]	43/90	89[a]
Haemangiosarcoma of the heart	M	0/70	0	0/70	0	1/70	2	5/70	13[a]	20/70	57[a]	6/90	53[a]
	F	0/70	0	0/70	0	0/70	0	1/70	3	20/70	64[a]	26/90	84[a]
Alveolar-bronchiolar adenoma and carcinoma[b]	M	22/70	46	23/70	48	20/70	45	33/70	72[a]	42/70	87[a]	12/90	73[a]
	F	4/70	8	15/70	32[a]	19/70	44[a]	27/70	61[a]	32/70	81[a]	25/90	83[a]
Forestomach papilloma and carcinoma	M	1/70	2	0/70	0	1/70	2	5/70	13	12/70	36[a]	13/90	75[a]
	F	2/70	4	2/70	4	3/70	8	4/70	12	7/70	31[a]	28/90	85[a]
Harderian gland adenoma and adenocarcinoma	M	6/70	13	7/70	15	11/70	25	24/70	53[a]	33/70	77[a]	7/90	58[a]
	F	9/70	18	10/70	21	7/70	17	16/70	40[a]	22/70	67[a]	7/90	48
Preputial gland adenoma and carcinoma	M	0/70	0	0/70	0	0/70	0	0/70	0	5/70	17[a]	0/90	0
Hepatocellular adenoma and carcinoma	M	31/70	55	27/70	54	35/70	68	32/70	69	40/70	87[a]	12/90	75
	F	17/70	35	20/70	41	23/70	52[a]	24/70	60[a]	20/70	68[a]	3/90	28
Adenocarcinoma of the mammary gland	F	0/70	0	2/70	4	2/70	5	6/70	16[a]	13/70	47[a]	13/90	66[a]
Benign and malignant granulosa-cell tumour of the ovary	F	1/70	2	0/70	0	0/70	0	9/70	24[a]	11/70	44[a]	6/90	44

From Melnick et al. (1990)

[a]Increased compared with chamber controls (0 ppm), $p < 0.05$, based on logistic regression analysis

[b]The Working Group noted that the incidence in control males and females was in the range of that in historical controls (Haseman et al., 1985).

(1380 mg/m^3) for 26 weeks. After the exposures were terminated, the animals were placed in control chambers for up to 104 weeks. A group of 70 males served as chamber controls (0 ppm). Survival was reduced in all treated groups; the numbers of survivors at the end of the study were 35 controls, nine exposed to 200 ppm, five exposed to 625 ppm for 13 weeks, one exposed to 312 ppm and none exposed to 625 ppm for 26 weeks. Tumours for which the rates were significantly increased by exposure to 1,3-butadiene are shown in Table 13 (Melnick *et al.*, 1990).

3.1.2 *Rat*

Groups of 100 male and 100 female Sprague–Dawley rats, five weeks of age, were exposed to 0, 1000 or 8000 ppm (2200 or 17 600 mg/m^3) 1,3-butadiene (minimal purity, 99.2%) for 6 h per day on five days per week for 111 weeks (males) or 105 weeks (females). Survival was reduced in low- and high-dose females and in high-dose males; the numbers of survivors were: males—45 control, 50 low-dose and 32 high-dose; females—46 control, 32 low-dose and 24 high-dose. Tumours that occurred at significantly increased incidence in males were exocrine adenomas and carcinomas of the pancreas (3 control, 1 low-dose, 11 ($p < 0.05$) high-dose) and Leydig-cell tumours of the testis (0 control, 3 low-dose, 8 ($p < 0.01$) high-dose). Those that occurred at significantly increased incidence (Fisher exact test) in females were follicular-cell adenomas and carcinomas of the thyroid gland (0 control, 4 low-dose, 11 ($p < 0.001$) high-dose) and benign and malignant mammary gland tumours (50 control, 79 low-dose and 81 high-dose, with a significant, dose-related trend ($p < 0.001$); most of the latter were fibroadenomas: 40 control, 75 ($p < 0.001$) low-dose, 67 ($p < 0.01$) high-dose. Tumours that occurred only with positive trends (Cochran–Armitage trend test) in females were sarcomas of the uterus ($p < 0.05$; 1 control, 4 low-dose, 5 high-dose) and carcinomas of the Zymbal gland ($p < 0.01$; 0 control, 0 low-dose, 4 high-dose) (Owen *et al.*, 1987; US Occupational Safety and Health Administration, 1990). [The Working Group noted that differences in tumour incidence between groups were not analysed using statistical methods that took into account differences in mortality between control and treated groups.]

3.2 Carcinogenicity of metabolites

Mouse: D,L-1,2:3,4-Diepoxybutane (IARC, 1976), an intermediate of 1,3-butadiene metabolism, induced 10/30 papillomas and 6/30 squamous-cell carcinomas of the skin when applied at 3 mg three times per week for life to the skin of female Swiss mice (Van Duuren *et al.*, 1965). 1,2-Epoxy-3-butene (vinyloxirane), another intermediate in 1,3-butadiene metabolism, induced 4/30 skin tumours when applied at 100 mg three times per week to the skin of male Swiss mice (Van Duuren *et al.*, 1963). Subcutaneous injection of D,L-1,2:3,4-diepoxybutane at 0.1 and 1.1 mg/animal in tricaprylin once per week for one year induced local fibrosarcomas in 5/50 and 5/30 female Swiss mice; no tumour was observed in three solvent-treated control groups. Administration of D,L-1,2:3,4-diepoxybutane at 1 mg/animal in tricaprylin once per week for one year induced local fibrosarcomas in 9/50 Sprague–Dawley rats, compared with none in controls (Van Duuren *et al.*, 1966).

Table 13. Tumour incidences (I) and percentage mortality-adjusted tumour rates (R) in male mice exposed to 1,3-butadiene in stop-exposure studies (After exposures were terminated, animals were placed in control chambers until the end of the study at 104 weeks.)

Tumour	Exposure									
	0		200 ppm, 40 wk		625 ppm, 13 wk		312 ppm, 52 wk		625 ppm, 26 wk	
	I	R	I	R	I	R	I	R	I	R
Lymphoma	4/70	8	12/50	35[a]	24/50	61[a]	15/50	55[a]	37/50	90[a]
Haemangiosarcoma of the heart	0/70	0	15/50	47[a]	7/50	31[a]	33/50	87[a]	13/50	76[a]
Alveolar–bronchiolar adenoma and carcinoma	22/70	46	35/50	88[a]	27/50	87[a]	32/50	88[a]	18/50	89[a]
Forestomach squamous-cell papilloma and carcinoma	1/70	2	6/50	20[a]	8/50	33[a]	13/50	52[a]	11/50	63[a]
Harderian gland adenoma and adenocarcinoma	6/70	13	27/50	72[a]	23/50	82[a]	28/50	86[a]	11/50	70[a]
Preputial gland carcinoma	0/70	0	1/50	3	5/50	21[a]	4/50	21[a]	3/50	31[a]
Renal tubular adenoma	0/70	0	5/50	16[a]	1/50	5	3/50	15[a]	1/50	11

From Melnick et al. (1990)

[a] Increased compared with chamber controls (0 ppm), $p < 0.05$, based on logistic regression analysis

3.3 Activated oncogenes

Tumours from the study of Melnick *et al.* (1990) were evaluated in independent studies for the presence of oncogenes. Activated K-*ras* oncogenes were detected in 6/9 lung adenocarcinomas, 3/12 hepatocellular carcinomas and 2/11 lymphomas obtained from B6C3F$_1$ mice exposed to 1,3-butadiene. A specific codon 13 mutation (guanine to cytosine transversion) was found in most of the activated K-*ras* genes (Goodrow *et al.*, 1990). Activated K-*ras* genes have not been found in spontaneously occurring liver tumours or lymphomas from B6C3F$_1$ mice (Reynolds *et al.*, 1987; Goodrow *et al.*, 1990) and were observed in only 1/10 spontaneous lung tumours in this strain of mice (Goodrow *et al.*, 1990).

4. Other Relevant Data

4.1 Absorption, distribution, metabolism and excretion

4.1.1 *Humans*

1,3-Butadiene was reported to be metabolized to 1,2-epoxy-3-butene by a single human postmitochondrial liver preparation; no metabolism was observed in a single lung sample (Schmidt & Loeser, 1985). [The Working Group was unable to determine whether the lung and the liver samples were from the same individual.] Incubations of 1,3-butadiene with human liver microsomes from four subjects produced the chiral antipodes 1,2-epoxy-3-butene at ratios of 52–56% *R*- to 44–48% *S*-epoxybutene (Wistuba *et al.*, 1989).

1,2-Epoxy-3-butene is further transformed by epoxide hydrolase and glutathione *S*-transferase, as measured by disappearance of the epoxide by human liver microsomes and cytosol (Kreuzer *et al.*, 1991).

4.1.2 *Experimental systems*

Male Sprague-Dawley rats were exposed in closed inhalation chambers to various initial concentrations of 1,3-butadiene to study the pharmacokinetic behaviour of the compound. Analysis of the resulting concentration decline curves of 1,3-butadiene in the gas phase revealed that its metabolism was saturable. At less than 800–1000 ppm [1800–2200 mg/m^3], 1,3-butadiene was metabolized according to first-order kinetics; at higher exposure concentrations (> 1500 ppm [> 3300 mg/m^3], saturation range), a maximal metabolic rate of 220 μmol/h per kg bw was observed; this was enhanced by pretreatment with Aroclor 1254 (Bolt *et al.*, 1984). In similar experiments in male B6C3F$_1$ mice, saturation of 1,3-butadiene metabolism was observed at higher exposure concentrations (> 2000 ppm [> 4400 mg/m^3]) at a maximal metabolic rate of 400 μmol/h per kg bw. Pharmacokinetic analysis of the data suggested that the species-related difference in the effect of 1,3-butadiene was due to more rapid uptake of the compound from the gas phase by mice (Kreiling *et al.*, 1986a).

1,3-Butadiene is converted to 1,2-epoxy-3-butene by mixed-function oxidases in rat liver microsomes *in vitro*. Pretreatment of rats with phenobarbital increases enzyme activity (Malvoisin *et al.*, 1979; Bolt *et al.*, 1983). 1,2-Epoxy-3-butene is further metabolized to 1,2:3,4-diepoxybutane and 3-butene-1,2-diol; the latter product is metabolized by mixed-function oxidases to 3,4-epoxy-1,2-butanediol (Malvoisin & Roberfroid, 1982) (Fig. 1).

Fig. 1. Possible pathways for metabolism of 1,3-butadiene by rat liver microsomes

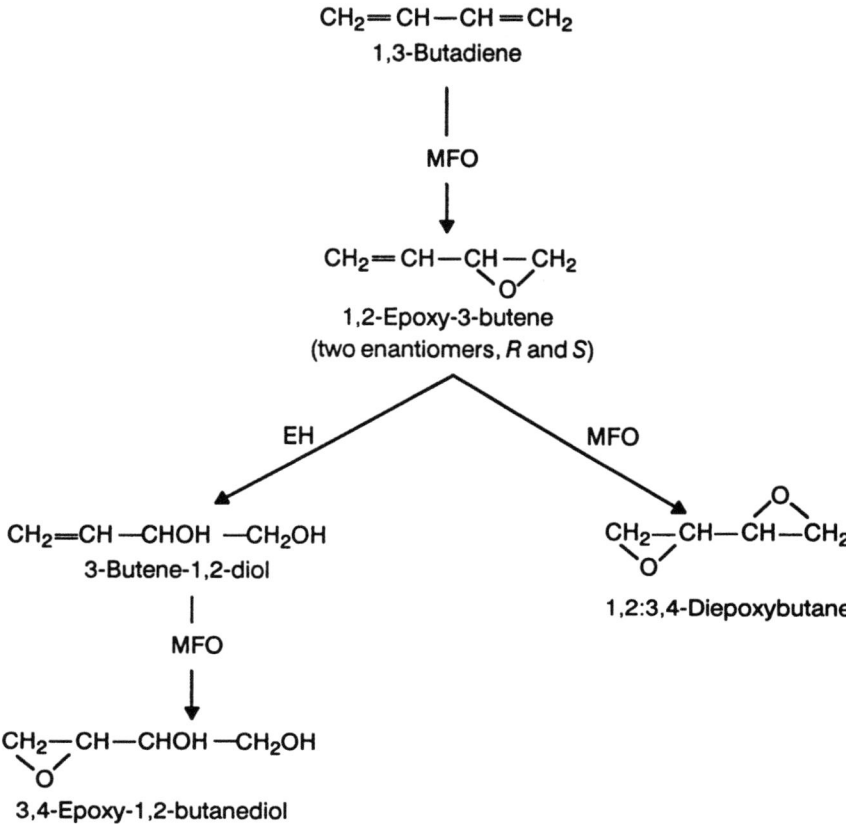

From Malvoisin and Roberfroid (1982); MFO, mixed-function oxidases; EH, epoxide hydrolase

Cytochrome P-450-mediated formation of 1,2-epoxy-3-butene from 1,3-butadiene also occurs in the presence of mouse liver microsomes, and crotonaldehyde has been shown to be a further metabolite (Elfarra et al., 1991).

1,2-Epoxy-3-butene is present in the expired air of rats and mice exposed to 1,3-butadiene (Bolt et al., 1983; Kreiling et al., 1987). When male Sprague-Dawley rats were exposed in closed exposure chambers to concentrations of 1,3-butadiene higher than 2000 ppm [4400 mg/m^3], which result in the maximum possible metabolic rate, about 4 ppm [8.8 mg/m^3] 1,2-epoxy-3-butene were measured in the gas phase under steady-state conditions. Kinetic analysis revealed that only 29% of the predicted value of 1,3-butadiene metabolite under these conditions was available systemically as 1,2-epoxy-3-butene, which was considered to be related to a first-pass metabolism of the 1,2-epoxy-3-butene originating in the liver (Filser & Bolt, 1984). The exhalation of 1,2-epoxy-3-butene by two male Sprague–Dawley rats and six male B6C3F$_1$ mice exposed in a closed system to 2000–4000 ppm [4400–8800 mg/m^3] 1,3-butadiene for 15 h was compared (Kreiling *et al.*, 1987). After about 2 h, rats had built up a constant concentration of 1,2-epoxy-3-butene at about 4 ppm [8 mg/m^3], with no sign of toxicity. 1,2-Epoxy-3-butene concentrations in the experiment with mice increased to about 10 ppm [22 mg/m^3] after 10 h; and after 12 h, animals showed signs of acute toxicity.

Studies on the disposition of inhaled (nose only) ^{14}C-labelled 1,3-butadiene in Sprague–Dawley rats and B6C3F$_1$ mice confirmed that mice metabolize 1,3-butadiene to a greater extent than rats. Radiolabelled metabolites present in blood were separated according to their volatility by vacuum line–cryogenic distillation (Dahl *et al.*, 1984). Blood samples taken from mice during exposure to 13 000 mg/m^3 (7100 ppm) (*sic*) for 6 h contained two to five times more radiolabelled 1,2-epoxy-3-butene than did the blood of rats (Bond *et al.*, 1987). Three male cynomolgus monkeys (*Macaca fascicularis*) were exposed by nose only to 10, 310 or 7760 ppm [22, 680 or 17 150 mg/m^3] ^{14}C-butadiene for 2 h. For exposures equivalent to those in mice and rats, the concentrations of total 1,3-butadiene metabolites in blood were 5–50 times lower in monkeys than in mice. The ranking of species was thus mice > rats > monkeys (Dahl *et al.*, 1991).

Metabolic species differences were also investigated *in vitro* using liver preparations from rats (Sprague–Dawley, Wistar), mice (NMRI and B6C3F$_1$), rhesus monkeys and humans (Schmidt & Loeser, 1985). The ranking of species for 1,2-epoxy-3-butene formation was: female mice > male mice > rats (humans) > monkeys. [The Working Group noted that the quantitative data on the human rate were derived from a single sample of liver.]

Repeated pretreatment of male Sprague–Dawley rats and male B6C3F$_1$ mice (inhalation by nose only) with 1,3-butadiene at 13 600 mg/m^3 (7600 ppm) for 6 h per day for five days had no effect on the ability of liver microsomes isolated from these animals to metabolize 1,3-butadiene. The metabolism of 1,3-butadiene *in vitro* was depressed significantly, however, in microsomes from lungs of pre-exposed rats and mice compared to unexposed controls (Bond *et al.*, 1988). Formation of 1,2-epoxy-3-butene was also observed after incubation of 1,3-butadiene with mouse and rat lung tissue but not after incubation with lung tissue from monkeys or humans (Schmidt & Loeser, 1985). [The Working Group noted that the quantitative data on the human rate were derived from a single sample of lung.]

The inhalation pharmacokinetics of the metabolite 1,2-epoxy-3-butene were studied in male Sprague–Dawley rats and male B6C3F$_1$ mice in closed chambers. Whereas in rats no indication of saturation kinetics could be obtained up to exposure concentrations of 5000 ppm [11 000 mg/m^3], saturation occurred in mice exposed to 500 ppm [1100 mg/m^3] or more (Kreiling *et al.*, 1987; Laib *et al.*, 1990).

4.2 Toxic effects

4.2.1 *Humans*

The toxic effects of combined exposures to 1,3-butadiene and other agents (e.g., styrene, chloroprene, hydrogen sulfide, acrylonitrile) have been reviewed (Parsons & Wilkins, 1976). Concentrations of several thousand parts per million of 1,3-butadiene irritate the skin, eyes, nose and throat (Carpenter *et al.*, 1944; Wilson *et al.*, 1948; Parsons & Wilkins, 1976).

Several studies have been reported on the effects of occupational exposure to 1,3-butadiene, mainly from the ex-USSR and Bulgaria. Few are substantiated by details on the atmospheric concentration or duration of exposure, and control data are generally not provided. The effects reported include haematological disorders (Batkina, 1966; Volkova & Bagdinov, 1969), kidney malfunction, laryngotracheitis, irritation of the upper respiratory tract, conjunctivitis, gastritis, various skin disorders, a variety of neuraesthenic symptoms (Parsons & Wilkins, 1976) and hypertension and neurological disorders (Spasovski *et al.*, 1986).

Checkoway and Williams (1982) reported minimal changes in haematological indices among eight workers exposed to about 20 ppm (44.2 mg/m^3) 1,3-butadiene, 14 ppm (59.5 mg/m^3) styrene and 0.03 ppm (0.1 mg/m^3) benzene, as compared to those among 145 workers exposed to less than 2 ppm (4.4 mg/m^3) 1,3-butadiene, 2 ppm (8.5 mg/m^3) styrene and 0.1 ppm (0.3 mg/m^3) benzene. Changes included a slight decrease in haemoglobin level and a slight increase in red-cell mean corpuscular volume. [The Working Group considered that these changes cannot be interpreted as an effect of 1,3-butadiene on the bone marrow, particularly as alcohol intake was not evaluated.]

4.2.2 *Experimental systems*

LC_{50} values for 1,3-butadiene were reported to be 270 000 mg/m^3 [122 170 ppm] in mice exposed for 2 h and 285 000 mg/m^3 [129 000 ppm] in rats exposed for 4 h; after 1 h of exposure, rats were in a state of deep narcosis (Shugaev, 1969). Oral LD_{50} values of 5.5 g/kg bw for rats and 3.2 g/kg bw for mice have been reported (US National Toxicology Program, 1984).

In female rats exposed to 1–30 mg/m^3 (0.45-14 ppm) 1,3-butadiene for 81 days, morphological changes were observed in liver, kidney, spleen, nasopharynx and heart (G.K. Ripp reported in Crouch *et al.*, 1979). In groups of 24 rats exposed to 600–6700 ppm [1300–14 800 mg/m^3] 1,3-butadiene for 7.5 h per day on six days per week for eight months, no adverse effect was noted, except for a slight retardation in growth with the highest concentration (Carpenter *et al.*, 1944). Rats exposed to 2200–17 600 mg/m^3 (1000–8000 ppm) 1,3-butadiene for 6 h per day on five days per week for three months showed no treatment-related effect other than increased salivation in females (Crouch *et al.*, 1979).

Groups of 110 male and 110 female CD Sprague–Dawley rats were exposed to atmospheres containing 0, 1000 or 8000 ppm [0, 2200 or 17 600 mg/m^3] 1,3-butadiene for 6 h per day on five days per week. The study was terminated when it was predicted that survival would drop to 20–25% (105 weeks for females, 111 weeks for males). Ten animals of each sex from each group were killed at 52 weeks. Treatment was associated with changes in clinical condition and lowering of body weight gain during the first 12 weeks, then nonsignificant changes, reduced survival and increases in certain organ weights and in the incidences of uncommon tumour types (for details, see p. 257). Increased mortality in high-dose males was accompanied by an increase in the severity of nephropathy (Owen *et al.*, 1987; Owen & Glaister, 1990).

B6C3F$_1$ mice exposed to 0, 625 or 1250 ppm [1380 or 2760 mg/m^3] 1,3-butadiene for 6 h per day on five days per week for 60–61 weeks had increased prevalences of atrophy of the ovary and testis, atrophy and metaplasia of the nasal epithelium, hyperplasia of the respiratory and forestomach epithelium and liver necrosis (see also pp. 254–255) (US National Toxicology Program, 1984).

Haematological changes in male B6C3F$_1$ mice exposed to 62.5, 200 or 625 ppm [138, 440 or 1375 mg/m^3] 1,3-butadiene for 6 h per day on five days per week for 40 weeks included decreased red blood cell count, haemoglobin concentration and packed red cell volume and increased mean corpuscular volume. Similar changes occurred in female mice exposed to 625 ppm [1375 mg/m^3] 1,3-butadiene (for details, see pp. 255–257) (Melnick et al., 1990).

The role of murine retroviruses on the induction of leukaemias and lymphomas following inhalation of 1,3-butadiene was evaluated in a series of studies reviewed by Irons (1990). Exposure of groups of male B6C3F$_1$ mice, which have the intact ecotropic murine leukaemia virus, to 1250 ppm [2750 mg/m^3] 1,3-butadiene for 6 h per day on 6 days per week for 6–24 weeks resulted in a decrease in the number of circulating erythrocytes, in total haemoglobin and in haematocrit and an increase in mean corpuscular volume. Leukopenia, due primarily to a decrease in the number of segmented neutrophils, and an increase in the number of circulating micronuclei were observed (Irons et al., 1986a). Persistent immunological defects were not detectable after this treatment (Thurmond et al., 1986). Exposure of male NIH Swiss mice, which do not possess intact endogenous ecotropic murine leukaemia virus, produced similar results (Irons et al., 1986b).

A further study was conducted to examine the expression and behaviour of endogenous retroviruses in these strains during the preleukaemic phase of 1,3-butadiene exposure. Chronic exposure of B6C3F$_1$ mice to 1,3-butadiene (1250 ppm [2740 mg/m^3]) for 6 h per day on five days per week for 3–21 weeks increased markedly the quantity of ecotropic retrovirus recoverable from the bone marrow, thymus and spleen. Expression of other endogenous retroviruses (xenotropic, MCF-ERV) was not enhanced. No virus of any type was found in similarly treated NIH Swiss mice (Irons et al., 1987a).

Enhanced susceptibility to 1,3-butadiene-induced leukaemogenesis as a result of the ability to express the retrovirus was suggested by the finding that exposure to 1250 ppm 1,3-butadiene for one year resulted in a 57% incidence of thymic lymphoma in B6C3F$_1$ mice (with expression of the virus) and a 14% incidence in NIH Swiss (without viral expression) (Irons et al., 1989).

4.3 Reproductive and developmental effects

4.3.1 *Humans*

No data were available to the Working Group.

4.3.2 *Experimental systems*

Fertility was reported to be unimpaired in mating studies in rats, guinea-pigs and rabbits exposed to 600, 2300 or 6700 ppm [1300, 5000 or 14 800 mg/m^3] 1,3-butadiene by inhalation for 7.5 h per day on six days per week for eight months (Carpenter et al., 1944). [The Working Group noted the incomplete reporting of this study].

Pregnant Sprague–Dawley rats (24–28 per group) and Swiss (CD-1) mice (18–22 per group) were exposed to atmospheric concentrations of 0, 40, 200 or 1000 ppm [0, 88, 440 or 2200 mg/m^3] 1,3-butadiene for 6 h per day on days 6–15 of gestation and killed on gestation day 18 (mice) or 20 (rats). Subsequently, the uterine contents were evaluated; individual fetal body weights were recorded; and external, visceral and skeletal examinations were performed. In rats, maternal toxicity was observed in the 1000-ppm group in the form of reduced extragestational weight gain and, during the first week of treatment, decreased body weight gain. Under these conditions, there was no evidence of developmental toxicity. Maternal toxicity was observed in mice given 200 and 1000 ppm 1,3-butadiene; 40 ppm and higher concentrations of 1,3-butadiene caused significant exposure-related reductions in the mean body weights of male fetuses. Mean body weights of female fetuses were reduced at the 200 and 1000 ppm exposure levels. No increased incidence of malformations was observed in either species. The frequency of fetal variations (supernumerary ribs, reduced sternebral ossification) was significantly increased in mice exposed to 200 and 1000 ppm. In a study of sperm-head morphology, groups of 20 male B6C3F$_1$ mice were exposed to atmospheric concentrations of 0, 200, 1000 or 5000 ppm [0, 440, 2200 or 11 000 mg/m^3] 1,3-butadiene for 6 h per day for five consecutive days. Small, concentration-related increases in the frequency of abnormal sperm morphology were seen five weeks after exposure (the only time of examination) (Hackett *et al.*, 1987; Morrissey *et al.*, 1990). [The Working Group noted that sequential examinations were not conducted after exposure to determine the effect of 1,3-butadiene on all stages of gamete development.]

4.4 Genetic and related effects

4.4.1 *Humans*

In an abstract of a study of workers engaged in the manufacture of 1,3-butadiene in Finland, cytogenetic analysis revealed no increase in the frequency of sister chromatid exchange, chromosomal aberrations or micronucleus formation in peripheral blood. The ambient air concentrations of 1,3-butadiene were generally < 1 ppm [< 2.2 mg/m^3], and the workers used protective clothing and respirators (Sorsa *et al.*, 1991).

4.4.2 *Experimental systems* (see also Tables 14–16 and Appendices 1 and 2)

The genetic toxicology of 1,3-butadiene has been reviewed (Rosenthal, 1985; de Meester, 1988; Brown, 1990). Additional information on 1,3-butadiene is included in a review by the Dutch Expert Committee for Occupational Standards (1990). The genetic and related effects of two main metabolites of 1,3-butadiene (1,2-epoxy-3-butene and 1,2:3,4-diepoxybutane) were reviewed by Ehrenberg and Hussain (1981) and de Meester (1988).

(a) *1,3-Butadiene*

1,3-Butadiene was mutagenic to *Salmonella typhimurium* TA1530 in the presence of liver S9 from phenobarbital- or Aroclor 1254-pretreated rats but was not mutagenic in the presence of uninduced rat liver S9 (de Meester *et al.*, 1980). It was also mutagenic to TA1535 in the presence of Arcolor 1254-induced rat S9, uninduced rat S9 and uninduced mouse S9 but was not mutagenic in the presence of uninduced human S9 (Arce *et al.*, 1990).

1,3-Butadiene gave negative results in tests for somatic mutation and recombination in *Drosophila melanogaster*.

1,3-Butadiene was not active in the L5178Y mouse lymphoma forward mutation assay. A weak positive response was reported for sister chromatid exchange induction in Chinese hamster ovary (CHO) cells.

In one study, sister chromatid exchange was induced weakly in human whole blood lymphocyte cultures after treatment with 1,3-butadiene in the presence and absence of Aroclor-1254-induced rat liver S9. No sister chromatid exchange was induced in another study in which S9 from a variety of sources was used, including mouse and human.

When B6C3F$_1$ mice and Wistar rats were exposed to ^{14}C-1,3-butadiene in a closed exposure system, radiolabel was associated with hepatic nucleoproteins and DNA from both species. The association of radiolabel with nucleoproteins was about two times stronger in mice than in rats, but the association with DNA was similar in the two species (Kreiling et al., 1986b). Acid hydrolysis of DNA isolated from the livers of mice exposed to ^{14}C-1,3-butadiene revealed the presence of two identifiable alkylation products: 7-N-(1-hydroxy-3-buten-2-yl)guanine and 7-N-(2,3,4-trihydroxybutyl)guanine. These were not found in similarly exposed rats (Jelitto et al., 1989).

After a 7-h exposure of mice and rats to 1,3-butadiene at 250, 500 or 1000 ppm (550, 1100 or 2200 mg/mg^3), alkaline elution profiles from the livers and lungs showed the occurrence of protein–DNA and DNA–DNA cross-links with all doses of 1,3-butadiene in mice but not in rats. This finding was interpreted as a biological effect in mice of the bifunctional alkylating metabolite, 1,2:3,4-diepoxybutane (Jelitto et al., 1989). In another study, there was no evidence of the formation of cross-links in DNA isolated from the livers of 1,3-butadiene-treated mice or rats (Ristau et al., 1990).

No unscheduled DNA synthesis was evident in the livers of either Sprague-Dawley rats or B6C3F$_1$ mice after exposure to 10 000 ppm [22 000 mg/m^3] 1,3-butadiene.

1,3-Butadiene increased the frequency of sister chromatid exchange in bone-marrow cells of mice, but not of rats, exposed *in vivo*. Chromosomal aberrations and micronuclei, but not aneuploidy, were induced in mice by 1,3-butadiene, but, in a single study, micronuclei were not induced in rats.

In a study of dominant lethal mutations, male Swiss CD-1 mice were exposed to 0, 70, 200, 1000 or 5000 ppm [155, 440, 2200 or 11 050 mg/m^3] 1,3-butadiene for 6 h per day for five days and then mated weekly for eight weeks. After one week, a significant increase was observed in the number of dead implants in females mated with males exposed to 1000 ppm (smaller increases were seen at 200 and 5000 ppm). Two weeks after exposure, the proportion of dead implants was increased in the 200- and 1000-ppm groups [details not given]. Sperm-head abnormalities were induced in exposed males (Morrissey et al., 1990).

(b) *1,2-Epoxy-3-butene*

1,2-Epoxy-3-butene reacts with DNA to give two main alkylated products, 7-(2-hydroxy-3-buten-1-yl)guanine and 7-(1-hydroxy-3-buten-2-yl)guanine (Citti et al., 1984).

1,2-Epoxy-3-butene was mutagenic to bacteria in the absence of an exogenous metabolic system. It did not induce unscheduled DNA synthesis in rat or mouse hepatocytes but induced sister chromatid exchange in CHO cells and in cultured human lymphocytes. In a single study, it induced sister chromatid exchange and chromosomal aberrations in mouse bone marrow *in vivo*.

(c) *1,2:3,4-Diepoxybutane*

1,2:3,4-Diepoxybutane induced interstrand cross-links in DNA by reaction at the $N7$ position of guanine (Lawley & Brookes, 1967).

Table 14. Genetic and related effects of 1,3-butadiene

Test system	Result[a] Without exogenous metabolic system	Result[a] With exogenous metabolic system	Dose[b] LED/HID	Reference
SA0, *Salmonella typhimurium* TA100, reverse mutation	–	–	1300.0000	Arce et al. (1990)
SA3, *Salmonella typhimurium* TA1530, reverse mutation	–	+	86.0000	de Meester et al. (1980)
SA5, *Salmonella typhimurium* TA1535, reverse mutation	–	(+)	650.0000	Arce et al. (1990)
SA9, *Salmonella typhimurium* TA98, reverse mutation	–	–	1300.0000	Arce et al. (1990)
SAS, *Salmonella typhimurium* TA97, reverse mutation	–	–	1300.0000	Arce et al. (1990)
DMM, *Drosophila melanogaster*, wing spot mutation		0	10000.0000	Victorin et al. (1990)
G5T, Gene mutation, mouse lymphoma L5178Y cells, *tk* locus	–	–	650.0000	McGregor et al. (1991)
SIC, Sister chromatid exchange, Chinese hamster ovary cells *in vitro*	–	(+)	1.3500	Sasiadek et al. (1991a)
SHL, Sister chromatid exchange, human lymphocytes *in vitro*	–	–	2160.0000	Arce et al. (1990)
SHL, Sister chromatid exchange, human lymphocytes *in vitro*	+	+	108.0000	Sasiadek et al. (1991b)
DVA, DNA-DNA cross-links, Sprague-Dawley rats *in vivo*	0		310.0000 inhal. 8 h/d, 7 d	Ristau et al. (1990)
DVA, DNA-DNA cross-links, B6C3F1 mice *in vivo*	0		3100.0000 inhal. 8 h/d, 7 d	Ristau et al. (1990)
BVD, DNA alkylation, male Wistar rat liver cells *in vivo*	0		550.0000	Jelitto et al. (1989)
BVD, DNA alkylation, male B6C3F1 mouse liver cells *in vivo*	+		680.0000	Jelitto et al. (1989)
DVA, DNA-DNA cross-links, Sprague-Dawley rat liver/lung *in vivo*	–		550.0000	Jelitto et al. (1989)
DVA, DNA-DNA cross-links, B6C3F1 mouse liver/lung *in vivo*	+		680.0000	Jelitto et al. (1989)
UPR, Unscheduled DNA synthesis, Sprague-Dawley rats *in vivo*	–		4000.0000 inhal.[c]	Arce et al. (1990)
UPR, Unscheduled DNA synthesis, Sprague-Dawley rats *in vivo*	–		4000.0000 inhal.[d]	Arce et al. (1990)
UVM, Unscheduled DNA synthesis, B6C3F1 mice *in vivo*	–		11600.0000 inhal.[c]	Arce et al. (1990)
UVM, Unscheduled DNA synthesis, B6C3F1 mice *in vivo*	–		11600.0000 inhal.[d]	Arce et al. (1990)
SVA, Sister chromatid exchange, male B6C3F1 mouse bone marrow *in vivo*	+	0	116.0000 inhal. 6 h/d[e]	Cunningham et al. (1986)
SVA, Sister chromatid exchange, male Sprague-Dawley rat bone marrow *in vivo*	–	0	4000.0000 inhal. 6 h/d[e]	Cunningham et al. (1986)
SVA, Sister chromatid exchange, male B6C3F1 mouse bone marrow *in vivo*	+	0	7.0000 inhal. 6 h/d, 10 d	Tice et al. (1987)
MVM, Micronucleus test, male B6C3F1 mouse bone marrow *in vivo*	+	0	116.0000 6 h/d[e]	Cunningham et al. (1986)
MVM, Micronucleus test, male B6C3F1 mouse peripheral blood *in vivo*	+	0	70.0000 inhal. 6 h/d, 10 d	Tice et al. (1987)
MVM, Micronucleus test, male B6C3F1 mouse peripheral blood *in vivo*	+	0	7.0000[f]	Jauhar et al. (1988)
MVM, Micronucleus test, NMRI mouse bone marrow *in vivo*	+	0	35.0000 inhal. 23 h	Victorin et al. (1990)

Table 14 (contd)

Test system	Result[a]		Dose[b] LED/HID	Reference
	Without exogenous metabolic system	With exogenous metabolic system		
MVR, Micronucleus test, male Sprague–Dawley rat bone marrow *in vivo*	–	0	4000.0000[e]	Cunningham *et al.* (1986)
CBA, Chromosomal aberrations, male B6C3F1 mouse bone marrow *in vivo*	+	0	1500.0000[g] inhal. 6 h[g]	Irons *et al.* (1987b)
CBA, Chromosomal aberrations, male NIH Swiss mouse bone marrow *in vivo*	+	0	1500.0000[g] inhal. 6 h[g]	Irons *et al.* (1987b)
CBA, Chromosomal aberrations, male B6C3F1 mouse bone-marrow *in vivo*	+	0	700.0000	Tice *et al.* (1987)
*Aneuploidy, male NIH Swiss mouse bone marrow *in vivo*	–	0	1500.0000 inhal. 6 h[g]	Irons *et al.* (1987b)
*Aneuploidy, male B6C3F1 mouse bone marrow *in vivo*	–	0	1500.0000 inhal. 6 h[g]	Irons *et al.* (1987b)
DLM, Dominant lethal test, Swiss CD–1 mouse	+	0	233.0000	Morrissey *et al.* (1990)
SPM, Sperm abnormality test, mouse	+	0	1165.0000	Morrissey *et al.* (1990)

[a]+, positive; (+), weakly positive; –, negative; 0, not tested; ?, inconclusive (variable response in several experiments within an adequate study)
[b]In-vitro tests, μg/ml; in-vivo tests, mg/kg bw
[c]6 h treatment on day 1, 3 h on day 2, liver sampled 2 h later
[d]6 h treatment on days 1 and 2, liver sampled 18 h later
[e]For two days, killed 24 h after the second exposure
[f]Five days/week for 13 weeks
[g]Killed at 24, 48, 72 and 96 h after cessation of exposure
*Data not displayed on profiles

Table 15. Genetic and related effects of 1,2-epoxy-3-butene

Test system	Result[a]		Dose[b] LED/HID	Reference
	Without exogenous metabolic system	With exogenous metabolic system		
SA0, *Salmonella typhimurium* TA100, reverse mutation	+	0	350.0000	de Meester et al. (1978)
SA0, *Salmonella typhimurium* TA100, reverse mutation	+	0	26.0000	Gervasi et al. (1985)
SA3, *Salmonella typhimurium* TA1530, reverse mutation	+	0	175.0000	de Meester et al. (1978)
SA5, *Salmonella typhimurium* TA1535, reverse mutation	+	0	1750.0000	de Meester et al. (1978)
SA7, *Salmonella typhimurium* TA1537, reverse mutation	−	0	8750.0000	de Meester et al. (1978)
SA8, *Salmonella typhimurium* TA1538, reverse mutation	−	0	8750.0000	de Meester et al. (1978)
SA9, *Salmonella typhimurium* TA98, reverse mutation	−	0	8750.0000	de Meester et al. (1978)
SA9, *Salmonella typhimurium* TA98, reverse mutation	+	0	105.0000	Gervasi et al. (1985)
ECW, *Escherichia coli* WP2 uvrA, reverse mutation	+	0	0.0000	Hemminki et al. (1980)
KPF, *Klebsiella pneumoniae*, fluctuation test	+	0	70.0000	Voogd et al. (1981)
URP, Unscheduled DNA synthesis, rat hepatocytes in vitro	−	0	1000.0000	Arce et al. (1990)
UIA, Unscheduled DNA synthesis, mouse hepatocytes in vitro	−	0	1000.0000	Arce et al. (1990)
SIC, Sister chromatid exchange, Chinese hamster ovary cells in vitro	+	+	0.0700	Sasiadek et al. (1991a)
SHL, Sister chromatid exchange, human lymphocytes in vitro	+	0	1.7500	Sasiadek et al. (1991b)
SVA, Sister chromatid exchange, male C57Bl/6 mouse bone marrow in vivo	+	0	25.0000	Sharief et al. (1986)
CBA, Chromosomal aberrations, male C57Bl/6 mouse bone marrow in vivo	+	0	25.0000	Sharief et al. (1986)

[a] +, positive; (+), weakly positive; −, negative; 0, not tested; ?, inconclusive (variable response in several experiments within an adequate study)
[b] In-vitro tests, μg/ml; in-vivo tests, mg/kg bw

Table 16. Genetic and related effects of 1,2,3,4-diepoxybutane

Test system	Result[a] Without exogenous metabolic system	With exogenous metabolic system	Dose[b] LED/HID	Reference
PRB, Prophage induction, *Bacillus megaterium*	+	0	0.0000	Lwoff (1953)
PRB, Prophage induction, *Pseudomonas pyocyanea*	+	0	0.0000	Lwoff (1953)
PRB, Prophage induction, *Escherichia coli* K-12	+	0	7.5000	Heinemann & Howard (1964)
ECB, *Escherichia coli* H540, DNA repair induction	+	0	2500.0000	Thielmann & Gersbach (1978)
SA0, *Salmonella typhimurium* TA100, reverse mutation	(+)	(+)	50.0000	Dunkel et al. (1984)
SA0, *Salmonella typhimurium* TA100, reverse mutation	+	0	20.0000	Gervasi et al. (1985)
SA5, *Salmonella typhimurium* TA1535, reverse mutation	+	0	25.0000	McCann et al. (1975)
SA5, *Salmonella typhimurium* TA1535, reverse mutation	+	+	5.0000	Rosenkranz & Poirier (1979)
SA5, *Salmonella typhimurium* TA1535, reverse mutation	+	+	5.0000	Dunkel et al. (1984)
SA7, *Salmonella typhimurium* TA1537, reverse mutation	–	–	167.0000	Dunkel et al. (1984)
SA8, *Salmonella typhimurium* TA1538, reverse mutation	–	–	50.0000	Rosenkranz & Poirier (1979)
SA8, *Salmonella typhimurium* TA1538, reverse mutation	–	–	167.0000	Dunkel et al. (1984)
SA9, *Salmonella typhimurium* TA98, reverse mutation	–	–	167.0000	Dunkel et al. (1984)
SA9, *Salmonella typhimurium* TA98, reverse mutation	–	0	60.0000	Gervasi et al. (1985)
ECW, *Escherichia coli* WP2 uvrA, reverse mutation	(+)	(+)	167.0000	Dunkel et al. (1984)
ECR, *Escherichia coli* B, reverse mutation	+	0	1720.0000	Glover (1956)
ECR, *Escherichia coli* B/r, reverse mutation	+	0	860.0000	Glover (1956)
KPF, *Klebsiella pneumoniae*, fluctuation test	+	0	4.0000	Voogd et al. (1981)
Saccharomyces cerevisiae D7, gene conversion	+	+	130.0000	Sandhu et al. (1984)
SCH, *Saccharomyces cerevisiae* D4, mitotic gene conversion	+	0	430.0000	Zimmermann (1971)
SCH, *Saccharomyces cerevisiae* D81, mitotic crossing-over	+	0	2000.0000	Zimmermann & Vig (1975)
SCH, *Saccharomyces cerevisiae* D3, mitotic recombination	+	+	400.0000	Simmon (1979)
Saccharomyces cerevisiae D7, mitotic crossing-over	+	+	130.0000	Sandhu et al. (1984)
Saccharomyces cerevisiae, reverse mutation	+	0	4000.0000	Polakowska & Putrament (1979)

Table 16 (contd)

Test system	Result[a]		Dose[b] LED/HID	Reference
	Without exogenous metabolic system	With exogenous metabolic system		
SCF, *Saccharomyces cerevisiae*, cytoplasmic petite mutation	–	0	4000.0000	Polakowska & Putrament (1979)
Saccharomyces cerevisiae, mitochondrial mutation	+	0	4000.0000	Polakowska & Putrament (1979)
Saccharomyces cerevisiae D7, reverse mutation	+	+	130.0000	Sandhu et al. (1984)
NCR, *Neurospora crassa*, reverse mutation	+	0	4300.0000	Kölmark & Westergaard (1953)
NCR, *Neurospora crassa*, reverse mutation	+	0	1720.0000	Pope et al. (1984)
DMM, *Drosophila melanogaster*, recombination and mutation, spot test	+	0	1000.0000	Graf et al. (1983)
DMX, *Drosophila melanogaster*, sex-linked recessive lethal mutation	+	0	100.0000	Bird & Fahmy (1953)
DMX, *Drosophila melanogaster*, sex-linked recessive lethal mutation	+	0	175.0000	Sankaranarayanan et al. (1983)
DMX, *Drosophila melanogaster*, sex-linked recessive lethal mutation	+	0	1000.0000	Fahmy & Fahmy (1970)
DMC, *Drosophila melanogaster*, chromosomal deletion	+	0	1000.0000	Fahmy & Fahmy (1970)
DIA, DNA–DNA cross-links, B6C3F1 mouse liver DNA *in vitro*	+	0	4.0000	Ristau et al. (1990)
GST, Gene mutation, mouse lymphoma L5178Y cells, *tk* locus	+	0	0.3000	McGregor et al. (1988)
SIC, Sister chromatid exchange, Chinese hamster CHO cells *in vitro*	+	0	0.0250	Perry & Evans (1975)
SIC, Sister chromatid exchange, Chinese hamster CHO cells *in vitro*	+	+	0.0100	Sasiadek et al. (1991a)
SHL, Sister chromatid exchange, human lymphocytes *in vitro*	+	0	0.1250	Wiencke et al. (1982)
SHL, Sister chromatid exchange, human lymphocytes[c] *in vitro*	–	0	0.0100	Porfirio et al. (1983)
SHL, Sister chromatid exchange, human lymphocytes *in vitro*	+	0	0.0100	Porfirio et al. (1983)
SHL, Sister chromatid exchange, human lymphocytes *in vitro*	+	+	0.0400	Sasiadek et al. (1991b)
CHF, Chromosomal aberrations, human skin fibroblasts[d] *in vitro*	+	0	0.0100	Auerbach & Wolman (1978)
CHF, Chromosomal aberrations, human skin fibroblasts *in vitro*	–	0	0.0100	Auerbach & Wolman (1978)
CHL, Chromosomal aberrations, human lymphoblastoid cell lines[e]	+	0	0.0100	Cohen et al. (1982)
CHL, Chromosomal aberrations, human lymphocytes[a] *in vitro*	+	0	0.1000	Marx et al. (1983)
CHL, Chromosomal aberrations, human lymphocytes *in vitro*	(+)	0	0.1000	Marx et al. (1983)
CHL, Chromosomal aberrations, human lymphocytes *in vitro*	–	0	0.0100	Porfirio et al. (1983)
CHL, Chromosomal aberrations, human lymphocytes[c] *in vitro*	+	0	0.0100	Porfirio et al. (1983)

Table 16 (contd)

Test system	Result[a]		Dose[b] LED/HID	Reference
	Without exogenous metabolic system	With exogenous metabolic system		
CIH, Chromosomal aberrations, human bone-marrow cells[c] *in vitro*	(+)	0	0.1000	Marx *et al.* (1983)
CIH, Chromosomal aberrations, normal human bone-marrow cells *in vitro*	(+)	0	0.1000	Marx *et al.* (1983)
HMM, Host-mediated assay, mutation, *S. typhimurium* TA1530 in mice	+	0	444.0000	Simmon (1979)?
HMM, Host-mediated assay, mitotic recombination, *S. cerevisiae* D3 in mice	−	0	56.0000	Simmon *et al.* (1979)
SVA, Sister chromatid exchange, mouse bone-marrow cells *in vivo*	+	0	1.0000	Conner *et al.* (1983)
SVA, Sister chromatid exchange, mouse alveolar macrophages *in vivo*	+	0	1.0000	Conner *et al.* (1983)
SVA, Sister chromatid exchange, mouse regenerating liver cells *in vivo*	+	0	1.0000	Conner *et al.* (1983)
SVA, Sister chromatid exchange, NMRI mouse bone-marrow cells *in vivo*	+	0	22.0000[f]	Walk *et al.* (1987)
SVA, Sister chromatid exchange, NMRI mouse bone-marrow cells *in vivo*	+	0	29.0000	Walk *et al.* (1987)
SVA, Sister chromatid exchange, Chinese hamster bone-marrow cells *in vivo*	+	0	34.0000[g]	Walk *et al.* (1987)
SVA, Sister chromatid exchange, Chinese hamster bone-marrow cells *in vivo*	+	0	32.0000	Walk *et al.* (1987)
CBA, Chromosomal aberrations, NMRI mouse bone marrow *in vivo*	+	0	22.0000[f]	Walk *et al.* (1987)
CBA, Chromosomal aberrations, NMRI mouse bone marrow *in vivo*	+	0	29.0000	Walk *et al.* (1987)
CBA, Chromosomal aberrations, Chinese hamster bone marrow *in vivo*	+	0	34.0000[g]	Walk *et al.* (1987)
CBA, Chromosomal aberrations, Chinese hamster bone marrow *in vivo*	+	0	32.0000	Walk *et al.* (1987)

[a] +, positive; (+), weakly positive; −, negative; 0, not tested; ?, inconclusive (variable response in several experiments within an adequate study)
[b] In-vitro tests, mg/ml; in-vivo tests, mg/kg bw
[c] Fanconi's anaemia (homozygotes and heterozygotes)
[d] Fanconi's anaemia (heterozygotes)
[e] Fanconi's anaemia (homozygotes and heterozygotes), ataxia telangiectasia, xeroderma pigmentosum, normal
[f] Calculated to give 22 (F) and 23 (M) mg/kg
[g] Calculated to give 34 (F) and 42 (M) mg/kg
[*] Not displayed on profile

Addition of an exogenous metabolic system was not required for genotoxic activity of this compound *in vitro*. In bacteria, it induced prophage, DNA repair and mutation. It induced mutation, gene conversion and mitotic recombination in yeast and mutation in fungi. In *Drosophila melanogaster*, it induced mutation and small chromosomal deletions.

1,2:3,4-Diepoxybutane induced DNA cross-links in mouse hepatocytes, dose-related increases in the frequency of sister chromatid exchange in cultured CHO cells and, in a single study, mutations in cultured mouse lymphoma L5178Y cells at the *tk* locus. It induced a dose-related increase in the frequency of sister chromatid exchange in cultured human lymphocytes from normal donors and from patients with a variety of solid tumours, but not from Fanconi's anaemia homozygotes or heterozygotes. It induced chromosomal aberrations in early-passage skin fibroblasts from Fanconi's anaemia heterozygotes, in primary lymphocytes from Fanconi's anaemia homozygotes and heterozygotes and in long-established lymphoblastoid cell lines from normal donors, Fanconi's anaemia homozygotes and heterozygotes and patients with xeroderma pigmentosum and ataxia telangiectasia. Bone-marrow cultures from Fanconi's anaemia patients and control individuals also showed increased frequencies of chromosomal aberrations after exposure to 1,2:3,4-diepoxybutane. Chromosomal aberrations were not induced in normal lymphocytes in two studies, but small increases were observed in another one.

1,2:3,4-Diepoxybutane induced mutations in *S. typhimurium* TA1530 in the mouse host-mediated assay, but it did not induce mitotic recombination in *Saccharomyces cerevisiae* D3.

Significant, dose-related increases in the frequency of sister chromatid exchange were observed in bone marrow and in alveolar macrophages from both intact and partially hepatectomized mice and in the regenerating liver of hepatectomized mice. 1,2:3,4-Diepoxybutane induced chromosomal aberrations and sister chromatid exchange in bone-marrow cells of male and female NMRI mice and Chinese hamsters exposed by inhalation or intraperitoneal injection.

5. Summary of Data Reported and Evaluation

5.1 Exposure data

1,3-Butadiene has been produced on a large scale since the 1930s. It is used to manufacture a wide range of polymers and copolymers, including styrene–butadiene rubber, polybutadiene, nitrile rubber, acrylonitrile–butadiene–styrene resins and styrene–butadiene latexes. It is also an intermediate in the production of various other chemicals.

Occupational exposure to 1,3-butadiene occurs in the production of monomeric 1,3-butadiene, of butadiene-based polymers and butadiene-derived products. The mean concentrations reported have usually been < 10 ppm (< 22 mg/m^3), although that level may be exceeded during some short-term activities. 1,3-Butadiene is not usually found at detectable levels in the manufacture of finished rubber and plastic products. Because gasoline contains 1,3-butadiene, loading of gasoline and other gasoline-related operations entail exposure to 1,3-butadiene.

1,3-Butadiene has also been detected in automobile exhaust and, at levels of < 0.02 ppm (< 0.04 mg/m^3), in urban air.

5.2 Human carcinogenicity data

One US cohort study of workers who manufactured 1,3-butadiene monomer showed a significant excess risk for lymphosarcoma and reticulosarcoma. Although there was no overall excess risk for leukaemia, there was a suggested increase in risk in a subgroup of workers with 'non-routine' exposure to 1,3-butadiene.

In a US study of workers employed in two styrene–butadiene rubber plants, there was a suggested increase of risk for leukaemia with exposure to 1,3-butadiene in one of the plants. No increase in risk was seen for cancers of the lymphatic and haematopoietic system other than leukaemia.

In a study of styrene–butadiene rubber workers in eight plants in the USA and Canada, there was no overall increased risk for leukaemia; however, a subgroup of production workers had a significantly increased risk. There was no apparent increased risk for 'other lymphatic system' cancers, although a significant risk was seen for production workers.

In a case–control study nested within this cohort of styrene–butadiene rubber workers, a large excess of leukaemia was found which was associated with exposure to 1,3-butadiene and not to styrene.

In a case–control study in the rubber industry, a large excess of lymphatic and haematopoietic cancers, including lymphatic leukaemia, was seen among workers employed in styrene-butadiene rubber production.

One study, therefore, specifically related increased risks for leukaemia to exposure to 1,3-butadiene and not to styrene. In other studies, the increased risks for leukaemia and other lymphatic cancers occurred among workers whose exposure had been in the manufacture of 1,3-butadiene or styrene–butadiene rubber.

5.3 Animal carcinogenicity data

1,3-Butadiene was tested for carcinogenicity by inhalation exposure in four experiments in mice and one in rats. Tumours were induced at all exposure concentrations studied, ranging from 6.25 to 8000 ppm (13.8–17 600 mg/m^3). 1,3-Butadiene produced tumours at multiple organ sites in animals of each sex of both species, including tumours of the haematopoietic system and an uncommon neoplasm of the heart in male and female mice. Neoplasms at multiple organ sites were induced in mice after only 13 weeks of exposure. 1,3-Butadiene induced dose-related increases in the incidence of tumours at many sites.

Two metabolites, 1,2-epoxy-3-butene and 1,2:3,4-diepoxybutane, were carcinogenic to mice and rats when administered by skin application or subcutaneous injection.

Activated K-*ras* oncogenes have been detected in lymphomas and in liver and lung tumours induced in mice by 1,3-butadiene.

5.4 Other relevant data

In rats, mice and monkeys, 1,3-butadiene is metabolized to an epoxide, 1,2-epoxy-3-butene, for which quantitative differences in metabolic rates (mice > rat > monkey) have been observed. Because 1,2-epoxy-3-butene is exhaled by rats and mice exposed to 1,3-butadiene, the epoxide must undergo systemic circulation. Two experiments with human liver tissue demonstrated conversion of 1,3-butadiene to 1,2-epoxy-3-butene, suggesting that humans are not qualitatively different from animals in terms of epoxide formation.

Developmental toxicity, in the form of reduced fetal weight and skeletal variations, has been observed in mice, but not rats, exposed by inhalation to 1,3-butadiene.

Genotoxic effects were generally observed in mice but not in rats *in vivo*. This apparent species difference was highlighted in a comparison of liver DNA adducts from the two species. 1,3-Butadiene induced dominant lethal effects, sperm-head abnormalities, chromosomal aberrations, micronucleus formation and sister chromatid exchange *in vivo* in mice; it did not induce micronuclei or sister chromatid exchange in rats. Unscheduled DNA synthesis was not induced in either rats or mice after exposure of 1,3-butadiene. The compound did not induce mutation in the mouse lymphoma forward mutation assay and was not genotoxic to *Drosophila melanogaster*. It induced mutation in bacteria in the presence of an exogenous metabolic system.

1,2-Epoxy-3-butene, one of the main metabolites of 1,3-butadiene, induced sister chromatid exchange and chromosomal aberrations in mice *in vivo* and sister chromatid exchange in cultured human lymphocytes and rodent cells. It did not induce unscheduled DNA synthesis in isolated rat or mouse hepatocytes. 1,2-Epoxy-3-butene induced point mutation in bacteria in the absence of exogenous metabolic systems. It also reacted with purified DNA.

1,2:3,4-Diepoxybutane, another metabolite of 1,3-butadiene, induced chromosomal aberrations and sister chromatid exchange in mice and Chinese hamsters exposed *in vivo*. It induced chromosomal aberrations and sister chromatid exchange in cultured human cells and both sister chromatid exchange and mutation in cultured mammalian cells. 1,2:3,4-Diepoxybutane induced chromosomal deletions and gene mutation in *Drosophila*. It was mutagenic to bacteria in a mouse host-mediated assay as well as *in vitro*. It induced bacterial prophage and DNA repair. In one study, it induced DNA–DNA cross-links in mouse liver DNA *in vitro*; it induced DNA interstrand cross-links *in vitro*.

5.5 Evaluation[1]

There is *limited evidence* for the carcinogenicity in humans of 1,3-butadiene.

There is *sufficient evidence* for the carcinogenicity in experimental animals of 1,3-butadiene.

Studies *in vitro* suggest that the metabolism of 1,3-butadiene is qualitatively similar in humans and experimental animals. 1,3-Butadiene is metabolized in mammals to epoxy metabolites which interact with DNA. Base-substitution mutations are induced in bacteria. Similar mutations in the K-*ras* oncogene have been reported in tumours induced in mice by 1,3-butadiene.

Overall evaluation

1,3-Butadiene is *probably carcinogenic to humans (Group 2A)*.

---

[1]For definition of the italicized terms, see Preamble, pp. 26–29.

6. References

Aldrich Chemical Co. (1990) *Aldrich Catalog/Handbook of Fine Chemicals 1990–1991*, Milwaukee, WI, p. 224

American Conference of Governmental Industrial Hygienists (1991) *1991–1992 Threshold Limit Values for Chemical Substances and Physical Agents and Biological Exposure Indices*, Cincinnati, OH, p. 13

Anon. (1984) Facts & figures for the chemical industry. *Chem. Eng. News*, **62**, 32–74

Anon. (1986) Facts & figures for the chemical industry. *Chem. Eng. News*, **64**, 32–86

Anon. (1988) Facts & figures for the chemical industry. *Chem. Eng. News*, **66**, 34–82

Anon. (1989) Facts & figures for the chemical industry. *Chem. Eng. News*, **67**, 36–90

Anon. (1991a) Chemical profile: butadiene. *Chem. Mark. Rep.*, **239**, 50

Anon. (1991b) Facts & figures for the chemical industry. *Chem. Eng. News*, **69**, 28–81

Arbetsmiljöfonden (Work Environment Fund) (1991) *Development and Evaluation of Biological and Chemical Methods for Exposure Assessment of 1,3-Butadiene* (Contract No. 88-0147), Helsinki, Institute of Occupational Health

Arce, G.T., Vincent, D.R., Cunningham, M.J., Choy, W.N. & Sarrif, A.M. (1990) In vitro and in vivo genotoxicity of 1,3-butadiene and metabolites. *Environ. Health Perspectives*, **86**, 75–78

Arnts, R.R. & Meeks, S.A. (1981) Biogenic hydrocarbon contribution to the ambient air of selected areas. *Atmos. Environ.*, **15**, 1643–1651

Auerbach, A.D. & Wolman, S.R. (1978) Carcinogen-induced chromosome breakage in Fanconi's anaemia heterozygous cells. *Nature*, **271**, 69–70

Batkina, I.P. (1966) Maximum permissible concentration of divinyl vapor in factory air. *Hyg. Sanit.*, **31**, 334–338

Belanger, P.L. & Elesh, E. (1980) *Health Hazard Evaluation Determination, Bell Helmets Inc., Norwalk, CA* (Report No. 79-36-656), Cincinnati, OH, National Institute for Occupational Safety and Health

Berg, S., Frostling, H. & Jacobsson, S. (1978) Chemical analysis of fire gases with gas chromatography–mass spectrometry. In: *Proceedings of an International Symposium on the Control of Air Pollution in the Work Environment, 1977*, Part 1, Stockholm, Arbetsskyddsfonden, pp. 309–321

Bird, M.J. & Fahmy, O.G. (1953) Cytogenetic analysis of the action of carcinogens and tumour inhibitors in *Drosophila melanogaster*. I. 1:2,3:4-Diepoxybutane. *Proc. R. Soc. B.*, **140**, 556–578

Bolt, H.M., Schmiedel, G., Filser, J.G., Rolzhäuser, H.P., Lieser, K., Wistuba, D. & Schurig, V. (1983) Biological activation of 1,3-butadiene to vinyl oxirane by rat liver microsomes and expiration of the reactive metabolite by exposed rats. *J. Cancer Res. clin. Oncol.*, **106**, 112–116

Bolt, H.M., Filser, J.G. & Störmer, F. (1984) Inhalation pharmacokinetics based on gas uptake studies. V. Comparative pharmacokinetics of ethylene and 1,3-butadiene in rats. *Arch. Toxicol.*, **55**, 213–218

Bond, J.A., Dahl, A.R., Henderson, R.F. & Birnbaum, L.S. (1987) Species differences in the distribution of inhaled butadiene in tissues. *Am. Ind. Hyg. Assoc. J.*, **48**, 867–872

Bond, J.A., Martin, O.S., Birnbaum, L.S., Dahl, A.R., Melnick, R.L. & Henderson, R.F. (1988) Metabolism of 1,3-butadiene by lung and liver microsomes of rats and mice repeatedly exposed by inhalation to 1,3-butadiene. *Toxicol. Lett.*, **44**, 143–151

Brown, J.P., ed. (1990) *Health Effects of 1,3-Butadiene*, Emeryville, CA, California Department of Health Services, Hazard Evaluation Section

Budavari, S., ed. (1989) *The Merck Index*, 11th ed., Rahway, NJ, Merck & Co., pp. 230–231

Burroughs, G.E. (1977) *Health Hazard Evaluation Determination, Firestone Synthetic Rubber Company, Akron, OH* (Report No. 77-1-426), Cincinnati, OH, National Institute for Occupational Safety and Health

Burroughs, G.E. (1979) *Health Hazard Evaluation Determination. Piper Aircraft Corporation, Vero Beach, FL* (Report No. 78-110-585), Cincinnati, OH, National Institute for Occupational Safety and Health

Carpenter, C.P., Shaffer, C.B., Weil, C.S. & Smyth, H.F., Jr (1944) Studies on the inhalation of 1:3-butadiene; with a comparison of its narcotic effects with benzol, toluol, and styrene, and a note on the elimination of styrene by the human. *J. ind. Hyg. Toxicol.*, **26**, 69–78

Checkoway, H. & Williams, T.M. (1982) A hematology survey of workers at a styrene–butadiene synthetic rubber manufacturing plant. *Am. ind. Hyg. Assoc. J.*, **43**, 164–169

Chemical Information Services (1988) *Directory of World Chemical Producers 1989/90 Edition*, Oceanside, NY, p. 104

Citti, L., Gervasi, P.G., Turchi, G., Bellucci, G. & Bianchini, R. (1984) The reaction of 3,4-epoxy-1-butene with deoxyguanosine and DNA in vitro: synthesis and characterization of the main adducts. *Carcinogenesis*, **5**, 47–52

Cohen, M.M., Fruchtman, C.E., Simpson, S.J. & Martin, A.O. (1982) The cytognetic response of Fanconi's anemia lymphoblastoid cell lines to various clastogens. *Cytogenet. Cell Genet.*, **34**, 230–240

CONCAWE (1987) *A Survey of Exposures to Gasoline Vapour* (Report No. 4/87), The Hague

Conner, M.K., Luo, J.E. & de Gotera, O.G. (1983) Induction and rapid repair of sister-chromatid exchanges in multiple murine tissues in vivo by diepoxybutane. *Mutat. Res.*, **108**, 251–263

Cook, W.A. (1987) *Occupational Exposure Limits—Worldwide*, Akron, OH, American Industrial Hygiene Association, pp. 118, 130, 166

Cote, I.L. & Bayard, S.P. (1990) Cancer risk assessment of 1,3-butadiene. *Environ. Health Perspectives*, **86**, 149–153

Crouch, C.N., Pullinger, D.H. & Gaunt, I.F. (1979) Inhalation toxicity studies with 1,3-butadiene. 2. 3 month toxicity study in rats. *Am. ind. Hyg. Assoc. J.*, **40**, 796–802

Cunningham, M.J., Choy, W.N., Arce, G.T., Rickard, L.B., Vlachos, D.A., Kinney, L.A. & Sarrif, A.M. (1986) In vivo sister chromatid exchange and micronucleus induction studies with 1,3-butadiene in $B6C3F_1$ mice and Sprague-Dawley rats. *Mutagenesis*, **1**, 449–452

Dahl, A.R., Benson, J.M., Hanson, R.L. & Rothenberg, S.J. (1984) The fractionation of environmental samples according to volatility by vacuum-line cryogenic distillation. *Am. ind. Hyg. Assoc. J.*, **45**, 193–198

Dahl, A.R., Sun, J.D., Birnbaum, L.S., Bond, J.A., Griffith, W.C., Jr, Mauderly, J.L., Muggenburg, B.A., Sabourin, P.J. & Henderson, R.F. (1991) Toxicokinetics of inhaled 1,3-butadiene in monkeys: comparison to toxicokinetics in rats and mice. *Toxicol. appl. Pharmacol.*, **110**, 9–19

Direktoratet for Arbeidstilsynet (Directorate of Labour Inspection) (1990) *Administrative Normer for Forurensning i Arbeidsatmosfaere* (Administrative Norms for Pollution in Work Atmosphere, 1990), Oslo, p. 7

Divine, B.J. (1990) An update on mortality among workers at a 1,3-butadiene facility—preliminary results. *Environ. Health Perspectives*, **86**, 119–128

Downs, T.D., Crane, M.M. & Kim, K.W. (1987) Mortality among workers at a butadiene facility. *Am. J. ind. Med.*, **12**, 311–329

Dunkel, V.C., Zeiger, E., Brusick, D., McCoy, E., McGregor, D., Mortelmans, K., Rosenkranz, H.S. & Simmon, V.F. (1984) Reproducibility of microbial mutagenicity assays. I. Tests with *Salmonella typhimurium* and *Escherichia coli* using a standardized protocol. *Environ. Mutag.*, **6** (Suppl. 2), 1–251

Dutch Expert Committee for Occupational Standards (1990) *Health-based Recommended Occupational Exposure Limits for 1,3-Butadiene* (ISSN 0921-9641), The Hague, Ministry of Social Affairs and Employment

Ehrenberg, L. & Hussain, S. (1981) Genetic toxicity of some important epoxides. *Mutat. Res.*, **86**, 1–113

Elfarra, A.A., Duescher, R.J. & Pasch, C.M. (1991) Mechanisms of 1,3-butadiene oxidations to butadiene monoxide and crotonaldehyde by mouse liver microsomes and chloroperoxidase. *Arch. Biochem. Biophys.*, **286**, 244–251

Eller, P.M., ed. (1987) *NIOSH Manual of Analytical Methods*, 3rd ed., Suppl. 2, (DHHS (NIOSH) Publ. No. 84-100), Washington DC, US Government Printing Office, pp. 1024-1–1024-9

Exxon Chemical Co. (1973) *Butadiene Specifications*, Houston, TX

Fahmy, O.G. & Fahmy, M.J. (1970) Gene elimination in carcinogenesis: reinterpretation of the somatic mutation theory. *Cancer Res.*, **30**, 195–205

Fajen, J.M. (1985a) *Industrial Hygiene Walk-through Survey Report of Texaco Chemical Company, Port Neches, TX* (Rep. No. 147.14), Cincinnati, OH, National Institute for Occupational Safety and Health

Fajen, J.M. (1985b) *Industrial Hygiene Walk-through Survey Report of Mobil Chemical Company, Beaumont, TX* (Rep. No. 147.11), Cincinnati, OH, National Institute for Occupational Safety and Health

Fajen, J.M. (1985c) *Industrial Hygiene Walk-through Survey Report of ARCO Chemical Company, Channelview, TX* (Rep. No. 147.12), Cincinnati, OH, National Institute for Occupational Safety and Health

Fajen, J.M. (1986a) *Industrial Hygiene Walk-through Survey Report of E.I. duPont deNemours and Company, LaPlace, LA* (Rep. No. 147.31), Cincinnati, OH, National Institute for Occupational Safety and Health

Fajen, J.M. (1986b) *Industrial Hygiene Walk-through Survey of the Goodyear Tire and Rubber Company, Houston, TX* (Rep. No. 147.34), Cincinnati, OH, National Institute for Occupational Safety and Health

Fajen, J.M. (1988) *Extent of Exposure Study: 1,3-Butadiene Polymer Production Industry*, Cincinnati, OH, National Institute for Occupational Safety and Health

Fajen, J.M., Roberts, D.R., Ungers, L.J. & Krishnan, E.R. (1990) Occupational exposure of workers to 1,3-butadiene. *Environ. Health Perspectives*, **86**, 11–18

Filser, J.G. & Bolt, H.M. (1984) Inhalation pharmacokinetics based on gas uptake studies. VI. Comparative evaluation of ethylene oxide and butadiene monoxide as exhaled reactive metabolites of ethylene and 1,3-butadiene in rats. *Arch. Toxicol.*, **55**, 219–223

Gervasi, P.G., Citti, L., Del Monte, M., Longo, V. & Benetti, D. (1985) Mutagenicity and chemical reactivity of epoxidic intermediates of the isoprene metabolism and other structurally related compounds. *Mutat. Res.*, **156**, 77–82

Glover, S.W. (1956) A comparative study of induced reversions in *Escherichia coli*. In: *Genetic Studies with Bacteria* (Carnegie Institution of Washington Publication 612), Washington DC, Carnegie Institution, pp. 121–136

Goodrow, T., Reynolds, S., Maronpot, R. & Anderson, M. (1990) Activation of K-*ras* by codon 13 mutations in C57Bl/6 × C3HF₁ mouse tumors induced by exposure to 1,3-butadiene. *Cancer Res.*, **50**, 4818–4823

Graf, U., Juon, H., Katz, A.J., Frei, H.J. & Würgler, F.E. (1983) A pilot study on a new *Drosophila* spot test. *Mutat. Res.*, **120**, 233–239

Grasselli, J.G. & Ritchey, W.M., eds (1975) *CRC Atlas of Spectral Data and Physical Constants for Organic Compounds*, Vol. 2, Cleveland, OH, CRC Press, Inc., p. 565

Greek, B.F. (1984) Elastomers finally recover growth. *Chem. Eng. News*, **62**, 35–56

Hackett, P.L., Sikov, M.R., Mast, T.J., Brown, M.G., Buschbom, R.L., Clark, M.L., Decker, J.R., Evanoff, J.J., Rommereim, R.L., Rowe, S.E. & Westerberg, R.B. (1987) *Inhalation Developmental Toxicology Studies of 1,3-Butadiene in the Rat* (Final Report No. NIH-401-ES-40131), Richland, WA, Pacific Northwest Laboratory

Harman, J.N. (1987) Infrared absorption spectroscopy. In: Lodge, J.P., ed., *Methods of Air Sampling and Analysis*, 3rd ed., Chelsea, MI, Lewis Publishers, pp. 78–83

Haseman, J.K., Huff, J.E., Rao, G.N., Arnold, J.E., Boorman, G.A. & McConnell, E.E. (1985) Neoplasms observed in untreated and corn oil gavage control groups of F344/N rats and (C57Bl/6N × C3H/HeN)F₁ (B6C3F₁) mice. *J. natl Cancer Inst.*, **75**, 975–984

Health and Safety Executive (1991) *Occupational Exposure Limits 1991* (Guidance Note EH 40/91), London, Her Majesty's Stationary Office, p. 9

Heiden Associates (1987) *Additional Industry Profile Data for Evaluating Compliance with Three Butadiene Workplace PEL Scenarios*, Washington DC

Heinemann, B. & Howard, A.J. (1964) Induction of lambda-bacteriophage in *Escherichia coli* as a screening test for potential antitumor agents. *Appl. Microbiol.*, **12**, 234–239

Hemminki, K., Falck, K. & Vainio, H. (1980) Comparison of alkylation rates and mutagenicity of directly acting industrial and laboratory chemicals. Epoxides, glycidyl ethers, methylating and ethylating agents, halogenated hydrocarbons, hydrazine derivatives, aldehydes, thiram and dithiocarbamate derivatives. *Arch. Toxicol.*, **46**, 277–285

Hendricks, W.D. & Schultz, G.R. (1986) A sampling and analytical method for monitoring low ppm air concentrations of 1,3-butadiene. *Appl. ind. Hyg.*, **1**, 186–190

Huff, J.E., Melnick, R.L., Solleveld, H.A., Haseman, J.K., Powers, M. & Miller, R.A. (1985) Multiple organ carcinogenicity of 1,3-butadiene in B6C3F₁ mice after 60 weeks of inhalation exposure. *Science*, **227**, 548–549

Hunt, W.F., Jr, Faoro, R.B. & Duggan, G.M. (1984) *Compilation of Air Toxic and Trace Metal Summary Statistics* (EPA-450/4-84-015), Research Triangle Park, NC, US Environmental Protection Agency, Office of Air and Radiation, Office of Air Quality Planning and Standards, pp. 4, 101

IARC (1976) *IARC Monographs on the Evaluation of Carcinogenic Risk of Chemicals to Man*, Vol. 11, *Cadmium, Nickel, Some Epoxides, Miscellaneous Industrial Chemicals and General Considerations on Volatile Anaesthetics*, Lyon, pp. 115–123

IARC (1979) *IARC Monographs on the Evaluation of the Carcinogenic Risk of Chemicals to Humans*, Vol. 19, *Some Monomers, Plastics and Synthetic Elastomers, and Acrolein*, Lyon, pp. 131–156

IARC (1982) *IARC Monographs on the Evaluation of the Carcinogenic Risk of Chemicals to Humans*, Vol. 28, *The Rubber Industry*, Lyon

IARC (1986a) *IARC Monographs on the Evaluation of the Carcinogenic Risk of Chemicals to Humans*, Vol. 39, *Some Chemicals Used in Plastics and Elastomers*, Lyon, pp. 155–179

IARC (1986b) *IARC Monographs on the Evaluation of the Carcinogenic Risk of Chemicals to Humans*, Vol. 39, *Some Chemicals Used in Plastics and Elastomers*, Lyon, pp. 181–192

IARC (1987a) *IARC Monographs on the Evaluation of the Carcinogenic Risk of Chemicals to Humans*, Vol. 42, *Silica and Some Silicates*, Lyon, p. 264

IARC (1987b) *IARC Monographs on the Evaluation of Carcinogenic Risks to Humans*, Suppl. 7, *Overall Evaluations of Carcinogenicity: An Updating of* IARC Monographs *Volumes 1 to 42*, Lyon, pp. 77–78, 79–80, 120–122, 136–137, 142–143, 252–254, 332–334, 345–347

IARC (1989) *IARC Monographs on the Evaluation of Carcinogenic Risks to Humans*, Vol. 47, *Some Organic Solvents, Resin Monomers and Related Compounds, Pigments and Occupational Exposures in Paint Manufacture and Painting*, Lyon, pp. 79–123

International Labour Office (1991) *Occupational Exposure Limits for Airborne Toxic Substances*, 3rd ed. (Occupational Safety and Health Series 37), Geneva, pp. 58–59

Irons, R.D. (1990) Studies on the mechanism of 1,3-butadiene-induced leukemogenesis: the potential role for endogenous murine leukemia virus. *Environ. Health Perspectives*, **86**, 49–55

Irons, R.D., Smith, C.N., Stillman, W.S., Shah, R.S., Steinhagen, W.H. & Leiderman, L.J. (1986a) Macrocytic–megaloblastic anemia in male B6C3F$_1$ mice following chronic exposure to 1,3-butadiene. *Toxicol. appl. Pharmacol.*, **83**, 95–100

Irons, R.D., Smith, C.N., Stillman, W.S., Shah, R.S., Steinhagen, W.H. & Leiderman, L.J. (1986b) Macrocytic–megaloblastic anemia in male HIN Swiss mice following repeated exposure to 1,3-butadiene. *Toxicol. appl. Pharmacol.*, **85**, 450–455

Irons, R.D., Stillman, W.S. & Cloyd, M.W. (1987a) Selective activation of endogenous ecotropic retrovirus in hematopoietic tissues of B6C3F$_1$ mice during the preleukemic phase of 1,3-butadiene exposure. *Virology*, **161**, 457–462

Irons, R.D., Oshimura, M. & Barrett, J.C. (1987b) Chromosome aberrations in mouse bone marrow cells following in vivo exposure to 1,3-butadiene. *Carcinogenesis*, **8**, 1711–1714

Irons, R.D., Cathro, H.P., Stillman, W.S., Steinhagen, W.H. & Shah, R.S. (1989) Susceptibility to 1,3-butadiene-induced leukemogenesis correlated with endogenous ecotropic retroviral background in the mouse. *Toxicol. appl. Pharmacol.*, **101**, 170–176

JACA Corp. (1987) *Draft Final Report. Preliminary Economic Analysis of the Proposed Revision to the Standard for 1,3-Butadiene: Phase II*, Fort Washington, PA

Jauhar, P.P., Henika, P.R., MacGregor, J.T., Wehr, C.M., Shelby, M.D., Murphy, S.A. & Margolin, B.H. (1988) 1,3-Butadiene: induction of micronucleated erythrocytes in the peripheral blood of B6C3F$_1$ mice exposed by inhalation for 13 weeks. *Mutat. Res.*, **209**, 171–176

Jelitto, B., Vangala, R.R. & Laib, R.J. (1989) Species differences in DNA damage by butadiene: role of diepoxybutane. *Arch. Toxicol.*, **Suppl. 13**, 246–249

Kirshenbaum, I. (1978) Butadiene. In: Mark, H.F., Othmer, D.F., Overberger, C.G. & Seaborg, G.T., eds, *Kirk–Othmer Encyclopedia of Chemical Technology*, 3rd ed., Vol. 4, New York, John Wiley & Sons, pp. 313–337

Kölmark, G. & Westergaard, M. (1953) Further studies on chemically-induced reversions at the adenine locus of *Neurospora. Hereditas*, **39**, 209–223

Kosaric, N., Duvnjak, Z., Farkas, A., Sahm, H., Bringer-Meyer, S., Goebel, O. & Mayer, D. (1987) Ethanol. In: Gerhartz, W., ed., *Ullmann's Encyclopedia of Industrial Chemistry*, 5th rev. ed., Vol. A9, New York, VCH Publishers, p. 590

Kraybill, H.F. (1980) Evaluation of public health aspects of carcinogenic/mutagenic biorefractories in drinking water. *Prev. Med.*, **9**, 212–218

Kreiling, R., Laib, R.J., Filser, J.G. & Bolt, H.M. (1986a) Species differences in butadiene metabolism between mice and rats evaluated by inhalation pharmacokinetics. *Arch. Toxicol.*, **58**, 235–238

Kreiling, R., Laib, R.J. & Bolt, H.M. (1986b) Alkylation of nuclear proteins and DNA after exposure of rats and mice to [1,4-^{14}C]1,3-butadiene. *Toxicol. Lett.*, **30**, 131–136

Kreiling, R., Laib, R.J., Filser, J.G. & Bolt, H.M. (1987) Inhalation pharmacokinetics of 1,2-epoxybutene-3 reveal species differences between rats and mice sensitive to butadiene-induced carcinogenesis. *Arch. Toxicol.*, **61**, 7–11

Kreuzer, P.E., Kessler, W., Welter, H.F., Baur, C. & Filser, J.G. (1991) Enzyme specific kinetics of 1,2-epoxybutene-3 in microsomes and cytosol from livers of mouse, rat, and man. *Arch. Toxicol.*, **65**, 59–67

Krishnan, E.R. & Corwin, T.K. (1987) Control of occupational exposure to 1,3-butadiene. In: *Proceedings of the 80th Annual Meeting of the Air Pollution Control Association, 1987*, Vol. 5 (Report 87-84A.14), Pittsburgh, PA, Air and Waste Management Association, pp. 2–14

Krishnan, E.R., Ungers, L.J., Morelli-Schroth, P.A. & Fajen, J.M. (1987) *Extent-of-exposure Study: 1,3-Butadiene Monomer Production Industry*, Cincinnati, OH, National Institute for Occupational Safety and Health

Kuney, J.H., ed. (1990) *Chemcyclopedia 91*, Vol. 9, Washington DC, American Chemical Society, p. 50

Laib, R.J., Filser, J.G., Kreiling, R., Vangala, R.R. & Bolt, H.M. (1990) Inhalation pharmacokinetics of 1,3-butadiene and 1,2-epoxybutene-3 in rats and mice. *Environ. Health Perspectives*, **86**, 57–63

Lawley, P.D. & Brookes, P. (1967) Interstrand cross-linking of DNA by difunctional alkylating agents. *J. mol. Biol.*, **25**, 143–160

Leviton, E.B. (1983) *Existing Chemical Market Review: 1,3-Butadiene*, Washington DC, US Environmental Protection Agency, Regulatory Impacts Branch

Locke, D.C., Feldstein, M., Bryan, R.J., Hyde, D.L., Levaggi, D.A., Rasmussen, R.A. & Warner, P.O. (1987) Determination of C_1 through C_5 atmospheric hydrocarbons. In: Lodge, J.P., ed., *Methods of Air Sampling and Analysis*, 3rd ed., Chelsea, MI, Lewis Publishers, pp. 243–248

Löfroth, G., Burton, R.M., Forehand, L., Hammond, S.K., Sella, R.L., Zweidinger, R.B. & Lewtas, J. (1989) Characterization of environmental tobacco smoke. *Environ. Sci. Technol.*, **23**, 610–614

Lunsford, R.A., Gagnon, Y.T., Palassis, J., Fajen, J.M., Roberts, D.R. & Eller, P.M. (1990) Determination of 1,3-butadiene down to sub-part-per-million levels in air by collection on charcoal and high resolution gas chromatography. *Appl. occup. environ. Hyg.*, **5**, 310–320

Lwoff, A. (1953) Lysogeny. *Bacteriol. Rev.*, **17**, 269–337

Lyondell Petrochemical Co. (1988) *Technical Data Sheet: Butadiene*, Houston, TX

Malvoisin, E. & Roberfroid, M. (1982) Hepatic microsomal metabolism of 1,3-butadiene. *Xenobiotica*, **12**, 137–144

Malvoisin, E., Lhoest, G., Poncelet, F., Roberfroid, M. & Mercier, M. (1979) Identification and quantitation of 1,2-epoxybutene-3 as the primary metabolite of 1,3-butadiene. *J. Chromatogr.*, **178**, 419–425

Marx, M.P., Smith, S., Heyns, A. du P. & van Tonder, I.Z. (1983) Fanconi's anemia: a cytogenetic study on lymphocyte and bone marrow cultures utilizing 1,2:3,4-diepoxybutane. *Cancer Genet. Cytogenet.*, **9**, 51–60

Matanoski, G.M. & Schwartz, L. (1987) Mortality of workers in styrene–butadiene polymer production. *J. occup. Med.*, **29**, 675–680

Matanoski, G.M., Santos-Burgoa, C. & Schwartz, L. (1990a) Mortality of a cohort of workers in the styrene–butadiene polymer manufacturing industry (1943–1982). *Environ. Health Perspectives*, **86**, 107–117

Matanoski, G.M., Santos-Burgoa, C., Zeger, S.L. & Schwarz, L. (1990b) Epidemiologic data related to health effects of 1,3-butadiene. In: Mohr, U., Bates, D.V., Dungworth, D.L., Lee, P.N., McClellan, R.O. & Roe, F.J.C., eds, *Assessment of Inhalation Hazards* (ILSI Monographs), New York, Springer-Verlag, pp. 201–214

McCann, J., Choi, E., Yamasaki, E. & Ames, B.N. (1975) Detection of carcinogens as mutagens in the *Salmonella*/microsome test: assay of 300 chemicals. *Proc. natl Acad. Sci. USA*, **72**, 5135–5139

McGregor, D.B., Brown, A., Cattanach, P., Edwards, I., McBride, D. & Caspary, W.J. (1988) Responses of the L5178Y tk$^+$/tk$^-$ mouse lymphoma cell forward mutation assay. II: 18 Coded chemicals. *Environ. mol. Mutag.*, **11**, 91–118

McGregor, D.B., Brown, A., Cattanach, P., Edwards, I., McBride, D., Riach, C., Shepherd, W. & Caspary, W.J. (1991) Responses of the L5178Y mouse lymphoma forward mutation assay. V. Gases and vapors. *Environ. mol. Mutag.*, **17**, 122–129

McMichael, A.J., Spirtas, R., Gamble, J.F. & Tousey, P.M. (1976) Mortality among rubber workers: relationship to specific jobs. *J. occup. Med.*, **18**, 178–185

de Meester, C. (1988) Genotoxic properties of 1,3-butadiene. *Mutat. Res.*, **195**, 273–281

de Meester, C., Poncelet, F., Roberfroid, M. & Mercier, M. (1978) Mutagenicity of butadiene and butadiene monoxide. *Biochem. biophys. Res. Commun.*, **80**, 298–305

de Meester, C., Poncelet, F., Roberfroid, M. & Mercier, M. (1980) The mutagenicity of butadiene towards *Salmonella typhimurium*. *Toxicol. Lett.*, **6**, 125–130

Meinhardt, T.J., Young, R.J. & Hartle, R.W. (1978) Epidemiologic investigations of styrene–butadiene rubber production and reinforced plastics production. *Scand. J. Work Environ. Health*, **4** (Suppl. 2), 240–246

Meinhardt, T.J., Lemen, R.A., Crandall, M.S. & Young, R.J. (1982) Environmental epidemiologic investigation of the styrene–butadiene rubber industry. Mortality patterns with discussion of the hematopoietic and lymphatic malignancies. *Scand. J. Work Environ. Health*, **8**, 250–259

Melnick, R.L., Huff, J., Chou, B.J. & Miller, R.A. (1990) Carcinogenicity of 1,3-butadiene in C57Bl/6 × C3HF$_1$ mice at low exposure concentrations. *Cancer Res.*, **50**, 6592–6599

Miller, L.M. (1978) *Investigation of Selected Potential Environmental Contaminants: Butadiene and Its Oligomers* (EPA-560/2-78-008; NTIS PB-291684), Washington DC, US Environmental Protection Agency, Office of Toxic Substances

Morrissey, R.E., Schwetz, B.A., Hackett, P.L., Sikov, M.R., Hardin, B.D., McClanahan, B.J., Decker, J.R. & Mast, T.J. (1990) Overview of reproductive and developmental toxicity studies of 1,3-butadiene in rodents. *Environ. Health Perspectives*, **86**, 79–84

Morrow, N.L. (1990) The industrial production and use of 1,3-butadiene. *Environ. Health Perspectives*, **86**, 7–8

Mullins, J.A. (1990) Industrial emissions of 1,3-butadiene. *Environ. Health Perspectives*, **86**, 9–10

Neligan, R.E. (1962) Hydrocarbons in the Los Angeles atmosphere. A comparison between the hydrocarbons in automobile exhaust and those found in the Los Angeles atmosphere. *Arch. environ. Health*, **5**, 581–591

Owen, P.E. & Glaister, J.R. (1990) Inhalation toxicity and carcinogenicity of 1,3-butadiene in Sprague-Dawley rats. *Environ. Health Perspectives*, **86**, 19–25

Owen, P.E., Glaister, J.R., Gaunt, I.F. & Pullinger, D.H. (1987) Inhalation toxicity studies with 1,3-butadiene. 3. Two year toxicity/carcinogenicity study in rats. *Am. ind. Hyg. Assoc. J.*, **48**, 407–413

Parsons, T.B. & Wilkins, G.E. (1976) *Biological Effects and Environmental Aspects of 1,3-Butadiene (Summary of the Published Literature)* (EPA-560/2-76-004), Washington DC, US Environmental Protection Agency

Perry, P. & Evans, H.J. (1975) Cytological detection of mutagen–carcinogen exposure by sister chromatid exchange. *Nature*, **258**, 121–125

Polakowska, R. & Putrament, A. (1979) Mitochondrial mutagenesis in *Saccharomyces cerevisiae*. II. Methyl methanesulphonate and diepoxybutane. *Mutat. Res.*, **61**, 207–213

Pope, S., Baker, J.M. & Parish, J.H. (1984) Assay of cytotoxicity and mutagenicity of alkylating agents by using *Neurospora* spheroplasts. *Mutat. Res.*, **125**, 43–53

Porfirio, B., Dallapiccola, B., Mokini, V., Alimena, G. & Gandini, E. (1983) Failure of diepoxybutane to enhance sister chromatid exchange levels in Fanconi's anemia patients and heterozygotes. *Hum. Genet.*, **63**, 117–120

Reynolds, S.H., Stowers, S.J., Patterson, R.M., Maronpot, R.R., Aaronson, S.A. & Anderson, M.W. (1987) Activated oncogenes in B6C3F$_1$ mouse liver tumors: implications for risk assessment. *Science*, **237**, 1309–1316

Ristau, C., Deutschmann, S., Laib, R.J. & Ottenwälder, H. (1990) Detection of diepoxybutane-induced DNA–DNA crosslinks by cesium trifluoroacetate (CsTFA) density-gradient centrifugation. *Arch. Toxicol.*, **64**, 343–344

Roberts, D.R. (1986) *Industrial Hygiene Walk-through Survey Report of Copolymer Rubber and Chemical Corporation, Baton Rouge, LA* (Rep. No. 147.22), Cincinnati, OH, National Institute for Occupational Safety and Health

Ropert, C.P., Jr (1976) *Health Hazard Evaluation Determination, Goodyear Tire and Rubber Company, Gadsden, AL* (Report No. 74-120-260), Cincinnati, OH, National Institute for Occupational Safety and Health

Rosenkranz, H.S. & Poirier, L.A. (1979) Evaluation of the mutagenicity and DNA-modifying activity of carcinogens and noncarcinogens in microbial systems. *J. natl Cancer Inst.*, **62**, 873–892

Rosenthal, S.L. (1985) The Reproductive Effects Assessment Group's report on the mutagenicity of 1,3-butadiene and its reactive metabolites. *Environ. Mutag.*, **7**, 933–945

Rubber Manufacturers' Association (1984) *Requests for Information Regarding 1,3-Butadiene, 49 Fed. Reg. 844 and 845 (Jan. 5, 1984)*, Washington DC

Ruhe, R.L. & Jannerfeldt, E.R. (1980) *Health Hazard Evaluation, Metamora Products Corporation, Elkland, PA* (Report No. HE-80-188-797), Cincinnati, OH, National Institute for Occupational Safety and Health

Sadtler Research Laboratories (1980) *The Sadtler Standard Spectra Collection, Cumulative Index*, Philadelphia, PA

Saltzman, B.E. & Harman, J.N. (1989) Direct reading colorimetric indicators. In: Lodge, J.P., Jr, ed., *Methods of Air Sampling and Analysis*, Chelsea, MI, Lewis Publishers, pp. 171–187

Sandhu, S.S., Waters, M.D., Mortelmans, K.E., Evans, E.L., Jotz, M.M., Mitchell, A.D. & Kasica, V. (1984) Evaluation of diallate and triallate herbicides for genotoxic effects in a battery of in vitro and short-term in vivo tests. *Mutat. Res.*, **136**, 173–183

Sankaranarayanan, K., Ferro, W. & Zijlstra, J.A. (1983) Studies on mutagen-sensitive strains of *Drosophila melanogaster*. III. A comparison of the mutagenic activities of the *ebony* (UV and X-ray sensitive) and *Canton*-S (wild-type) strains to MMS, ENU, DEB, DEN and 2,4,6-Cl$_3$-PDMT. *Mutat. Res.*, **110**, 59–70

Santodonato, J. (1985) *Monograph on Human Exposure to Chemicals in the Workplace: 1,3-Butadiene* (PB86-147261), Washington DC, US National Technical Information Service

Santos-Burgoa, C. (1988) *Case–Control Study of Lympho-hematopoietic Malignant Neoplasms Within a Cohort of Styrene–Butadiene Polymerization Workers*, Doctoral thesis, Baltimore, MD, Johns Hopkins School of Hygiene and Public Health

Sasiadek, M., Järventaus, H. & Sorsa, M. (1991a) Sister-chromatid exchanges induced by 1,3-butadiene and its epoxides in CHO cells. *Mutat. Res.*, **263**, 47–50

Sasiadek, M., Norppa, H. & Sorsa, M. (1991b) 1,3-Butadiene and its epoxides induce sister-chromatid exchanges in human lymphocytes in vitro. *Mutat. Res.*, **261**, 117–121

Sax, N.I. & Lewis, R.J., Sr (1987) *Hawley's Condensed Chemical Dictionary*, 11th ed., New York, Van Nostrand Reinhold, p. 177

Schmidt, U. & Loeser, E. (1985) Species differences in the formation of butadiene monoxide from 1,3-butadiene. *Arch. Toxicol.*, **57**, 222–225

Sharief, Y., Brown, A.M., Backer, L.C., Campbell, J.A., Westbrook-Collins, B., Stead, A.G. & Allen, J.W. (1986) Sister chromatid exchange and chromosome aberration analyses in mice after in vivo exposure to acrylonitrile, styrene, or butadiene monoxide. *Environ. Mutag.*, **8**, 439–448

Shugaev, B.B. (1969) Concentrations of hydrocarbons in tissues as a measure of toxicity. *Arch. environ. Health*, **18**, 878–882

Siddiqi, A.A. & Worley, F.L., Jr (1977) Urban and industrial air pollution in Houston, Texas. I. Hydrocarbons. *Atmos. Environ.*, **11**, 131–143

Siematycki, J., ed. (1991) *Risk Factors for Cancer in the Workplace*, Boca Raton, FL, CRC Press

Simmon, V.F. (1979) In vitro assays for recombinogenic activity of chemical carcinogens and related compounds with *Saccharomyces cerevisiae* D3. *J. natl Cancer Inst.*, **62**, 901–909

Simmon, V.F., Rosenkranz, H.S., Zeiger, E. & Poirier, L.A. (1979) Mutagenic activity of chemical carcinogens and related compounds in the intraperitoneal host-mediated assay. *J. natl Cancer Inst.*, **62**, 911–918

Sorsa, M., Osterman-Golkar, S., Sasiadek, M. & Peltonen, K. (1991) Genetic toxicology and biological monitoring of exposure to 1,3-butadiene (Abstract No. 14). *Mutat. Res.*, **252**, 172

Spasovski, M., Dimitrova, M., Ginčeva, N., Hristeva, V., Muhtarova, M., Benčev, I., Bajnova, A., Hinkova, L., Halkova, Z., Nosko, M., Handžieva, M., Pernov, K., Nikolov, C. & Kajtaska, M. (1986) New data on the epidemiological study in divinyl production (Bulg.). *Probl. Khig.*, **11**, 81–89

Startin, J.R. & Gilbert, J. (1984) Single ion monitoring of butadiene in plastics and foods by coupled mass spectrometry–automatic headspace gas chromatography. *J. Chromatogr.*, **294**, 427–430

Thielmann, H.W. & Gersbach, H. (1978) Carcinogen-induced DNA repair in nucleotide-permeable *Escherichia coli* cells. Analysis of DNA repair induced by carcinogenic K-region epoxides and 1,2:3,4-diepoxybutane. *Z. Krebsforsch.*, **92**, 157–176

Thurmond, L.M., Lauer, L.D., House, R.V., Stillman, W.S., Irons, R.D., Steinhagen, W.H. & Dean, J.H. (1986) Effect of short-term inhalation exposure to 1,3-butadiene on murine immune functions. *Toxicol. appl. Pharmacol.*, **86**, 170–179

Tice, R.R., Boucher, R., Luke, C.A. & Shelby, M.D. (1987) Comparative cytogenetic analysis of bone marrow damage induced in male $B6C3F_1$ mice by multiple exposures to gaseous 1,3-butadiene. *Environ. Mutag.*, **9**, 235–250

Union Carbide Corp. (1987) *Product Specification: Crude Butadiene—Taft Grade*, South Charleston, WV

US Environmental Protection Agency (1978) Interim primary drinking water regulations. *Fed. Regist.*, **43**, 20135–29150

US Environmental Protection Agency (1987) *Episodic Emissions Data Summary. Final Report* (EPA Report No. EPA-450/3-87-016; US NTIS PB87-228409), Research Triangle Park, NC, Office of Air Quality Planning and Standards, pp. 6-1–6-9, 7-1–7-9, 8-1–8-9, 9-1–9-13, 10-1–10-7

US Environmental Protection Agency (1989) *Nonmethane Organic Compound Monitoring Program* (Final Report 1988), Vol. 2, *Urban Air Toxics Monitoring Program* (PB90-146697), Washington DC

US Environmental Protection Agency (1990) *Cancer Risk from Outdoor Exposure to Air Toxics*, Vol. II, *Appendices* (EPA-450/1-90-004b), Washington DC

US Food and Drug Administration (1987) 1,3-Butadiene. In: Fazio, T. & Sherma, J., eds, *Food Additives Analytical Manual*, Vol. II, *A Collection of Analytical Methods for Selected Food Additives*, Arlington, VA, Association of Official Analytical Chemists, pp. 58–68

US Food and Drug Administration (1989) Food and drugs. *US Code fed. Regul.*, **Title 21**, Parts 175.300, 176.170, 177.1010, 177.1210, 177.2800, pp. 145–304

US National Institute for Occupational Safety and Health (1990) *National Occupational Exposure Survey (1981–1983)*, Cincinnati, OH

US National Institutes of Health/Environmental Protection Agency Chemical Information System (1983) *Carbon-13 NMR Spectral Search System, Mass Spectral Search System*, and *Infrared Spectral Search System*, Arlington, VA, Information Consultants, Inc.

US National Library of Medicine (1991) *Toxic Chemical Release Inventory (TRI) Data Bank*, Bethesda, MD

US National Toxicology Program (1984) *Toxicology and Carcinogenesis Studies of 1,3-Butadiene (CAS No. 106-99-0) in B6C3F$_1$ Mice (Inhalation Studies)* (Tech. Rep. Ser. No. 288), Research Triangle Park, NC

US Occupational Safety and Health Administration (1989) Air contaminants—permissible exposure limits. *Code fed. Regul.*, **Title 29**, Part 1910.1000

US Occupational Safety and Health Administration (1990) Occupational exposure to 1,3-butadiene. *Fed. Regist.*, **55**, 32736–32826

Van Duuren, B.L., Nelson, N., Orris, L., Palmes, E.D. & Schmitt, F.L. (1963) Carcinogenicity of epoxides, lactones, and peroxy compounds. *J. natl Cancer Inst.*, **31**, 41–55

Van Duuren, B.L., Orris, L. & Nelson, N. (1965) Carcinogenicity of epoxides, lactones, and peroxy compounds. Part II. *J. natl Cancer Inst.*, **35**, 707–717

Van Duuren, B.L., Langseth, L., Orris, L., Teebor, G., Nelson, N. & Kuschner, M. (1966) Carcinogenicity of epoxides, lactones, and peroxy compounds. IV. Tumor response in epithelial and connective tissue in mice and rats. *J. natl Cancer Inst.*, **37**, 825–838

Verschueren, K. (1983) *Handbook of Environmental Data on Organic Chemicals*, 2nd ed., New York, Van Nostrand Reinhold, pp. 295–297

Victorin, K., Busk, L., Cederberg, H. & Magnusson, J. (1990) Genotoxic activity of 1,3-butadiene and nitrogen dioxide and their photochemical reaction products in *Drosophila* and in the mouse bone marrow micronucleus assay. *Mutat. Res.*, **228**, 203–209

Vista Chemical Co. (1985) *Butadiene Concentrate*, Houston, TX

Vogt, H. (1988) Reliability of analytical methods for verifying migration data. *Food Addit. Contam.*, **5** (Suppl. 1), 455–465

Volkova, Z.A. & Bagdinov, Z.M. (1969) Problems of labor hygiene in rubber vulcanization. *Hyg. Sanit.*, **34**, 326–333

Voogd, C.E., van der Stel, J.J. & Jacobs, J.J.J.A.A. (1981) The mutagenic action of aliphatic epoxides. *Mutat. Res.*, **89**, 269–282

Walk, R.-A., Jenderny, J., Röhrborn, G. & Hackenberg, U. (1987) Chromosomal abnormalities and sister-chromatid exchange in bone marrow cells of mice and Chinese hamsters after inhalation and intraperitoneal administration: I. Diepoxybutane. *Mutat. Res.*, **182**, 333–342

Weast, R.C., ed. (1989) *CRC Handbook of Chemistry and Physics*, 70th ed., Boca Raton, FL, CRC Press, p. C-160

Wiencke, J.K., Vosika, J., Johnson, P., Wang, N. & Garry, V.F. (1982) Differential induction of sister chromatid exchange by chemical carcinogens in lymphocytes cultured from patients with solid tumors. *Pharmacology*, **24**, 67–73

Wilson, R.H., Hough, G.V. & McCormick, W.E. (1948) Medical problems encountered in the manufacture of American-made rubber. *Ind. Med.*, **17**, 199–207

Wistuba, D., Nowotny, H.-P., Träger, O. & Schurig, V. (1989) Cytochrome P-450-catalyzed asymmetric epoxidation of simple prochiral and chiral aliphatic alkenes: species dependence and effect of enzyme induction on enantioselective oxirane formation. *Chirality*, **1**, 127–136

Zimmermann, F.K. (1971) Induction of mitotic gene conversion by mutagens. *Mutat. Res.*, **11**, 327–337

Zimmermann, F.K. & Vig, B.K. (1975) Mutagen specificity in the induction of mitotic crossing-over in *Saccharomyces cerevisiae*. *Mol. gen. Genet.*, **139**, 255–268

SUMMARY OF FINAL EVALUATIONS

Agent	Degree of evidence of carcinogenicity		Overall evaluation of carcinogenicity to humans
	Human	Animal	
Bisulfites	I	I	3
1,3-Butadiene	L	S	2A
Diethyl sulfate	I	S	2A
Diisopropyl sulfate	I	S	2B
Hydrochloric acid	I	I	3
Metabisulfites	I	I	3
Occupational exposures to strong-inorganic-acid mists containing sulfuric acid	S	–	1
Sulfites	I	I	3
Sulfur dioxide	I	L	3

APPENDIX 1

SUMMARY TABLES OF
GENETIC AND RELATED EFFECTS

APPENDIX 1

Summary table of genetic and related effects of strong acid mists and acid pH, including sulfuric acid

Nonmammalian systems															Mammalian systems																			
Prokaryotes		Lower eukaryotes				Plants				Insects					In vitro													In vivo						
															Animal cells							Human cells						Animals[a]				Humans		
D	G	D	R	G	A	A	D	G	C	R	G	C	A		A	D	G	S	M	C	A	T	I	D	G	S	M	C	A	T	D	G	S	M	C	A	DL	A	D	S	M	C	A
−		+[1]	−								+							+[1]			+	+																	+[1]	+[1]	+[1]		

A, aneuploidy; C, chromosomal aberrations; D, DNA damage; DL, dominant lethal mutation; G, gene mutation; I, inhibition of intercellular communication; M, micronuclei; R, mitotic recombination and gene conversion; S, sister chromatid exchange; T, cell transformation

In completing the tables, the following symbols indicate the consensus of the Working Group with regard to the results for each endpoint:

+ considered to be positive for the specific endpoint and level of biological complexity
+[1] considered to be positive, but only one valid study was available to the Working Group
− considered to be negative
−[1] considered to be negative, but only one valid study was available to the Working Group
? considered to be equivocal or inconclusive (e.g., there were contradictory results from different laboratories; there were confounding exposures; the results were equivocal)

[a]Chromosomal aberrations, sea urchins, +

Summary table of genetic and related effects of sulfur dioxide and sodium bisulfite

Nonmammalian systems														Mammalian systems																					
Prokaryotes		Lower eukaryotes			Plants				Insects					In vitro														In vivo							
														Animal cells							Human cells							Animals							Humans
D	G	D	G	R	A	D	G	C	C	R	G	C	A	D	G	S	M	C	A	T	D	G	S	M	C	A	T	D	G	S	M	C	DL	A	D S M C A
+		$-^1$	+			$+^1$	+							$-^1$	-	+					$-^1$		+					$+^1$							- - - $-^1$?

A, aneuploidy; C, chromosomal aberrations; D, DNA damage; DL, dominant lethal mutation; G, gene mutation; I, inhibition of intercellular communication; M, micronuclei; R, mitotic recombination and gene conversion; S, sister chromatid exchange; T, cell transformation

In completing the tables, the following symbols indicate the consensus of the Working Group with regard to the results for each endpoint:

+ considered to be positive for the specific endpoint and level of biological complexity
$+^1$ considered to be positive, but only one valid study was available to the Working Group
– considered to be negative
$-^1$ considered to be negative, but only one valid study was available to the Working Group
? considered to be equivocal or inconclusive (e.g., there were contradictory results from different laboratories; there were confounding exposures; the results were equivocal)

APPENDIX 1

Summary table of genetic and related effects of hydrochloric acid

Nonmammalian systems				Mammalian systems		
Proka-ryotes	Lower eukaryotes	Plants	Insects	In vitro		In vivo
				Animal cells	Human cells	Animals / Humans

Proka-ryotes		Lower eukaryotes				Plants			Insects				Animal cells					Human cells								Animals								Humans				
D	G	D	R	G	A	D	G	C	R	G	C	A	D	G	S	M	C	D	G	S	M	C	A	T	I	D	G	S	M	C	DL	A	D	S	M	C	A
	−¹									+						+¹																					

A, aneuploidy; C, chromosomal aberrations; D, DNA damage; DL, dominant lethal mutation; G, gene mutation; I, inhibition of intercellular communication; M, micronuclei; R, mitotic recombination and gene conversion; S, sister chromatid exchange; T, cell transformation

In completing the tables, the following symbols indicate the consensus of the Working Group with regard to the results for each endpoint:

+ considered to be positive for the specific endpoint and level of biological complexity
+¹ considered to be positive, but only one valid study was available to the Working Group; sperm abnormality, mouse
− considered to be negative
−¹ considered to be negative, but only one valid study was available to the Working Group
? considered to be equivocal or inconclusive (e.g., there were contradictory results from different laboratories; there were confounding exposures; the results were equivocal)

Summary table of genetic and related effects of diethyl sulfate

Nonmammalian systems																Mammalian systems																		
Prokaryotes		Lower eukaryotes					Plants				Insects					In vitro												In vivo						
																Animal cells									Human cells					Animals					Humans			
D	G	D	R	G	A	D	G	C	R	G	C	A	D	G	S	M	C	A	T	D	G	S	M	C	A	T	D	G	S	M	C	DL	A	D	S	M	C	A
+	+	+¹	+¹			+¹	+¹	+¹	+	+¹	+	−¹	+	+	+¹	+	+¹	+		+¹			+¹	+			+	+¹ᵃ		+	+¹	+¹						

A, aneuploidy; C, chromosomal aberrations; D, DNA damage; DL, dominant lethal mutation; G, gene mutation; I, inhibition of intercellular communication; M, micronuclei; R, mitotic recombination and gene conversion; S, sister chromatid exchange; T, cell transformation

In completing the tables, the following symbols indicate the consensus of the Working Group with regard to the results for each endpoint:

+   considered to be positive for the specific endpoint and level of biological complexity
+¹   considered to be positive, but only one valid study was available to the Working Group; sperm abnormality, mouse
−   considered to be negative
−¹   considered to be negative, but only one valid study was available to the Working Group
?   considered to be equivocal or inconclusive (e.g., there were contradictory results from different laboratories; there were confounding exposures; the results were equivocal)

ᵃInconclusive result in the mouse spot test and weakly positive at one dose in the mouse specific locus test without dose–dependence

APPENDIX 1

Summary table of genetic and related effects of 1,3-butadiene and metabolites

Nonmammalian systems															Mammalian systems																						
Prokaryotes		Lower eukaryotes				Plants				Insects					In vitro														In vivo								
															Animal cells							Human cells							Animals							Humans				
D	G	D	R	G	A	D	G	C	A	C	R	G	C	A	D	G	S	M	C	A	T	D	G	S	M	C	A	T	D	G	S	M	C	DL	A	D	S	M	C	A
1,3-Butadiene																																								
+											-¹						-¹	+¹						?					+		+	+	+	+¹	-					
1,2-Epoxy-3-butene																																								
+																	-¹	+¹						+¹							+¹	+¹						+	+	
1,2,3,4-Diepoxybutane																																								
+	+									+¹	+	+¹			+¹	+¹	+						+	+													+	+		

A, aneuploidy; C, chromosomal aberrations; D, DNA damage; DL, dominant lethal mutation; G, gene mutation; I, inhibition of intercellular communication; M, micronuclei; R, mitotic recombination and gene conversion; S, sister chromatid exchange; T, cell transformation

In completing the tables, the following symbols indicate the consensus of the Working Group with regard to the results for each endpoint:

+   considered to be positive for the specific endpoint and level of biological complexity
+¹   considered to be positive, but only one valid study was available to the Working Group; sperm abnormality, mouse
−   considered to be negative
−¹   considered to be negative, but only one valid study was available to the Working Group
?   considered to be equivocal or inconclusive (e.g., there were contradictory results from different laboratories; there were confounding exposures; the results were equivocal)

ªSperm abnormality, mouse +¹

APPENDIX 2

ACTIVITY PROFILES FOR GENETIC AND RELATED EFFECTS

APPENDIX 2

ACTIVITY PROFILES FOR
GENETIC AND RELATED EFFECTS

Methods

The x-axis of the activity profile (Waters *et al.*, 1987, 1988) represents the bioassays in phylogenetic sequence by endpoint, and the values on the y-axis represent the logarithmically transformed lowest effective doses (LED) and highest ineffective doses (HID) tested. The term 'dose', as used in this report, does not take into consideration length of treatment or exposure and may therefore be considered synonymous with concentration. In practice, the concentrations used in all the in-vitro tests were converted to μg/ml, and those for in-vivo tests were expressed as mg/kg bw. Because dose units are plotted on a log scale, differences in molecular weights of compounds do not, in most cases, greatly influence comparisons of their activity profiles. Conventions for dose conversions are given below.

Profile-line height (the magnitude of each bar) is a function of the LED or HID, which is associated with the characteristics of each individual test system—such as population size, cell-cycle kinetics and metabolic competence. Thus, the detection limit of each test system is different, and, across a given activity profile, responses will vary substantially. No attempt is made to adjust or relate responses in one test system to those of another.

Line heights are derived as follows: for negative test results, the highest dose tested without appreciable toxicity is defined as the HID. If there was evidence of extreme toxicity, the next highest dose is used. A single dose tested with a negative result is considered to be equivalent to the HID. Similarly, for positive results, the LED is recorded. If the original data were analysed statistically by the author, the dose recorded is that at which the response was significant ($p < 0.05$). If the available data were not analysed statistically, the dose required to produce an effect is estimated as follows: when a dose-related positive response is observed with two or more doses, the lower of the doses is taken as the LED; a single dose resulting in a positive response is considered to be equivalent to the LED.

In order to accommodate both the wide range of doses encountered and positive and negative responses on a continuous scale, doses are transformed logarithmically, so that effective (LED) and ineffective (HID) doses are represented by positive and negative numbers, respectively. The response, or logarithmic dose unit (LDU_{ij}), for a given test system i and chemical j is represented by the expressions

$LDU_{ij} = -\log_{10}$ (dose), for HID values; LDU ≤ 0
and (1)
$LDU_{ij} = -\log_{10}$ (dose $\times$ 10^{-5}), for LED values; LDU ≥ 0.

These simple relationships define a dose range of 0 to -5 logarithmic units for ineffective doses (1–100 000 µg/ml or mg/kg bw) and 0 to $+8$ logarithmic units for effective doses (100 000–0.001 µg/ml or mg/kg bw). A scale illustrating the LDU values is shown in Figure 1. Negative responses at doses less than 1 µg/ml (mg/kg bw) are set equal to 1. Effectively, an LED value $\geq$100 000 or an HID value $\leq$1 produces an LDU = 0; no quantitative information is gained from such extreme values. The dotted lines at the levels of log dose units 1 and -1 define a 'zone of uncertainty' in which positive results are reported at such high doses (between 10 000 and 100 000 µg/ml or mg/kg bw) or negative results are reported at such low dose levels (1 to 10 µg/ml or mg/kg bw) as to call into question the adequacy of the test.

Fig. 1. Scale of log dose units used on the y-axis of activity profiles

Positive (µg/ml or mg/kg bw)		Log dose units	
0.001	....	8	——
0.01	....	7	—
0.1	....	6	—
1.0	....	5	—
10	....	4	—
100	....	3	—
1000	....	2	—
10 000	....	1	—
100 000	.... 1	0	——
	.... 10	-1	—
	.... 100	-2	—
	.... 1000	-3	—
	.... 10 000	-4	—
	.... 100 000	-5	——
	Negative (µg/ml or mg/kg bw)		

LED and HID are expressed as µg/ml or mg/kg bw.

In practice, an activity profile is computer generated. A data entry programme is used to store abstracted data from published reports. A sequential file (in ASCII) is created for each compound, and a record within that file consists of the name and Chemical Abstracts Service number of the compound, a three-letter code for the test system (see below), the qualitative test result (with and without an exogenous metabolic system), dose (LED or HID), citation number and additional source information. An abbreviated citation for each publication is stored in a segment of a record accessing both the test data file and the citation file. During processing of the data file, an average of the logarithmic values of the data subset is calculated, and the length of the profile line represents this average value. All dose values are plotted for each profile line, regardless of whether results are positive or negative. Results obtained in the absence of an exogenous metabolic system are indicated by a bar (–), and results obtained in the presence of an exogenous metabolic system are indicated by an upward-directed arrow (↑). When all results for a given assay are either positive or negative, the mean of the LDU values is plotted as a solid line; when conflicting data are reported for the same assay (i.e., both positive and negative results), the majority data are shown by a solid line and the minority data by a dashed line (drawn to the extreme conflicting response). In the few cases in which the numbers of positive and negative results are equal, the solid line is drawn in the positive direction and the maximal negative response is indicated with a dashed line.

Profile lines are identified by three-letter code words representing the commonly used tests. Code words for most of the test systems in current use in genetic toxicology were defined for the US Environmental Protection Agency's GENE-TOX Program (Waters, 1979; Waters & Auletta, 1981). For *IARC Monographs* Supplement 6, Volume 44 and subsequent volumes, including this publication, codes were redefined in a manner that should facilitate inclusion of additional tests. Naming conventions are described below.

Data listings are presented in the text and include endpoint and test codes, a short test code definition, results [either with (M) or without (NM) an exogenous activation system], the associated LED or HID value and a short citation. Test codes are organized phylogenetically and by endpoint from left to right across each activity profile and from top to bottom of the corresponding data listing. Endpoints are defined as follows: A, aneuploidy; C, chromosomal aberrations; D, DNA damage; F, assays of body fluids; G, gene mutation; H, host-mediated assays; I, inhibition of intercellular communication; M, micronuclei; P, sperm morphology; R, mitotic recombination or gene conversion; S, sister chromatid exchange; and T, cell transformation.

Dose conversions for activity profiles

Doses are converted to µg/ml for in-vitro tests and to mg/kg bw per day for in-vivo experiments.

1. In-vitro test systems
   (a) Weight/volume converts directly to µg/ml.
   (b) Molar (M) concentration × molecular weight = mg/ml = 10^3 µg/ml; mM concentration × molecular weight = µg/ml.
   (c) Soluble solids expressed as % concentration are assumed to be in units of mass per volume (i.e., 1% = 0.01 g/ml = 10 000 µg/ml; also, 1 ppm = 1 µg/ml).
   (d) Liquids and gases expressed as % concentration are assumed to be given in units of volume per volume. Liquids are converted to weight per volume using the density (D) of the solution (D = g/ml). Gases are converted from volume to mass using the ideal gas law, PV = nRT. For exposure at 20–37°C at standard atmospheric pressure, 1% (v/v) = 0.4 µg/ml × molecular weight of the gas. Also, 1 ppm (v/v) = 4×10^{-5} µg/ml × molecular weight.

(e) In microbial plate tests, it is usual for the doses to be reported as weight/plate, whereas concentrations are required to enter data on the activity profile chart. While remaining cognisant of the errors involved in the process, it is assumed that a 2-ml volume of top agar is delivered to each plate and that the test substance remains in solution within it; concentrations are derived from the reported weight/plate values by dividing by this arbitrary volume. For spot tests, a 1-ml volume is used in the calculation.

(f) Conversion of particulate concentrations given in $\mu g/cm^2$ are based on the area (A) of the dish and the volume of medium per dish; i.e., for a 100-mm dish: $A = \pi R^2 = \pi \times (5\ cm)^2 = 78.5\ cm^2$. If the volume of medium is 10 ml, then $78.5\ cm^2 = 10$ ml and $1\ cm^2 = 0.13$ ml.

2. In-vitro systems using in-vivo activation

For the body fluid–urine (BF–) test, the concentration used is the dose (in mg/kg bw) of the compound administered to test animals or patients.

3. In-vivo test systems

(a) Doses are converted to mg/kg bw per day of exposure, assuming 100% absorption. Standard values are used for each sex and species of rodent, including body weight and average intake per day, as reported by Gold *et al.* (1984). For example, in a test using male mice fed 50 ppm of the agent in the diet, the standard food intake per day is 12% of body weight, and the conversion is dose = 50 ppm × 12% = 6 mg/kg bw per day.

Standard values used for humans are: weight—males, 70 kg; females, 55 kg; surface area, 1.7 m²; inhalation rate, 20 l/min for light work, 30 l/min for mild exercise.

(b) When reported, the dose at the target site is used. For example, doses given in studies of lymphocytes of humans exposed *in vivo* are the measured blood concentrations in $\mu g/ml$.

Codes for test systems

For specific nonmammalian test systems, the first two letters of the three-symbol code word define the test organism (e.g., SA– for *Salmonella typhimurium*, EC– for *Escherichia coli*). If the species is not known, the convention used is –S–. The third symbol may be used to define the tester strain (e.g., SA8 for *S. typhimurium* TA1538, ECW for *E. coli* WP2*uvr*A). When strain designation is not indicated, the third letter is used to define the specific genetic endpoint under investigation (e.g., ––D for differential toxicity, ––F for forward mutation, ––G for gene conversion or genetic crossing-over, ––N for aneuploidy, ––R for reverse mutation, ––U for unscheduled DNA synthesis). The third letter may also be used to define the general endpoint under investigation when a more complete definition is not possible or relevant (e.g., ––M for mutation, ––C for chromosomal aberration).

For mammalian test systems, the first letter of the three-letter code word defines the genetic endpoint under investigation: A–– for aneuploidy, B–– for binding, C–– for chromosomal aberration, D–– for DNA strand breaks, G–– for gene mutation, I–– for inhibition of intercellular communication, M–– for micronucleus formation, R–– for DNA repair, S— for sister chromatid exchange, T— for cell transformation and U— for unscheduled DNA synthesis.

For animal (i.e., non-human) test systems *in vitro*, when the cell type is not specified, the code letters –IA are used. For such assays *in vivo*, when the animal species is not specified, the code letters –VA are used. Commonly used animal species are identified by the third letter (e.g., —C for Chinese hamster, —M for mouse, —R for rat, —S for Syrian hamster).

For test systems using human cells *in vitro*, when the cell type is not specified, the code letters –IH are used. For assays on humans *in vivo*, when the cell type is not specified, the code letters –VH are used. Otherwise, the second letter specifies the cell type under investigation (e.g., -BH for bone marrow, -LH for lymphocytes).

Some other specific coding conventions used for mammalian systems are as follows: BF– for body fluids, HM– for host-mediated, —L for leukocytes or lymphocytes *in vitro* (-AL, animals; -HL, humans), -L- for leukocytes *in vivo* (-LA, animals; -LH, humans), —T for transformed cells.

Note that these are examples of major conventions used to define the assay code words. The alphabetized listing of codes must be examined to confirm a specific code word. As might be expected from the limitation to three symbols, some codes do not fit the naming conventions precisely. In a few cases, test systems are defined by first-letter code words, for example: MST, mouse spot test; SLP, mouse specific locus test, postspermatogonia; SLO, mouse specific locus test, other stages; DLM, dominant lethal test in mice; DLR, dominant lethal test in rats; MHT, mouse heritable translocation test.

The genetic activity profiles and listings were prepared in collaboration with Environmental Health Research and Testing Inc. (EHRT) under contract to the US Environmental Protection Agency; EHRT also determined the doses used. The references cited in each genetic activity profile listing can be found in the list of references in the appropriate monograph.

References

Garrett, N.E., Stack, H.F., Gross, M.R. & Waters, M.D. (1984) An analysis of the spectra of genetic activity produced by known or suspected human carcinogens. *Mutat. Res.*, 134, 89–111

Gold, L.S., Sawyer, C.B., Magaw, R., Backman, G.M., de Veciana, M., Levinson, R., Hooper, N.K., Havender, W.R., Bernstein, L., Peto, R., Pike, M.C. & Ames, B.N. (1984) A carcinogenic potency database of the standardized results of animal bioassays. *Environ. Health Perspect.*, 58, 9–319

Waters, M.D. (1979) *The GENE-TOX program*. In: Hsie, A.W., O'Neill, J.P. & McElheny, V.K., eds, *Mammalian Cell Mutagenesis: The Maturation of Test Systems* (Banbury Report 2), Cold Spring Harbor, NY, CSH Press, pp. 449–467

Waters, M.D. & Auletta, A. (1981) The GENE-TOX program: genetic activity evaluation. *J. chem. Inf. comput. Sci.*, 21, 35–38

Waters, M.D., Stack, H.F., Brady, A.L., Lohman, P.H.M., Haroun, L. & Vainio, H. (1987) Appendix 1: Activity profiles for genetic and related tests. In: *IARC Monographs on the Evaluation of the Carcinogenic Risk of Chemicals to Humans*, Suppl. 6, *Genetic and Related Effects: An Updating of Selected* IARC Monographs *from Volumes 1 to 42*, Lyon, IARC, pp. 687–696

Waters, M.D., Stack, H.F., Brady, A.L., Lohman, P.H.M., Haroun, L. & Vainio, H. (1988) Use of computerized data listings and activity profiles of genetic and related effects in the review of 195 compounds. *Mutat. Res.*, *205*, 295–312

APPENDIX 2

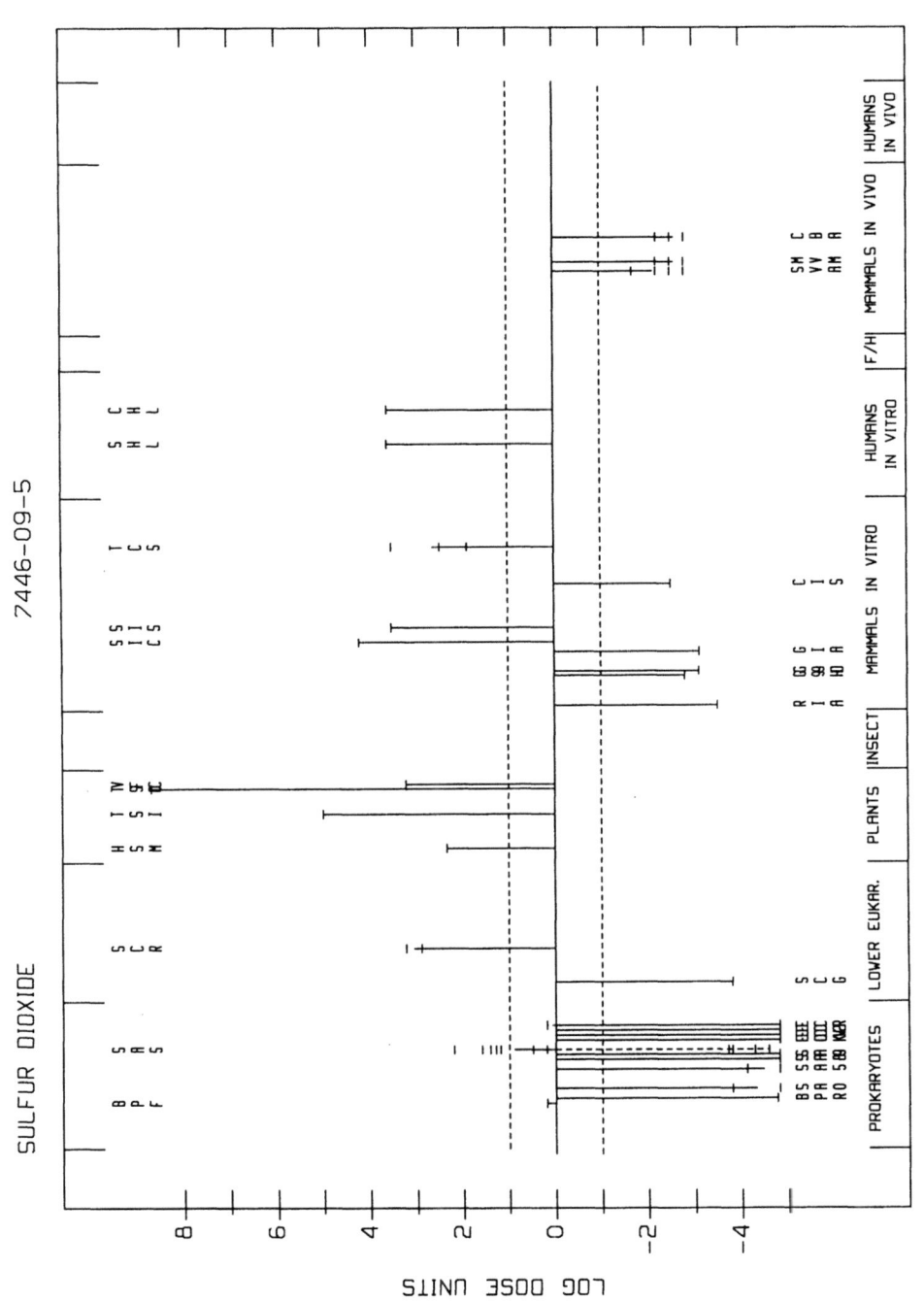

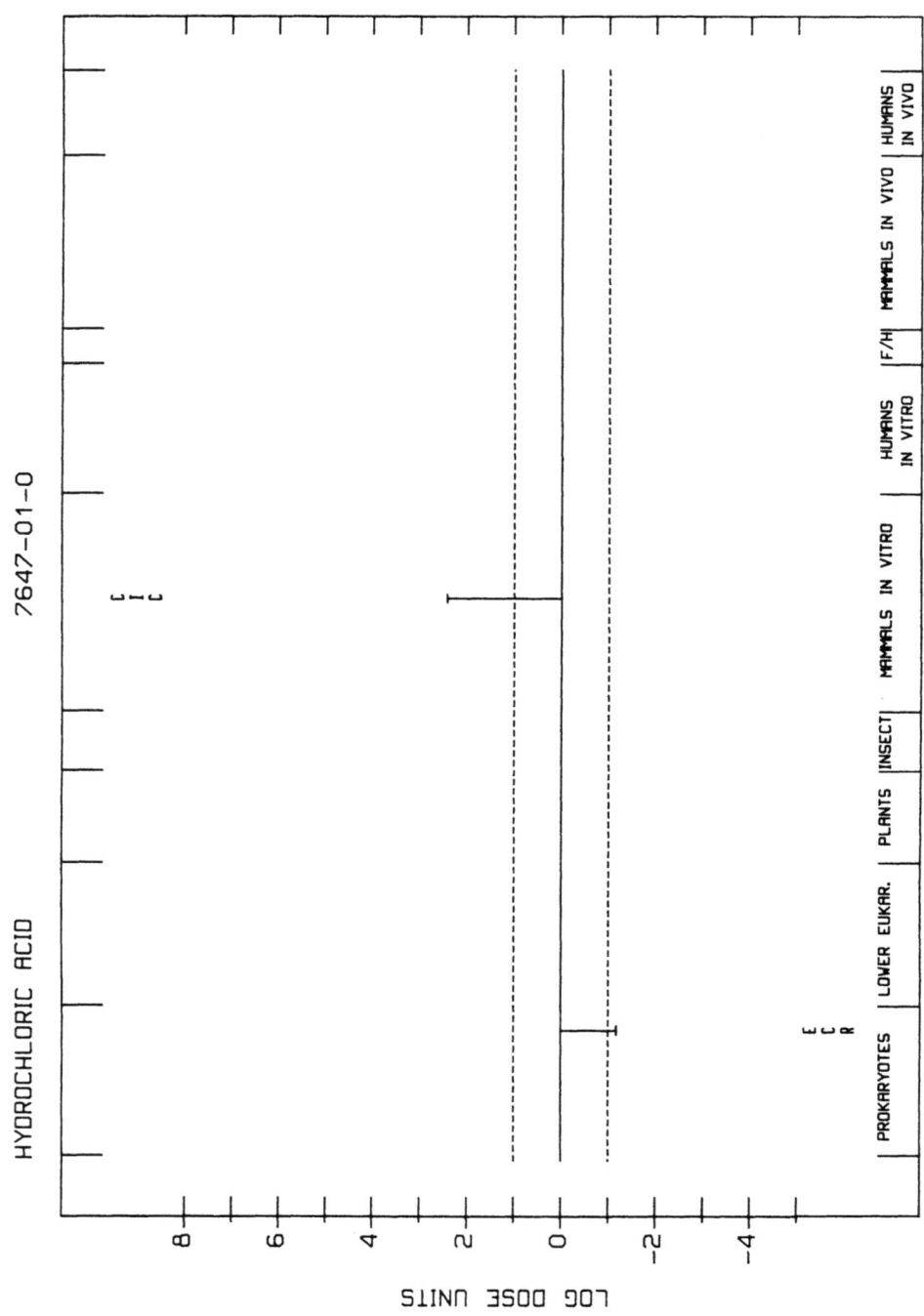

APPENDIX 2

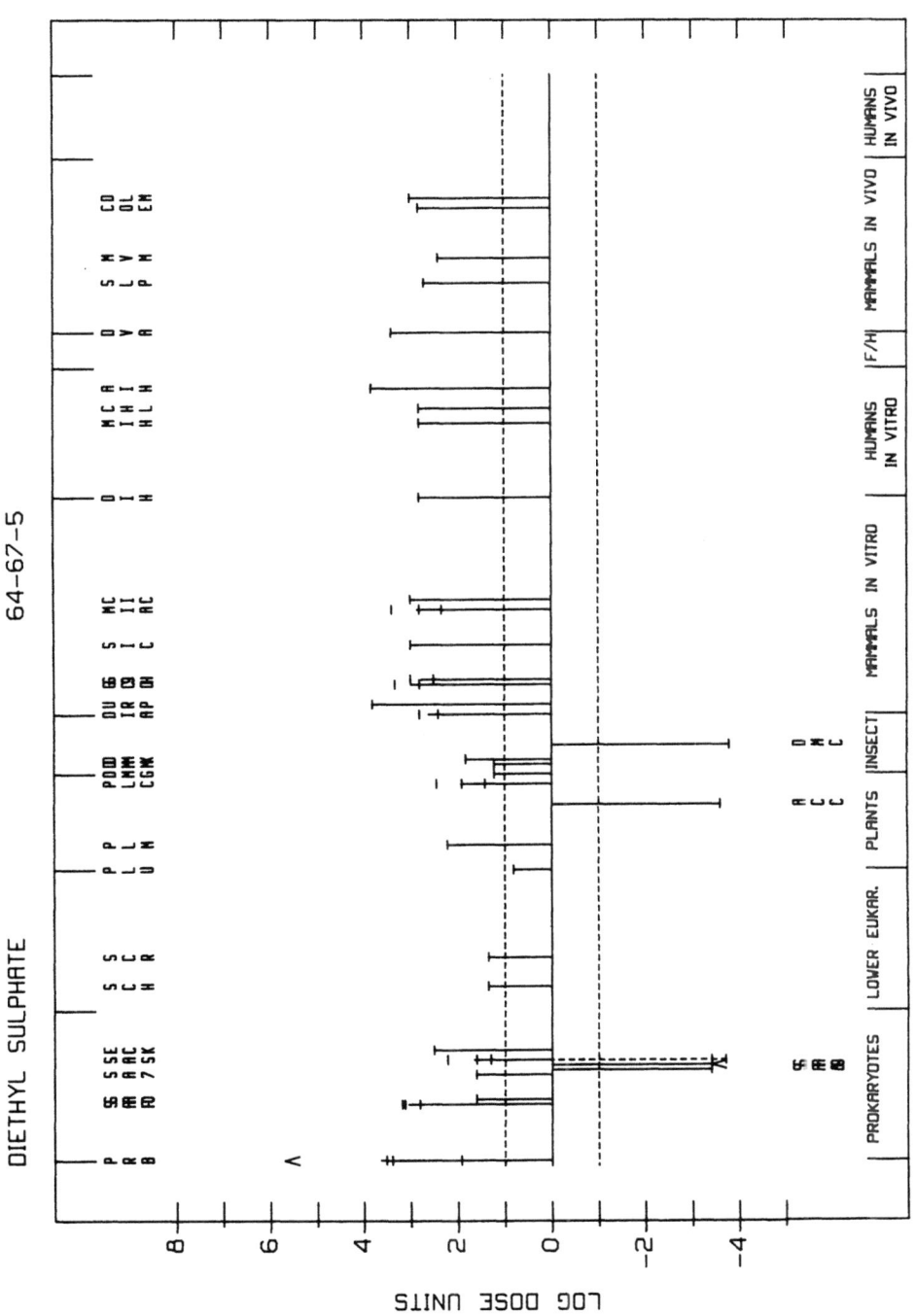

308   IARC MONOGRAPHS VOLUME 54

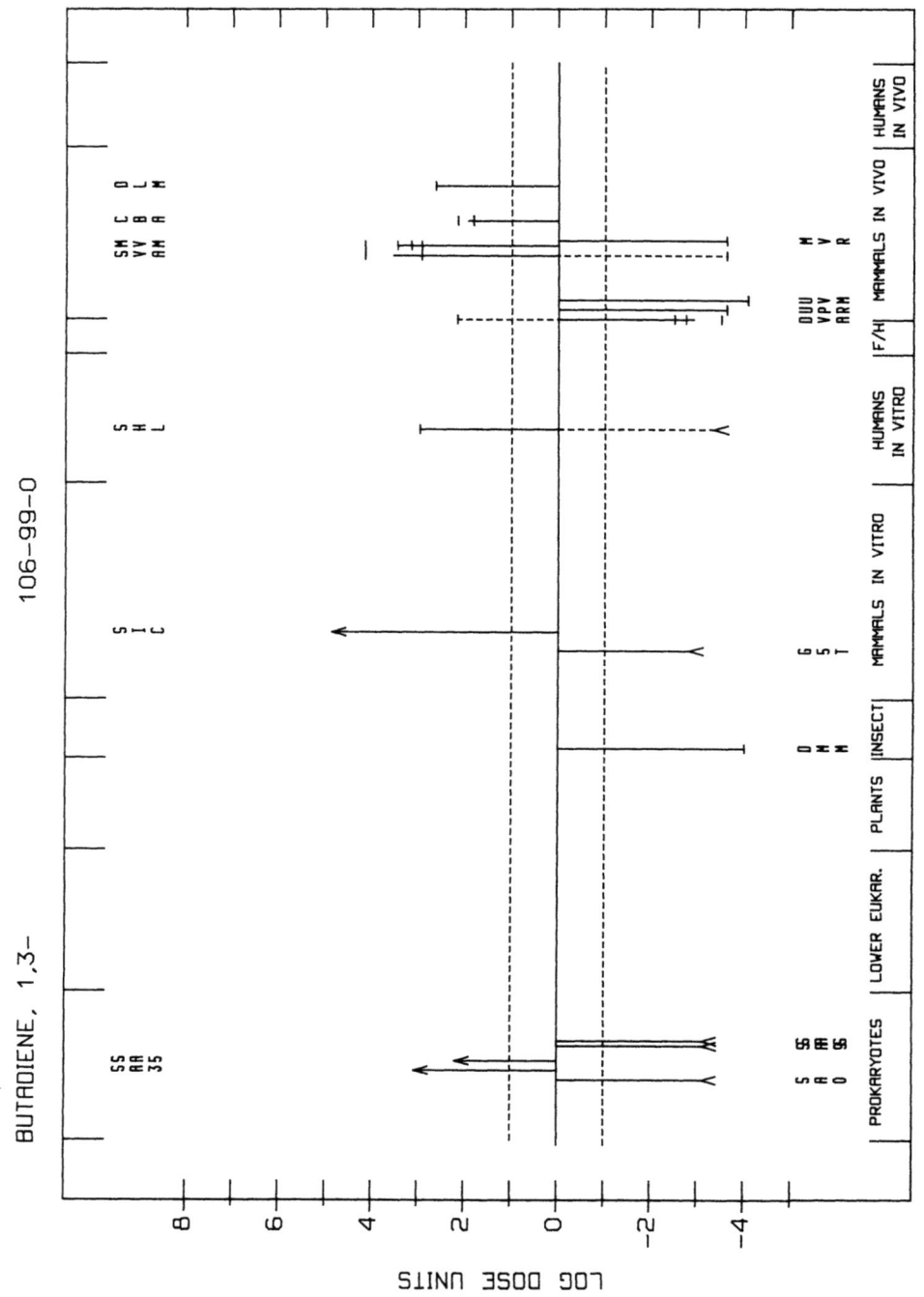

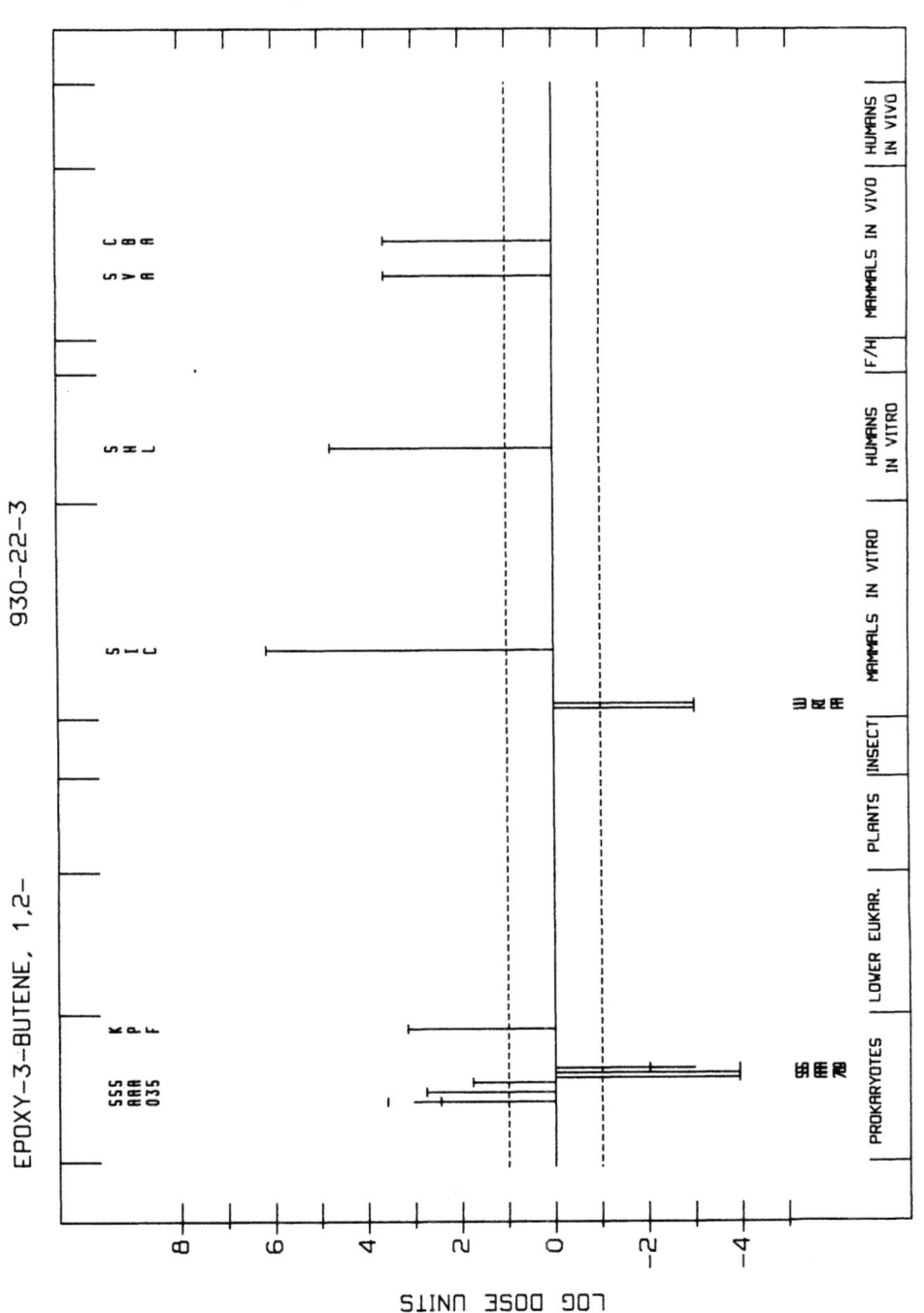

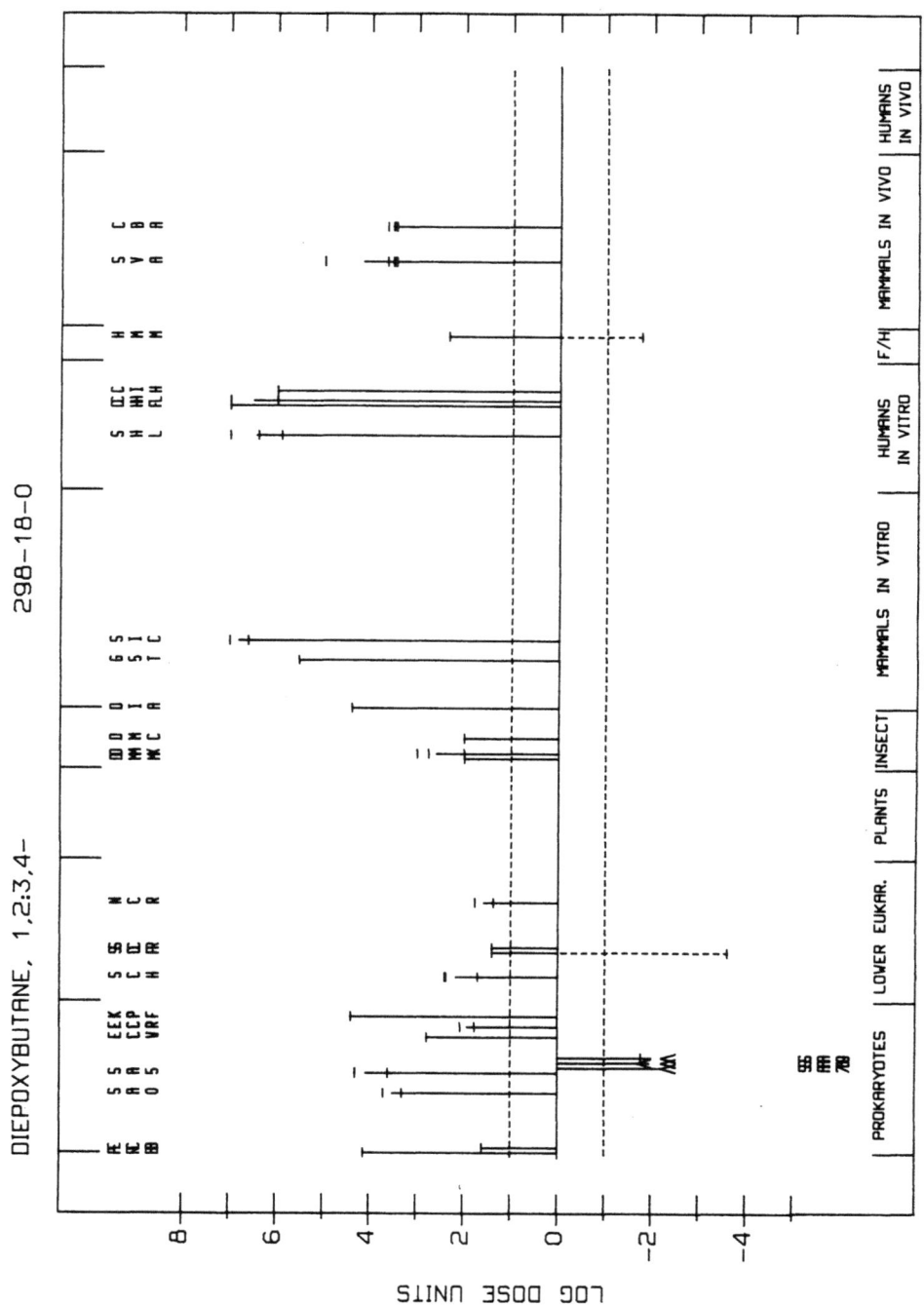

CUMULATIVE CROSS INDEX TO *IARC MONOGRAPHS ON THE EVALUATION OF CARCINOGENIC RISKS TO HUMANS*

The volume, page and year are given. References to corrigenda are given in parentheses.

A

A-α-C	*40*, 245 (1986); *Suppl. 7*, 56 (1987)
Acetaldehyde	*36*, 101 (1985) (*corr. 42*, 263); *Suppl. 7*, 77 (1987)
Acetaldehyde formylmethylhydrazone (*see* Gyromitrin)	
Acetamide	*7*, 197 (1974); *Suppl. 7*, 389 (1987)
Acetaminophen (*see* Paracetamol)	
Acridine orange	*16*, 145 (1978); *Suppl. 7*, 56 (1987)
Acriflavinium chloride	*13*, 31 (1977); *Suppl. 7*, 56 (1987)
Acrolein	*19*, 479 (1979); *36*, 133 (1985); *Suppl. 7*, 78 (1987)
Acrylamide	*39*, 41 (1986); *Suppl. 7*, 56 (1987)
Acrylic acid	*19*, 47 (1979); *Suppl. 7*, 56 (1987)
Acrylic fibres	*19*, 86 (1979); *Suppl. 7*, 56 (1987)
Acrylonitrile	*19*, 73 (1979); *Suppl. 7*, 79 (1987)
Acrylonitrile–butadiene–styrene copolymers	*19*, 91 (1979); *Suppl. 7*, 56 (1987)
Actinolite (*see* Asbestos)	
Actinomycins	*10*, 29 (1976) (*corr. 42*, 255); *Suppl. 7*, 80 (1987)
Adriamycin	*10*, 43 (1976); *Suppl. 7*, 82 (1987)
AF-2	*31*, 47 (1983); *Suppl. 7*, 56 (1987)
Aflatoxins	*1*, 145 (1972) (*corr. 42*, 251); *10*, 51 (1976); *Suppl. 7*, 83 (1987)
Aflatoxin B$_1$ (*see* Aflatoxins)	
Aflatoxin B$_2$ (*see* Aflatoxins)	
Aflatoxin G$_1$ (*see* Aflatoxins)	
Aflatoxin G$_2$ (*see* Aflatoxins)	
Aflatoxin M$_1$ (*see* Aflatoxins)	
Agaritine	*31*, 63 (1983); *Suppl. 7*, 56 (1987)
Alcohol drinking	*44* (1988)
Aldicarb	*53*, 93 (1991)
Aldrin	*5*, 25 (1974); *Suppl. 7*, 88 (1987)
Allyl chloride	*36*, 39 (1985); *Suppl. 7*, 56 (1987)
Allyl isothiocyanate	*36*, 55 (1985); *Suppl. 7*, 56 (1987)
Allyl isovalerate	*36*, 69 (1985); *Suppl. 7*, 56 (1987)
Aluminium production	*34*, 37 (1984); *Suppl. 7*, 89 (1987)
Amaranth	*8*, 41 (1975); *Suppl. 7*, 56 (1987)
5-Aminoacenaphthene	*16*, 243 (1978); *Suppl. 7*, 56 (1987)

2-Aminoanthraquinone	27, 191 (1982); *Suppl. 7*, 56 (1987)
para-Aminoazobenzene	8, 53 (1975); *Suppl. 7*, 390 (1987)
ortho-Aminoazotoluene	8, 61 (1975) *(corr. 42*, 254); *Suppl. 7*, 56 (1987)
para-Aminobenzoic acid	16, 249 (1978); *Suppl. 7*, 56 (1987)
4-Aminobiphenyl	*1*, 74 (1972) *(corr. 42*, 251); *Suppl. 7*, 91 (1987)
2-Amino-3,4-dimethylimidazo[4,5-*f*]quinoline (*see* MeIQ)	
2-Amino-3,8-dimethylimidazo[4,5-*f*]quinoxaline (*see* MeIQx)	
3-Amino-1,4-dimethyl-5*H*-pyrido[4,3-*b*]indole (*see* Trp-P-1)	
2-Aminodipyrido[1,2-*a*:3′,2′-*d*]imidazole (*see* Glu-P-2)	
1-Amino-2-methylanthraquinone	27, 199 (1982); *Suppl. 7*, 57 (1987)
2-Amino-3-methylimidazo[4,5-*f*]quinoline (*see* IQ)	
2-Amino-6-methyldipyrido[1,2-*a*:3′,2′-*d*]imidazole (*see* Glu-P-1)	
2-Amino-3-methyl-9*H*-pyrido[2,3-*b*]indole (*see* MeA-α-C)	
3-Amino-1-methyl-5*H*-pyrido[4,3-*b*]indole (*see* Trp-P-2)	
2-Amino-5-(5-nitro-2-furyl)-1,3,4-thiadiazole	7, 143 (1974); *Suppl. 7*, 57 (1987)
4-Amino-2-nitrophenol	16, 43 (1978); *Suppl. 7*, 57 (1987)
2-Amino-5-nitrothiazole	31, 71 (1983); *Suppl. 7*, 57 (1987)
2-Amino-9*H*-pyrido[2,3-*b*]indole (*see* A-α-C)	
11-Aminoundecanoic acid	39, 239 (1986); *Suppl. 7*, 57 (1987)
Amitrole	7, 31 (1974); *41*, 293 (1986) *(corr. 52*, 513; *Suppl. 7*, 92 (1987)
Ammonium potassium selenide (*see* Selenium and selenium compounds)	
Amorphous silica (*see also* Silica)	42, 39 (1987); *Suppl. 7*, 341 (1987)
Amosite (*see* Asbestos)	
Ampicillin	*50*, 153 (1990)
Anabolic steroids (*see* Androgenic (anabolic) steroids)	
Anaesthetics, volatile	*11*, 285 (1976); *Suppl. 7*, 93 (1987)
Analgesic mixtures containing phenacetin (*see also* Phenacetin)	*Suppl. 7*, 310 (1987)
Androgenic (anabolic) steroids	*Suppl. 7*, 96 (1987)
Angelicin and some synthetic derivatives (*see also* Angelicins)	40, 291 (1986)
Angelicin plus ultraviolet radiation (*see also* Angelicin and some synthetic derivatives)	*Suppl. 7*, 57 (1987)
Angelicins	*Suppl. 7*, 57 (1987)
Aniline	*4*, 27 (1974) *(corr. 42*, 252); 27, 39 (1982); *Suppl. 7*, 99 (1987)
ortho-Anisidine	27, 63 (1982); *Suppl. 7*, 57 (1987)
para-Anisidine	27, 65 (1982); *Suppl. 7*, 57 (1987)
Anthanthrene	32, 95 (1983); *Suppl. 7*, 57 (1987)
Anthophyllite (*see* Asbestos)	
Anthracene	32, 105 (1983); *Suppl. 7*, 57 (1987)
Anthranilic acid	16, 265 (1978); *Suppl. 7*, 57 (1987)
Antimony trioxide	47, 291 (1989)
Antimony trisulfide	47, 291 (1989)
ANTU (*see* 1-Naphthylthiourea)	
Apholate	9, 31 (1975); *Suppl. 7*, 57 (1987)
Aramite®	5, 39 (1974); *Suppl. 7*, 57 (1987)
Areca nut (*see* Betel quid)	
Arsanilic acid (*see* Arsenic and arsenic compounds)	
Arsenic and arsenic compounds	*1*, 41 (1972); 2, 48 (1973); 23, 39 (1980); *Suppl. 7*, 100 (1987)

Arsenic pentoxide (*see* Arsenic and arsenic compounds)
Arsenic sulfide (*see* Arsenic and arsenic compounds)
Arsenic trioxide (*see* Arsenic and arsenic compounds)
Arsine (*see* Arsenic and arsenic compounds)
Asbestos   *2*, 17 (1973) (*corr. 42*, 252);
                                                                  14 (1977) (*corr. 42*, 256); Suppl. 7,
                                                                  106 (1987) (*corr. 45*, 283)
Atrazine   *53*, 441 (1991)
Attapulgite   *42*, 159 (1987); *Suppl. 7*, 117 (1987)
Auramine (technical-grade)   *1*, 69 (1972) (*corr. 42*, 251); *Suppl.
                                                                  7*, 118 (1987)
Auramine, manufacture of (*see also* Auramine, technical-grade)   *Suppl. 7*, 118 (1987)
Aurothioglucose   *13*, 39 (1977); *Suppl. 7*, 57 (1987)
Azacitidine   *26*, 37 (1981); *Suppl. 7*, 57 (1987);
                                                                  50, 47 (1990)
5-Azacytidine (*see* Azacitidine)
Azaserine   *10*, 73 (1976) (*corr. 42*, 255);
                                                                  Suppl. 7, 57 (1987)
Azathioprine   *26*, 47 (1981); *Suppl. 7*, 119 (1987)
Aziridine   *9*, 37 (1975); *Suppl. 7*, 58 (1987)
2-(1-Aziridinyl)ethanol   *9*, 47 (1975); *Suppl. 7*, 58 (1987)
Aziridyl benzoquinone   *9*, 51 (1975); *Suppl. 7*, 58 (1987)
Azobenzene   *8*, 75 (1975); *Suppl. 7*, 58 (1987)

B

Barium chromate (*see* Chromium and chromium compounds)
Basic chromic sulphate (*see* Chromium and chromium compounds)
BCNU (*see* Bischloroethyl nitrosourea)
Benz[*a*]acridine   *32*, 123 (1983); *Suppl. 7*, 58 (1987)
Benz[*c*]acridine   *3*, 241 (1973); *32*, 129 (1983);
                                                                  Suppl. 7, 58 (1987)
Benzal chloride (*see also* α-Chlorinated toluenes)   *29*, 65 (1982); *Suppl. 7*, 148 (1987)
Benz[*a*]anthracene   *3*, 45 (1973); *32*, 135 (1983);
                                                                  Suppl. 7, 58 (1987)
Benzene   *7*, 203 (1974) (*corr. 42*, 254); *29*, 93,
                                                                  391 (1982); *Suppl. 7*, 120 (1987)
Benzidine   *1*, 80 (1972); *29*, 149, 391 (1982);
                                                                  Suppl. 7, 123 (1987)
Benzidine-based dyes   *Suppl. 7*, 125 (1987)
Benzo[*b*]fluoranthene   *3*, 69 (1973); *32*, 147 (1983);
                                                                  Suppl. 7, 58 (1987)
Benzo[*j*]fluoranthene   *3*, 82 (1973); *32*, 155 (1983); *Suppl.
                                                                  7*, 58 (1987)
Benzo[*k*]fluoranthene   *32*, 163 (1983); *Suppl. 7*, 58 (1987)
Benzo[*ghi*]fluoranthene   *32*, 171 (1983); *Suppl. 7*, 58 (1987)
Benzo[*a*]fluorene   *32*, 177 (1983); *Suppl. 7*, 58 (1987)
Benzo[*b*]fluorene   *32*, 183 (1983); *Suppl. 7*, 58 (1987)
Benzo[*c*]fluorene   *32*, 189 (1983); *Suppl. 7*, 58 (1987)
Benzo[*ghi*]perylene   *32*, 195 (1983); *Suppl. 7*, 58 (1987)
Benzo[*c*]phenanthrene   *32*, 205 (1983); *Suppl. 7*, 58 (1987)

Benzo[a]pyrene	3, 91 (1973); 32, 211 (1983); Suppl. 7, 58 (1987)
Benzo[e]pyrene	3, 137 (1973); 32, 225 (1983); Suppl. 7, 58 (1987)
para-Benzoquinone dioxime	29, 185 (1982); Suppl. 7, 58 (1987)
Benzotrichloride (see also α-Chlorinated toluenes)	29, 73 (1982); Suppl. 7, 148 (1987)
Benzoyl chloride	29, 83 (1982) (corr. 42, 261); Suppl. 7, 126 (1987)
Benzoyl peroxide	36, 267 (1985); Suppl. 7, 58 (1987)
Benzyl acetate	40, 109 (1986); Suppl. 7, 58 (1987)
Benzyl chloride (see also α-Chlorinated toluenes)	11, 217 (1976) (corr. 42, 256); 29, 49 (1982); Suppl. 7, 148 (1987)
Benzyl violet 4B	16, 153 (1978); Suppl. 7, 58 (1987)
Bertrandite (see Beryllium and beryllium compounds)	
Beryllium and beryllium compounds	1, 17 (1972); 23, 143 (1980) (corr. 42, 260); Suppl. 7, 127 (1987)
Beryllium acetate (see Beryllium and beryllium compounds)	
Beryllium acetate, basic (see Beryllium and beryllium compounds)	
Beryllium–aluminium alloy (see Beryllium and beryllium compounds)	
Beryllium carbonate (see Beryllium and beryllium compounds)	
Beryllium chloride (see Beryllium and beryllium compounds)	
Beryllium–copper alloy (see Beryllium and beryllium compounds)	
Beryllium–copper–cobalt alloy (see Beryllium and beryllium compounds)	
Beryllium fluoride (see Beryllium and beryllium compounds)	
Beryllium hydroxide (see Beryllium and beryllium compounds)	
Beryllium–nickel alloy (see Beryllium and beryllium compounds)	
Beryllium oxide (see Beryllium and beryllium compounds)	
Beryllium phosphate (see Beryllium and beryllium compounds)	
Beryllium silicate (see Beryllium and beryllium compounds)	
Beryllium sulfate (see Beryllium and beryllium compounds)	
Beryl ore (see Beryllium and beryllium compounds)	
Betel quid	37, 141 (1985); Suppl. 7, 128 (1987)
Betel-quid chewing (see Betel quid)	
BHA (see Butylated hydroxyanisole)	
BHT (see Butylated hydroxytoluene)	
Bis(1-aziridinyl)morpholinophosphine sulphide	9, 55 (1975); Suppl. 7, 58 (1987)
Bis(2-chloroethyl)ether	9, 117 (1975); Suppl. 7, 58 (1987)
N,N-Bis(2-chloroethyl)-2-naphthylamine	4, 119 (1974) (corr. 42, 253); Suppl. 7, 130 (1987)
Bischloroethyl nitrosourea (see also Chloroethyl nitrosoureas)	26, 79 (1981); Suppl. 7, 150 (1987)
1,2-Bis(chloromethoxy)ethane	15, 31 (1977); Suppl. 7, 58 (1987)
1,4-Bis(chloromethoxymethyl)benzene	15, 37 (1977); Suppl. 7, 58 (1987)
Bis(chloromethyl)ether	4, 231 (1974) (corr. 42, 253); Suppl. 7, 131 (1987)
Bis(2-chloro-1-methylethyl)ether	41, 149 (1986); Suppl. 7, 59 (1987)
Bis(2,3-epoxycyclopentyl)ether	47, 231 (1989)
Bisphenol A diglycidyl ether (see Glycidyl ethers)	
Bisulfites (see Sulfur dioxide and some sulfites, bisulfites and metabisulfites)	
Bitumens	35, 39 (1985); Suppl. 7, 133 (1987)
Bleomycins	26, 97 (1981); Suppl. 7, 134 (1987)
Blue VRS	16, 163 (1978); Suppl. 7, 59 (1987)
Boot and shoe manufacture and repair	25, 249 (1981); Suppl. 7, 232 (1987)

Bracken fern	*40*, 47 (1986); *Suppl. 7*, 135 (1987)
Brilliant Blue FCF, disodium salt	*16*, 171 (1978) (*corr. 42*, 257); *Suppl. 7*, 59 (1987)
Bromochloroacetonitrile (*see* Halogenated acetonitriles)	
Bromodichloromethane	*52*, 179 (1991)
Bromoethane	*52*, 299 (1991)
Bromoform	*52*, 213 (1991)
1,3-Butadiene	*39*, 155 (1986) (*corr. 42*, 264); *Suppl. 7*, 136 (1987); *54*, 237 (1992)
1,4-Butanediol dimethanesulfonate	*4*, 247 (1974); *Suppl. 7*, 137 (1987)
n-Butyl acrylate	*39*, 67 (1986); *Suppl. 7*, 59 (1987)
Butylated hydroxyanisole	*40*, 123 (1986); *Suppl. 7*, 59 (1987)
Butylated hydroxytoluene	*40*, 161 (1986); *Suppl. 7*, 59 (1987)
Butyl benzyl phthalate	*29*, 193 (1982) (*corr. 42*, 261); *Suppl. 7*, 59 (1987)
β-Butyrolactone	*11*, 225 (1976); *Suppl. 7*, 59 (1987)
γ-Butyrolactone	*11*, 231 (1976); *Suppl. 7*, 59 (1987)

C

Cabinet-making (*see* Furniture and cabinet-making)	
Cadmium acetate (*see* Cadmium and cadmium compounds)	
Cadmium and cadmium compounds	*2*, 74 (1973); *11*, 39 (1976) (*corr. 42*, 255); *Suppl. 7*, 139 (1987)
Cadmium chloride (*see* Cadmium and cadmium compounds)	
Cadmium oxide (*see* Cadmium and cadmium compounds)	
Cadmium sulfate (*see* Cadmium and cadmium compounds)	
Cadmium sulfide (*see* Cadmium and cadmium compounds)	
Caffeine	*51*, 291 (1991)
Calcium arsenate (*see* Arsenic and arsenic compounds)	
Calcium chromate (*see* Chromium and chromium compounds)	
Calcium cyclamate (*see* Cyclamates)	
Calcium saccharin (*see* Saccharin)	
Cantharidin	*10*, 79 (1976); *Suppl. 7*, 59 (1987)
Caprolactam	*19*, 115 (1979) (*corr. 42*, 258); *39*, 247 (1986) (*corr. 42*, 264); *Suppl. 7*, 390 (1987)
Captafol	*53*, 353 (1991)
Captan	*30*, 295 (1983); *Suppl. 7*, 59 (1987)
Carbaryl	*12*, 37 (1976); *Suppl. 7*, 59 (1987)
Carbazole	*32*, 239 (1983); *Suppl. 7*, 59 (1987)
3-Carbethoxypsoralen	*40*, 317 (1986); *Suppl. 7*, 59 (1987)
Carbon blacks	*3*, 22 (1973); *33*, 35 (1984); *Suppl. 7*, 142 (1987)
Carbon tetrachloride	*1*, 53 (1972); *20*, 371 (1979); *Suppl. 7*, 143 (1987)
Carmoisine	*8*, 83 (1975); *Suppl. 7*, 59 (1987)
Carpentry and joinery	*25*, 139 (1981); *Suppl. 7*, 378 (1987)
Carrageenan	*10*, 181 (1976) (*corr. 42*, 255); *31*, 79 (1983); *Suppl. 7*, 59 (1987)
Catechol	*15*, 155 (1977); *Suppl. 7*, 59 (1987)

CCNU (see 1-(2-Chloroethyl)-3-cyclohexyl-1-nitrosourea)
Ceramic fibres (see Man-made mineral fibres)
Chemotherapy, combined, including alkylating agents (see MOPP and other combined chemotherapy including alkylating agents)

Chlorambucil	9, 125 (1975); 26, 115 (1981); Suppl. 7, 144 (1987)
Chloramphenicol	10, 85 (1976); Suppl. 7, 145 (1987); 50, 169 (1990)
Chlorendic acid	48, 45 (1990)
Chlordane (see also Chlordane/Heptachlor)	20, 45 (1979) (corr. 42, 258)
Chlordane/Heptachlor	Suppl. 7, 146 (1987); 53, 115 (1991)
Chlordecone	20, 67 (1979); Suppl. 7, 59 (1987)
Chlordimeform	30, 61 (1983); Suppl. 7, 59 (1987)
Chlorinated dibenzodioxins (other than TCDD)	15, 41 (1977); Suppl. 7, 59 (1987)
Chlorinated drinking-water	52, 45 (1991)
Chlorinated paraffins	48, 55 (1990)
α-Chlorinated toluenes	Suppl. 7, 148 (1987)
Chlormadinone acetate (see also Progestins; Combined oral contraceptives)	6, 149 (1974); 21, 365 (1979)

Chlornaphazine (see N,N-Bis(2-chloroethyl)-2-naphthylamine)
Chloroacetonitrile (see Halogenated acetonitriles)

Chlorobenzilate	5, 75 (1974); 30, 73 (1983); Suppl. 7, 60 (1987)
Chlorodibromomethane	52, 243 (1991)
Chlorodifluoromethane	41, 237 (1986) (corr. 51, 483); Suppl. 7, 149 (1987)
Chloroethane	52, 315 (1991)
1-(2-Chloroethyl)-3-cyclohexyl-1-nitrosourea (see also Chloroethyl nitrosoureas)	26, 137 (1981) (corr. 42, 260); Suppl. 7, 150 (1987)
1-(2-Chloroethyl)-3-(4-methylcyclohexyl)-1-nitrosourea (see also Chloroethyl nitrosoureas)	Suppl. 7, 150 (1987)
Chloroethyl nitrosoureas	Suppl. 7, 150 (1987)
Chlorofluoromethane	41, 229 (1986); Suppl. 7, 60 (1987)
Chloroform	1, 61 (1972); 20, 401 (1979); Suppl. 7, 152 (1987)
Chloromethyl methyl ether (technical-grade) (see also Bis(chloromethyl)ether)	4, 239 (1974); Suppl. 7, 131 (1987)

(4-Chloro-2-methylphenoxy)acetic acid (see MCPA)

Chlorophenols	Suppl. 7, 154 (1987)
Chlorophenols (occupational exposures to)	41, 319 (1986)
Chlorophenoxy herbicides	Suppl. 7, 156 (1987)
Chlorophenoxy herbicides (occupational exposures to)	41, 357 (1986)
4-Chloro-ortho-phenylenediamine	27, 81 (1982); Suppl. 7, 60 (1987)
4-Chloro-meta-phenylenediamine	27, 82 (1982); Suppl. 7, 60 (1987)
Chloroprene	19, 131 (1979); Suppl. 7, 160 (1987)
Chloropropham	12, 55 (1976); Suppl. 7, 60 (1987)
Chloroquine	13, 47 (1977); Suppl. 7, 60 (1987)
Chlorothalonil	30, 319 (1983); Suppl. 7, 60 (1987)
para-Chloro-ortho-toluidine and its strong acid salts (see also Chlordimeform)	16, 277 (1978); 30, 65 (1983); Suppl. 7, 60 (1987); 48, 123 (1990)
Chlorotrianisene (see also Nonsteroidal oestrogens)	21, 139 (1979)
2-Chloro-1,1,1-trifluoroethane	41, 253 (1986); Suppl. 7, 60 (1987)

Chlorozotocin	*50*, 65 (1990)
Cholesterol	*10*, 99 (1976); *31*, 95 (1983); *Suppl. 7*, 161 (1987)
Chromic acetate (*see* Chromium and chromium compounds)	
Chromic chloride (*see* Chromium and chromium compounds)	
Chromic oxide (*see* Chromium and chromium compounds)	
Chromic phosphate (*see* Chromium and chromium compounds)	
Chromite ore (*see* Chromium and chromium compounds)	
Chromium and chromium compounds	*2*, 100 (1973); *23*, 205 (1980); *Suppl. 7*, 165 (1987); *49*, 49 (1990) (*corr. 51*, 483)
Chromium carbonyl (*see* Chromium and chromium compounds)	
Chromium potassium sulfate (*see* Chromium and chromium compounds)	
Chromium sulfate (*see* Chromium and chromium compounds)	
Chromium trioxide (*see* Chromium and chromium compounds)	
Chrysazin (*see* Dantron)	
Chrysene	*3*, 159 (1973); *32*, 247 (1983); *Suppl. 7*, 60 (1987)
Chrysoidine	*8*, 91 (1975); *Suppl. 7*, 169 (1987)
Chrysotile (*see* Asbestos)	
Ciclosporin	*50*, 77 (1990)
CI Disperse Yellow 3	*8*, 97 (1975); *Suppl. 7*, 60 (1987)
Cimetidine	*50*, 235 (1990)
Cinnamyl anthranilate	*16*, 287 (1978); *31*, 133 (1983); *Suppl. 7*, 60 (1987)
Cisplatin	*26*, 151 (1981); *Suppl. 7*, 170 (1987)
Citrinin	*40*, 67 (1986); *Suppl. 7*, 60 (1987)
Citrus Red No. 2	*8*, 101 (1975) (*corr. 42*, 254); *Suppl. 7*, 60 (1987)
Clofibrate	*24*, 39 (1980); *Suppl. 7*, 171 (1987)
Clomiphene citrate	*21*, 551 (1979); *Suppl. 7*, 172 (1987)
Coal gasification	*34*, 65 (1984); *Suppl. 7*, 173 (1987)
Coal-tar pitches (*see also* Coal-tars)	*35*, 83 (1985); *Suppl. 7*, 174 (1987)
Coal-tars	*35*, 83 (1985); *Suppl. 7*, 175 (1987)
Cobalt[III] acetate (*see* Cobalt and cobalt compounds)	
Cobalt–aluminium–chromium spinel (*see* Cobalt and cobalt compounds)	
Cobalt and cobalt compounds	*52*, 363 (1991)
Cobalt[II] chloride (*see* Cobalt and cobalt compounds)	
Cobalt–chromium alloy (*see* Chromium and chromium compounds)	
Cobalt–chromium–molybdenum alloys (*see* Cobalt and cobalt compounds)	
Cobalt metal powder (*see* Cobalt and cobalt compounds)	
Cobalt naphthenate (*see* Cobalt and cobalt compounds)	
Cobalt[II] oxide (*see* Cobalt and cobalt compounds)	
Cobalt[II,III] oxide (*see* Cobalt and cobalt compounds)	
Cobalt[II] sulfide (*see* Cobalt and cobalt compounds)	
Coffee	*51*, 41 (1991) (*corr. 52*, 513)
Coke production	*34*, 101 (1984); *Suppl. 7*, 176 (1987)
Combined oral contraceptives (*see also* Oestrogens, progestins and combinations)	*Suppl. 7*, 297 (1987)
Conjugated oestrogens (*see also* Steroidal oestrogens)	*21*, 147 (1979)

Contraceptives, oral (see Combined oral contraceptives;
    Sequential oral contraceptives)
Copper 8-hydroxyquinoline   15, 103 (1977); Suppl. 7, 61 (1987)
Coronene   32, 263 (1983); Suppl. 7, 61 (1987)
Coumarin   10, 113 (1976); Suppl. 7, 61 (1987)
Creosotes (see also Coal-tars)   35, 83 (1985); Suppl. 7, 177 (1987)
meta-Cresidine   27, 91 (1982); Suppl. 7, 61 (1987)
para-Cresidine   27, 92 (1982); Suppl. 7, 61 (1987)
Crocidolite (see Asbestos)
Crude oil   45, 119 (1989)
Crystalline silica (see also Silica)   42, 39 (1987); Suppl. 7, 341 (1987)
Cycasin   1, 157 (1972) (corr. 42, 251); 10,
                                                     121 (1976); Suppl. 7, 61 (1987)
Cyclamates   22, 55 (1980); Suppl. 7, 178 (1987)
Cyclamic acid (see Cyclamates)
Cyclochlorotine   10, 139 (1976); Suppl. 7, 61 (1987)
Cyclohexanone   47, 157 (1989)
Cyclohexylamine (see Cyclamates)
Cyclopenta[cd]pyrene   32, 269 (1983); Suppl. 7, 61 (1987)
Cyclopropane (see Anaesthetics, volatile)
Cyclophosphamide   9, 135 (1975); 26, 165 (1981);
                                                     Suppl. 7, 182 (1987)

D

2,4-D (see also Chlorophenoxy herbicides; Chlorophenoxy   15, 111 (1977)
    herbicides, occupational exposures to)
Dacarbazine   26, 203 (1981); Suppl. 7, 184 (1987)
Dantron   50, 265 (1990)
D & C Red No. 9   8, 107 (1975); Suppl. 7, 61 (1987)
Dapsone   24, 59 (1980); Suppl. 7, 185 (1987)
Daunomycin   10, 145 (1976); Suppl. 7, 61 (1987)
DDD (see DDT)
DDE (see DDT)
DDT   5, 83 (1974) (corr. 42, 253);
                                                     Suppl. 7, 186 (1987); 53, 179 (1991)
Decabromodiphenyl oxide   48, 73 (1990)
Deltamethrin   53, 251 (1991)
Diacetylaminoazotoluene   8, 113 (1975); Suppl. 7, 61 (1987)
N,N'-Diacetylbenzidine   16, 293 (1978); Suppl. 7, 61 (1987)
Dichlorvos   53, 267 (1991)
Diallate   12, 69 (1976); 30, 235 (1983);
                                                     Suppl. 7, 61 (1987)
2,4-Diaminoanisole   16, 51 (1978); 27, 103 (1982);
                                                     Suppl. 7, 61 (1987)
4,4'-Diaminodiphenyl ether   16, 301 (1978); 29, 203 (1982);
                                                     Suppl. 7, 61 (1987)
1,2-Diamino-4-nitrobenzene   16, 63 (1978); Suppl. 7, 61 (1987)
1,4-Diamino-2-nitrobenzene   16, 73 (1978); Suppl. 7, 61 (1987)
2,6-Diamino-3-(phenylazo)pyridine (see Phenazopyridine
    hydrochloride)
2,4-Diaminotoluene (see also Toluene diisocyanates) 16, 83 (1978); Suppl. 7, 61 (1987)

2,5-Diaminotoluene (see also Toluene diisocyanates)	16, 97 (1978); Suppl. 7, 61 (1987)
ortho-Dianisidine (see 3,3'-Dimethoxybenzidine)	
Diazepam	13, 57 (1977); Suppl. 7, 189 (1987)
Diazomethane	7, 223 (1974); Suppl. 7, 61 (1987)
Dibenz[a,h]acridine	3, 247 (1973); 32, 277 (1983); Suppl. 7, 61 (1987)
Dibenz[a,j]acridine	3, 254 (1973); 32, 283 (1983); Suppl. 7, 61 (1987)
Dibenz[a,c]anthracene	32, 289 (1983) (corr. 42, 262); Suppl. 7, 61 (1987)
Dibenz[a,h]anthracene	3, 178 (1973) (corr. 43, 261); 32, 299 (1983); Suppl. 7, 61 (1987)
Dibenz[a,j]anthracene	32, 309 (1983); Suppl. 7, 61 (1987)
7H-Dibenzo[c,g]carbazole	3, 260 (1973); 32, 315 (1983); Suppl. 7, 61 (1987)
Dibenzodioxins, chlorinated (other than TCDD) [see Chlorinated dibenzodioxins (other than TCDD)]	
Dibenzo[a,e]fluoranthene	32, 321 (1983); Suppl. 7, 61 (1987)
Dibenzo[h,rst]pentaphene	3, 197 (1973); Suppl. 7, 62 (1987)
Dibenzo[a,e]pyrene	3, 201 (1973); 32, 327 (1983); Suppl. 7, 62 (1987)
Dibenzo[a,h]pyrene	3, 207 (1973); 32, 331 (1983); Suppl. 7, 62 (1987)
Dibenzo[a,i]pyrene	3, 215 (1973); 32, 337 (1983); Suppl. 7, 62 (1987)
Dibenzo[a,l]pyrene	3, 224 (1973); 32, 343 (1983); Suppl. 7, 62 (1987)
Dibromoacetonitrile (see Halogenated acetonitriles)	
1,2-Dibromo-3-chloropropane	15, 139 (1977); 20, 83 (1979); Suppl. 7, 191 (1987)
Dichloroacetonitrile (see Halogenated acetonitriles)	
Dichloroacetylene	39, 369 (1986); Suppl. 7, 62 (1987)
ortho-Dichlorobenzene	7, 231 (1974); 29, 213 (1982); Suppl. 7, 192 (1987)
para-Dichlorobenzene	7, 231 (1974); 29, 215 (1982); Suppl. 7, 192 (1987)
3,3'-Dichlorobenzidine	4, 49 (1974); 29, 239 (1982); Suppl. 7, 193 (1987)
trans-1,4-Dichlorobutene	15, 149 (1977); Suppl. 7, 62 (1987)
3,3'-Dichloro-4,4'-diaminodiphenyl ether	16, 309 (1978); Suppl. 7, 62 (1987)
1,2-Dichloroethane	20, 429 (1979); Suppl. 7, 62 (1987)
Dichloromethane	20, 449 (1979); 41, 43 (1986); Suppl. 7, 194 (1987)
2,4-Dichlorophenol (see Chlorophenols; Chlorophenols, occupational exposures to)	
(2,4-Dichlorophenoxy)acetic acid (see 2,4-D)	
2,6-Dichloro-para-phenylenediamine	39, 325 (1986); Suppl. 7, 62 (1987)
1,2-Dichloropropane	41, 131 (1986); Suppl. 7, 62 (1987)
1,3-Dichloropropene (technical-grade)	41, 113 (1986); Suppl. 7, 195 (1987)
Dichlorvos	20, 97 (1979); Suppl. 7, 62 (1987); 53, 267 (1991)
Dicofol	30, 87 (1983); Suppl. 7, 62 (1987)

Dicyclohexylamine (see Cyclamates)
Dieldrin   5, 125 (1974); Suppl. 7, 196 (1987)
Dienoestrol (see also Nonsteroidal oestrogens)   21, 161 (1979)
Diepoxybutane   11, 115 (1976) (corr. 42, 255); Suppl.
                                                       7, 62 (1987)
Diesel and gasoline engine exhausts   46, 41 (1989)
Diesel fuels   45, 219 (1989) (corr. 47, 505)
Diethyl ether (see Anaesthetics, volatile)
Di(2-ethylhexyl)adipate   29, 257 (1982); Suppl. 7, 62 (1987)
Di(2-ethylhexyl)phthalate   29, 269 (1982) (corr. 42, 261); Suppl.
                                                       7, 62 (1987)
1,2-Diethylhydrazine   4, 153 (1974); Suppl. 7, 62 (1987)
Diethylstilboestrol   6, 55 (1974); 21, 173 (1979)
                                                       (corr. 42, 259); Suppl. 7, 273 (1987)
Diethylstilboestrol dipropionate (see Diethylstilboestrol)
Diethyl sulfate   4, 277 (1974); Suppl. 7, 198 (1987);
                                                       54, 213 (1992)
Diglycidyl resorcinol ether   11, 125 (1976); 36, 181 (1985);
                                                       Suppl. 7, 62 (1987)
Dihydrosafrole   1, 170 (1972); 10, 233 (1976);
                                                       Suppl. 7, 62 (1987)
1,8-Dihydroxyanthraquinone (see Dantron)
Dihydroxybenzenes (see Catechol; Hydroquinone; Resorcinol)
Dihydroxymethylfuratrizine   24, 77 (1980); Suppl. 7, 62 (1987)
Diisopropyl sulfate   54, 229 (1992)
Dimethisterone (see also Progestins; Sequential oral   6, 167 (1974); 21, 377 (1979)
  contraceptives)
Dimethoxane   15, 177 (1977); Suppl. 7, 62 (1987)
3,3'-Dimethoxybenzidine   4, 41 (1974); Suppl. 7, 198 (1987)
3,3'-Dimethoxybenzidine-4,4'-diisocyanate   39, 279 (1986); Suppl. 7, 62 (1987)
para-Dimethylaminoazobenzene   8, 125 (1975); Suppl. 7, 62 (1987)
para-Dimethylaminoazobenzenediazo sodium sulfonate   8, 147 (1975); Suppl. 7, 62 (1987)
trans-2-[(Dimethylamino)methylimino]-5-[2-(5-nitro-2-furyl)- 7, 147 (1974) (corr. 42, 253); Suppl. 7,
  vinyl]-1,3,4-oxadiazole   62 (1987)
4,4'-Dimethylangelicin plus ultraviolet radiation (see also Suppl. 7, 57 (1987)
  Angelicin and some synthetic derivatives)
4,5'-Dimethylangelicin plus ultraviolet radiation (see also Suppl. 7, 57 (1987)
  Angelicin and some synthetic derivatives)
Dimethylarsinic acid (see Arsenic and arsenic compounds)
3,3'-Dimethylbenzidine   1, 87 (1972); Suppl. 7, 62 (1987)
Dimethylcarbamoyl chloride   12, 77 (1976); Suppl. 7, 199 (1987)
Dimethylformamide   47, 171 (1989)
1,1-Dimethylhydrazine   4, 137 (1974); Suppl. 7, 62 (1987)
1,2-Dimethylhydrazine   4, 145 (1974) (corr. 42, 253); Suppl. 7,
                                                       62 (1987)
Dimethyl hydrogen phosphite   48, 85 (1990)
1,4-Dimethylphenanthrene   32, 349 (1983); Suppl. 7, 62 (1987)
Dimethyl sulfate   4, 271 (1974); Suppl. 7, 200 (1987)
3,7-Dinitrofluoranthene   46, 189 (1989)
3,9-Dinitrofluoranthene   46, 195 (1989)
1,3-Dinitropyrene   46, 201 (1989)
1,6-Dinitropyrene   46, 215 (1989)

1,8-Dinitropyrene	*33*, 171 (1984); *Suppl. 7*, 63 (1987); *46*, 231 (1989)
Dinitrosopentamethylenetetramine	*11*, 241 (1976); *Suppl. 7*, 63 (1987)
1,4-Dioxane	*11*, 247 (1976); *Suppl. 7*, 201 (1987)
2,4'-Diphenyldiamine	*16*, 313 (1978); *Suppl. 7*, 63 (1987)
Direct Black 38 (*see also* Benzidine-based dyes)	*29*, 295 (1982) (*corr. 42*, 261)
Direct Blue 6 (*see also* Benzidine-based dyes)	*29*, 311 (1982)
Direct Brown 95 (*see also* Benzidine-based dyes)	*29*, 321 (1982)
Disperse Blue 1	*48*, 139 (1990)
Disperse Yellow 3	*48*, 149 (1990)
Disulfiram	*12*, 85 (1976); *Suppl. 7*, 63 (1987)
Dithranol	*13*, 75 (1977); *Suppl. 7*, 63 (1987)
Divinyl ether (*see* Anaesthetics, volatile)	
Dulcin	*12*, 97 (1976); *Suppl. 7*, 63 (1987)

E

Endrin	*5*, 157 (1974); *Suppl. 7*, 63 (1987)
Enflurane (*see* Anaesthetics, volatile)	
Eosin	*15*, 183 (1977); *Suppl. 7*, 63 (1987)
Epichlorohydrin	*11*, 131 (1976) (*corr. 42*, 256); *Suppl. 7*, 202 (1987)
1,2-Epoxybutane	*47*, 217 (1989)
1-Epoxyethyl-3,4-epoxycyclohexane	*11*, 141 (1976); *Suppl. 7*, 63 (1987)
3,4-Epoxy-6-methylcyclohexylmethyl-3,4-epoxy-6-methyl-cyclohexane carboxylate	*11*, 147 (1976); *Suppl. 7*, 63 (1987)
cis-9,10-Epoxystearic acid	*11*, 153 (1976); *Suppl. 7*, 63 (1987)
Erionite	*42*, 225 (1987); *Suppl. 7*, 203 (1987)
Ethinyloestradiol (*see also* Steroidal oestrogens)	*6*, 77 (1974); *21*, 233 (1979)
Ethionamide	*13*, 83 (1977); *Suppl. 7*, 63 (1987)
Ethyl acrylate	*19*, 57 (1979); *39*, 81 (1986); *Suppl. 7*, 63 (1987)
Ethylene	*19*, 157 (1979); *Suppl. 7*, 63 (1987)
Ethylene dibromide	*15*, 195 (1977); *Suppl. 7*, 204 (1987)
Ethylene oxide	*11*, 157 (1976); *36*, 189 (1985) (*corr. 42*, 263); *Suppl. 7*, 205 (1987)
Ethylene sulfide	*11*, 257 (1976); *Suppl. 7*, 63 (1987)
Ethylene thiourea	*7*, 45 (1974); *Suppl. 7*, 207 (1987)
Ethyl methanesulfonate	*7*, 245 (1974); *Suppl. 7*, 63 (1987)
N-Ethyl-*N*-nitrosourea	*1*, 135 (1972); *17*, 191 (1978); *Suppl. 7*, 63 (1987)
Ethyl selenac (*see also* Selenium and selenium compounds)	*12*, 107 (1976); *Suppl. 7*, 63 (1987)
Ethyl tellurac	*12*, 115 (1976); *Suppl. 7*, 63 (1987)
Ethynodiol diacetate (*see also* Progestins; Combined oral contraceptives)	*6*, 173 (1974); *21*, 387 (1979)
Eugenol	*36*, 75 (1985); *Suppl. 7*, 63 (1987)
Evans blue	*8*, 151 (1975); *Suppl. 7*, 63 (1987)

F

Fast Green FCF	*16*, 187 (1978); *Suppl. 7*, 63 (1987)
Fenvalerate	*53*, 309

Ferbam	12, 121 (1976) (corr. 42, 256); Suppl. 7, 63 (1987)
Ferric oxide	1, 29 (1972); Suppl. 7, 216 (1987)
Ferrochromium (see Chromium and chromium compounds)	
Fluometuron	30, 245 (1983); Suppl. 7, 63 (1987)
Fluoranthene	32, 355 (1983); Suppl. 7, 63 (1987)
Fluorene	32, 365 (1983); Suppl. 7, 63 (1987)
Fluorides (inorganic, used in drinking-water)	27, 237 (1982); Suppl. 7, 208 (1987)
5-Fluorouracil	26, 217 (1981); Suppl. 7, 210 (1987)
Fluorspar (see Fluorides)	
Fluosilicic acid (see Fluorides)	
Fluroxene (see Anaesthetics, volatile)	
Formaldehyde	29, 345 (1982); Suppl. 7, 211 (1987)
2-(2-Formylhydrazino)-4-(5-nitro-2-furyl)thiazole	7, 151 (1974) (corr. 42, 253); Suppl. 7, 63 (1987)
Frusemide (see Furosemide)	
Fuel oils (heating oils)	45, 239 (1989) (corr. 47, 505)
Furazolidone	31, 141 (1983); Suppl. 7, 63 (1987)
Furniture and cabinet-making	25, 99 (1981); Suppl. 7, 380 (1987)
Furosemide	50, 277 (1990)
2-(2-Furyl)-3-(5-nitro-2-furyl)acrylamide (see AF-2)	
Fusarenon-X	11, 169 (1976); 31, 153 (1983); Suppl. 7, 64 (1987)

G

Gasoline	45, 159 (1989) (corr. 47, 505)
Gasoline engine exhaust (see Diesel and gasoline engine exhausts)	
Glass fibres (see Man-made mineral fibres)	
Glasswool (see Man-made mineral fibres)	
Glass filaments (see Man-made mineral fibres)	
Glu-P-1	40, 223 (1986); Suppl. 7, 64 (1987)
Glu-P-2	40, 235 (1986); Suppl. 7, 64 (1987)
L-Glutamic acid, 5-[2-(4-hydroxymethyl)phenylhydrazide] (see Agaratine)	
Glycidaldehyde	11, 175 (1976); Suppl. 7, 64 (1987)
Glycidyl ethers	47, 237 (1989)
Glycidyl oleate	11, 183 (1976); Suppl. 7, 64 (1987)
Glycidyl stearate	11, 187 (1976); Suppl. 7, 64 (1987)
Griseofulvin	10, 153 (1976); Suppl. 7, 391 (1987)
Guinea Green B	16, 199 (1978); Suppl. 7, 64 (1987)
Gyromitrin	31, 163 (1983); Suppl. 7, 391 (1987)

H

Haematite	1, 29 (1972); Suppl. 7, 216 (1987)
Haematite and ferric oxide	Suppl. 7, 216 (1987)
Haematite mining, underground, with exposure to radon	1, 29 (1972); Suppl. 7, 216 (1987)
Hair dyes, epidemiology of	16, 29 (1978); 27, 307 (1982)
Halogenated acetonitriles	52, 269 (1991)
Halothane (see Anaesthetics, volatile)	
α-HCH (see Hexachlorocyclohexanes)	

β-HCH (see Hexachlorocyclohexanes)
γ-HCH (see Hexachlorocyclohexanes)
Heating oils (see Fuel oils)
Heptachlor (see also Chlordane/Heptachlor) — 5, 173 (1974); 20, 129 (1979)
Hexachlorobenzene — 20, 155 (1979); Suppl. 7, 219 (1987)
Hexachlorobutadiene — 20, 179 (1979); Suppl. 7, 64 (1987)
Hexachlorocyclohexanes — 5, 47 (1974); 20, 195 (1979) (corr. 42, 258); Suppl. 7, 220 (1987)

Hexachlorocyclohexane, technical-grade (see Hexachlorocyclohexanes)
Hexachloroethane — 20, 467 (1979); Suppl. 7, 64 (1987)
Hexachlorophene — 20, 241 (1979); Suppl. 7, 64 (1987)
Hexamethylphosphoramide — 15, 211 (1977); Suppl. 7, 64 (1987)
Hexoestrol (see Nonsteroidal oestrogens)
Hycanthone mesylate — 13, 91 (1977); Suppl. 7, 64 (1987)
Hydralazine — 24, 85 (1980); Suppl. 7, 222 (1987)
Hydrazine — 4, 127 (1974); Suppl. 7, 223 (1987)
Hydrochloric acid — 54, 189 (1992)
Hydrochlorothiazide — 50, 293 (1990)
Hydrogen peroxide — 36, 285 (1985); Suppl. 7, 64 (1987)
Hydroquinone — 15, 155 (1977); Suppl. 7, 64 (1987)
4-Hydroxyazobenzene — 8, 157 (1975); Suppl. 7, 64 (1987)
17α-Hydroxyprogesterone caproate (see also Progestins) — 21, 399 (1979) (corr. 42, 259)
8-Hydroxyquinoline — 13, 101 (1977); Suppl. 7, 64 (1987)
8-Hydroxysenkirkine — 10, 265 (1976); Suppl. 7, 64 (1987)
Hypochlorite salts — 52, 159 (1991)

I

Indeno[1,2,3-cd]pyrene — 3, 229 (1973); 32, 373 (1983); Suppl. 7, 64 (1987)

Inorganic acids (see Sulfuric acid and other strong inorganic acids, occupational exposures to mists and vapours from)
Insecticides, occupational exposures in spraying and application of — 53, 45 (1991)
IQ — 40, 261 (1986); Suppl. 7, 64 (1987)
Iron and steel founding — 34, 133 (1984); Suppl. 7, 224 (1987)
Iron-dextran complex — 2, 161 (1973); Suppl. 7, 226 (1987)
Iron-dextrin complex — 2, 161 (1973) (corr. 42, 252); Suppl. 7, 64 (1987)

Iron oxide (see Ferric oxide)
Iron oxide, saccharated (see Saccharated iron oxide)
Iron sorbitol–citric acid complex — 2, 161 (1973); Suppl. 7, 64 (1987)
Isatidine — 10, 269 (1976); Suppl. 7, 65 (1987)
Isoflurane (see Anaesthetics, volatile)
Isoniazid (see Isonicotinic acid hydrazide)
Isonicotinic acid hydrazide — 4, 159 (1974); Suppl. 7, 227 (1987)
Isophosphamide — 26, 237 (1981); Suppl. 7, 65 (1987)
Isopropyl alcohol — 15, 223 (1977); Suppl. 7, 229 (1987)
Isopropyl alcohol manufacture (strong-acid process) — Suppl. 7, 229 (1987)
    (see also Isopropyl alcohol; Sulfuric acid and other strong inorganic acids, occupational exposures to mists and vapours from)
Isopropyl oils — 15, 223 (1977); Suppl. 7, 229 (1987)

Isosafrole	*1*, 169 (1972); *10*, 232 (1976); Suppl. 7, 65 (1987)

J

Jacobine	*10*, 275 (1976); Suppl. 7, 65 (1987)
Jet fuel	*45*, 203 (1989)
Joinery (*see* Carpentry and joinery)	

K

Kaempferol	31, 171 (1983); Suppl. 7, 65 (1987)
Kepone (*see* Chlordecone)	

L

Lasiocarpine	*10*, 281 (1976); Suppl. 7, 65 (1987)
Lauroyl peroxide	*36*, 315 (1985); Suppl. 7, 65 (1987)
Lead acetate (*see* Lead and lead compounds)	
Lead and lead compounds	*1*, 40 (1972) (*corr.* 42, 251); *2*, 52, 150 (1973); *12*, 131 (1976); *23*, 40, 208, 209, 325 (1980); Suppl. 7, 230 (1987)
Lead arsenate (*see* Arsenic and arsenic compounds)	
Lead carbonate (*see* Lead and lead compounds)	
Lead chloride (*see* Lead and lead compounds)	
Lead chromate (*see* Chromium and chromium compounds)	
Lead chromate oxide (*see* Chromium and chromium compounds)	
Lead naphthenate (*see* Lead and lead compounds)	
Lead nitrate (*see* Lead and lead compounds)	
Lead oxide (*see* Lead and lead compounds)	
Lead phosphate (*see* Lead and lead compounds)	
Lead subacetate (*see* Lead and lead compounds)	
Lead tetroxide (*see* Lead and lead compounds)	
Leather goods manufacture	*25*, 279 (1981); Suppl. 7, 235 (1987)
Leather industries	*25*, 199 (1981); Suppl. 7, 232 (1987)
Leather tanning and processing	*25*, 201 (1981); Suppl. 7, 236 (1987)
Ledate (*see also* Lead and lead compounds)	*12*, 131 (1976)
Light Green SF	*16*, 209 (1978); Suppl. 7, 65 (1987)
Lindane (*see* Hexachlorocyclohexanes)	
The lumber and sawmill industries (including logging)	*25*, 49 (1981); Suppl. 7, 383 (1987)
Luteoskyrin	*10*, 163 (1976); Suppl. 7, 65 (1987)
Lynoestrenol (*see also* Progestins; Combined oral contraceptives)	*21*, 407 (1979)

M

Magenta	*4*, 57 (1974) (*corr.* 42, 252); Suppl. 7, 238 (1987)
Magenta, manufacture of (*see also* Magenta)	Suppl. 7, 238 (1987)
Malathion	*30*, 103 (1983); Suppl. 7, 65 (1987)
Maleic hydrazide	*4*, 173 (1974) (*corr.* 42, 253); Suppl. 7, 65 (1987)

Malonaldehyde	36, 163 (1985); *Suppl. 7*, 65 (1987)
Maneb	12, 137 (1976); *Suppl. 7*, 65 (1987)
Man-made mineral fibres	43, 39 (1988)
Mannomustine	9, 157 (1975); *Suppl. 7*, 65 (1987)
Mate	51, 273 (1991)
MCPA (*see also* Chlorophenoxy herbicides; Chlorophenoxy herbicides, occupational exposures to)	30, 255 (1983)
MeA-α-C	40, 253 (1986); *Suppl. 7*, 65 (1987)
Medphalan	9, 168 (1975); *Suppl. 7*, 65 (1987)
Medroxyprogesterone acetate	6, 157 (1974); *21*, 417 (1979) (*corr. 42*, 259); *Suppl. 7*, 289 (1987)
Megestrol acetate (*see* also Progestins; Combined oral contraceptives)	
MeIQ	40, 275 (1986); *Suppl. 7*, 65 (1987)
MeIQx	40, 283 (1986); *Suppl. 7*, 65 (1987)
Melamine	39, 333 (1986); *Suppl. 7*, 65 (1987)
Melphalan	9, 167 (1975); *Suppl. 7*, 239 (1987)
6-Mercaptopurine	26, 249 (1981); *Suppl. 7*, 240 (1987)
Merphalan	9, 169 (1975); *Suppl. 7*, 65 (1987)
Mestranol (*see also* Steroidal oestrogens)	6, 87 (1974); *21*, 257 (1979) (*corr. 42*, 259)
Metabisulfites (*see* Sulfur dioxide and some sulfites, bisulfites and metabisulfites)	
Methanearsonic acid, disodium salt (*see* Arsenic and arsenic compounds)	
Methanearsonic acid, monosodium salt (*see* Arsenic and arsenic compounds	
Methotrexate	26, 267 (1981); *Suppl. 7*, 241 (1987)
Methoxsalen (*see* 8-Methoxypsoralen)	
Methoxychlor	5, 193 (1974); *20*, 259 (1979); *Suppl. 7*, 66 (1987)
Methoxyflurane (*see* Anaesthetics, volatile)	
5-Methoxypsoralen	40, 327 (1986); *Suppl. 7*, 242 (1987)
8-Methoxypsoralen (*see also* 8-Methoxypsoralen plus ultraviolet radiation)	24, 101 (1980)
8-Methoxypsoralen plus ultraviolet radiation	*Suppl. 7*, 243 (1987)
Methyl acrylate	19, 52 (1979); *39*, 99 (1986); *Suppl. 7*, 66 (1987)
5-Methylangelicin plus ultraviolet radiation (*see also* Angelicin and some synthetic derivatives)	*Suppl. 7*, 57 (1987)
2-Methylaziridine	9, 61 (1975); *Suppl. 7*, 66 (1987)
Methylazoxymethanol acetate	1, 164 (1972); *10*, 131 (1976); *Suppl. 7*, 66 (1987)
Methyl bromide	41, 187 (1986) (*corr. 45*, 283); *Suppl. 7*, 245 (1987)
Methyl carbamate	12, 151 (1976); *Suppl. 7*, 66 (1987)
Methyl-CCNU [*see* 1-(2-Chloroethyl)-3-(4-methylcyclohexyl)-1-nitrosourea]	
Methyl chloride	41, 161 (1986); *Suppl. 7*, 246 (1987)
1-, 2-, 3-, 4-, 5- and 6-Methylchrysenes	32, 379 (1983); *Suppl. 7*, 66 (1987)
N-Methyl-*N*,4-dinitrosoaniline	1, 141 (1972); *Suppl. 7*, 66 (1987)
4,4′-Methylene bis(2-chloroaniline)	4, 65 (1974) (*corr. 42*, 252);

	Suppl. 7, 246 (1987)
4,4'-Methylene bis(*N,N*-dimethyl)benzenamine	*27*, 119 (1982); *Suppl. 7*, 66 (1987)
4,4'-Methylene bis(2-methylaniline)	*4*, 73 (1974); *Suppl. 7*, 248 (1987)
4,4'-Methylenedianiline	*4*, 79 (1974) (*corr. 42, 252*); *39*, 347 (1986); *Suppl. 7*, 66 (1987)
4,4'-Methylenediphenyl diisocyanate	*19*, 314 (1979); *Suppl. 7*, 66 (1987)
2-Methylfluoranthene	*32*, 399 (1983); *Suppl. 7*, 66 (1987)
3-Methylfluoranthene	*32*, 399 (1983); *Suppl. 7*, 66 (1987)
Methylglyoxal	*51*, 443 (1991)
Methyl iodide	*15*, 245 (1977); *41*, 213 (1986); *Suppl. 7*, 66 (1987)
Methyl methacrylate	*19*, 187 (1979); *Suppl. 7*, 66 (1987)
Methyl methanesulfonate	*7*, 253 (1974); *Suppl. 7*, 66 (1987)
2-Methyl-1-nitroanthraquinone	*27*, 205 (1982); *Suppl. 7*, 66 (1987)
N-Methyl-*N'*-nitro-*N*-nitrosoguanidine	*4*, 183 (1974); *Suppl. 7*, 248 (1987)
3-Methylnitrosaminopropionaldehyde [*see* 3-(*N*-Nitrosomethylamino)-propionaldehyde]	
3-Methylnitrosaminopropionitrile [*see* 3-(*N*-Nitrosomethylamino)-propionitrile]	
4-(Methylnitrosamino)-4-(3-pyridyl)-1-butanal [*see* 4-(*N*-Nitrosomethylamino)-4-(3-pyridyl)-1-butanal]	
4-(Methylnitrosamino)-1-(3-pyridyl)-1-butanone [*see* 4-(*N*-Nitrosomethylamino)-1-(3-pyridyl)-1-butanone]	
N-Methyl-*N*-nitrosourea	*1*, 125 (1972); *17*, 227 (1978); *Suppl. 7*, 66 (1987)
N-Methyl-*N*-nitrosourethane	*4*, 211 (1974); *Suppl. 7*, 66 (1987)
Methyl parathion	*30*, 131 (1983); *Suppl. 7*, 392 (1987)
1-Methylphenanthrene	*32*, 405 (1983); *Suppl. 7*, 66 (1987)
7-Methylpyrido[3,4-*c*]psoralen	*40*, 349 (1986); *Suppl. 7*, 71 (1987)
Methyl red	*8*, 161 (1975); *Suppl. 7*, 66 (1987)
Methyl selenac (*see also* Selenium and selenium compounds)	*12*, 161 (1976); *Suppl. 7*, 66 (1987)
Methylthiouracil	*7*, 53 (1974); *Suppl. 7*, 66 (1987)
Metronidazole	*13*, 113 (1977); *Suppl. 7*, 250 (1987)
Mineral oils	*3*, 30 (1973); *33*, 87 (1984) (*corr. 42, 262*); *Suppl. 7*, 252 (1987)
Mirex	*5*, 203 (1974); *20*, 283 (1979) (*corr. 42, 258*); *Suppl. 7*, 66 (1987)
Mitomycin C	*10*, 171 (1976); *Suppl. 7*, 67 (1987)
MNNG [*see N*-Methyl-*N'*-nitro-*N*-nitrosoguanidine]	
MOCA [*see* 4,4'-Methylene bis(2-chloroaniline)]	
Modacrylic fibres	*19*, 86 (1979); *Suppl. 7*, 67 (1987)
Monocrotaline	*10*, 291 (1976); *Suppl. 7*, 67 (1987)
Monuron	*12*, 167 (1976); *Suppl. 7*, 67 (1987); *53*, 467 (1991)
MOPP and other combined chemotherapy including alkylating agents	*Suppl. 7*, 254 (1987)
Morpholine	*47*, 199 (1989)
5-(Morpholinomethyl)-3-[(5-nitrofurfurylidene)amino]-2-oxazolidinone	*7*, 161 (1974); *Suppl. 7*, 67 (1987)
Mustard gas	*9*, 181 (1975) (*corr. 42, 254*); *Suppl. 7*, 259 (1987)
Myleran (*see* 1,4-Butanediol dimethanesulfonate)	

N

Nafenopin	24, 125 (1980); Suppl. 7, 67 (1987)
1,5-Naphthalenediamine	27, 127 (1982); Suppl. 7, 67 (1987)
1,5-Naphthalene diisocyanate	19, 311 (1979); Suppl. 7, 67 (1987)
1-Naphthylamine	4, 87 (1974) (corr. 42, 253); Suppl. 7, 260 (1987)
2-Naphthylamine	4, 97 (1974); Suppl. 7, 261 (1987)
1-Naphthylthiourea	30, 347 (1983); Suppl. 7, 263 (1987)
Nickel acetate (see Nickel and nickel compounds)	
Nickel ammonium sulfate (see Nickel and nickel compounds)	
Nickel and nickel compounds	2, 126 (1973) (corr. 42, 252); 11, 75 (1976); Suppl. 7, 264 (1987) (corr. 45, 283); 49, 257 (1990)
Nickel carbonate (see Nickel and nickel compounds)	
Nickel carbonyl (see Nickel and nickel compounds)	
Nickel chloride (see Nickel and nickel compounds)	
Nickel–gallium alloy (see Nickel and nickel compounds)	
Nickel hydroxide (see Nickel and nickel compounds)	
Nickelocene (see Nickel and nickel compounds)	
Nickel oxide (see Nickel and nickel compounds)	
Nickel subsulfide (see Nickel and nickel compounds)	
Nickel sulfate (see Nickel and nickel compounds)	
Niridazole	13, 123 (1977); Suppl. 7, 67 (1987)
Nithiazide	31, 179 (1983); Suppl. 7, 67 (1987)
Nitrilotriacetic acid and its salts	48, 181 (1990)
5-Nitroacenaphthene	16, 319 (1978); Suppl. 7, 67 (1987)
5-Nitro-ortho-anisidine	27, 133 (1982); Suppl. 7, 67 (1987)
9-Nitroanthracene	33, 179 (1984); Suppl. 7, 67 (1987)
7-Nitrobenz[a]anthracene	46, 247 (1989)
6-Nitrobenzo[a]pyrene	33, 187 (1984); Suppl. 7, 67 (1987); 46, 255 (1989)
4-Nitrobiphenyl	4, 113 (1974); Suppl. 7, 67 (1987)
6-Nitrochrysene	33, 195 (1984); Suppl. 7, 67 (1987); 46, 267 (1989)
Nitrofen (technical-grade)	30, 271 (1983); Suppl. 7, 67 (1987)
3-Nitrofluoranthene	33, 201 (1984); Suppl. 7, 67 (1987)
2-Nitrofluorene	46, 277 (1989)
Nitrofural	7, 171 (1974); Suppl. 7, 67 (1987); 50, 195 (1990)
5-Nitro-2-furaldehyde semicarbazone (see Nitrofural)	
Nitrofurantoin	50, 211 (1990)
Nitrofurazone (see Nitrofural)	
1-[(5-Nitrofurfurylidene)amino]-2-imidazolidinone	7, 181 (1974); Suppl. 7, 67 (1987)
N-[4-(5-Nitro-2-furyl)-2-thiazolyl]acetamide	1, 181 (1972); 7, 185 (1974); Suppl. 7, 67 (1987)
Nitrogen mustard	9, 193 (1975); Suppl. 7, 269 (1987)
Nitrogen mustard N-oxide	9, 209 (1975); Suppl. 7, 67 (1987)
1-Nitronaphthalene	46, 291 (1989)
2-Nitronaphthalene	46, 303 (1989)
3-Nitroperylene	46, 313 (1989)
2-Nitropropane	29, 331 (1982); Suppl. 7, 67 (1987)

1-Nitropyrene	*33*, 209 (1984); *Suppl. 7*, 67 (1987); *46*, 321 (1989)
2-Nitropyrene	*46*, 359 (1989)
4-Nitropyrene	*46*, 367 (1989)
N-Nitrosatable drugs	*24*, 297 (1980) *(corr. 42*, 260)
N-Nitrosatable pesticides	*30*, 359 (1983)
N'-Nitrosoanabasine	*37*, 225 (1985); *Suppl. 7*, 67 (1987)
N'-Nitrosoanatabine	*37*, 233 (1985); *Suppl. 7*, 67 (1987)
N-Nitrosodi-n-butylamine	*4*, 197 (1974); *17*, 51 (1978); *Suppl. 7*, 67 (1987)
N-Nitrosodiethanolamine	*17*, 77 (1978); *Suppl. 7*, 67 (1987)
N-Nitrosodiethylamine	*1*, 107 (1972) *(corr. 42*, 251); *17*, 83 (1978) *(corr. 42*, 257); *Suppl. 7*, 67 (1987)
N-Nitrosodimethylamine	*1*, 95 (1972); *17*, 125 (1978) *(corr. 42*, 257); *Suppl. 7*, 67 (1987)
N-Nitrosodiphenylamine	*27*, 213 (1982); *Suppl. 7*, 67 (1987)
para-Nitrosodiphenylamine	*27*, 227 (1982) *(corr. 42*, 261); *Suppl. 7*, 68 (1987)
N-Nitrosodi-n-propylamine	*17*, 177 (1978); *Suppl. 7*, 68 (1987)
N-Nitroso-N-ethylurea (see N-Ethyl-N-nitrosourea)	
N-Nitrosofolic acid	*17*, 217 (1978); *Suppl. 7*, 68 (1987)
N-Nitrosoguvacine	*37*, 263 (1985); *Suppl. 7*, 68 (1987)
N-Nitrosoguvacoline	*37*, 263 (1985); *Suppl. 7*, 68 (1987)
N-Nitrosohydroxyproline	*17*, 304 (1978); *Suppl. 7*, 68 (1987)
3-(N-Nitrosomethylamino)propionaldehyde	*37*, 263 (1985); *Suppl. 7*, 68 (1987)
3-(N-Nitrosomethylamino)propionitrile	*37*, 263 (1985); *Suppl. 7*, 68 (1987)
4-(N-Nitrosomethylamino)-4-(3-pyridyl)-1-butanal	*37*, 205 (1985); *Suppl. 7*, 68 (1987)
4-(N-Nitrosomethylamino)-1-(3-pyridyl)-1-butanone	*37*, 209 (1985); *Suppl. 7*, 68 (1987)
N-Nitrosomethylethylamine	*17*, 221 (1978); *Suppl. 7*, 68 (1987)
N-Nitroso-N-methylurea (see N-Methyl-N-nitrosourea)	
N-Nitroso-N-methylurethane (see N-Methyl-N-methylurethane)	
N-Nitrosomethylvinylamine	*17*, 257 (1978); *Suppl. 7*, 68 (1987)
N-Nitrosomorpholine	*17*, 263 (1978); *Suppl. 7*, 68 (1987)
N'-Nitrosonornicotine	*17*, 281 (1978); *37*, 241 (1985); *Suppl. 7*, 68 (1987)
N-Nitrosopiperidine	*17*, 287 (1978); *Suppl. 7*, 68 (1987)
N-Nitrosoproline	*17*, 303 (1978); *Suppl. 7*, 68 (1987)
N-Nitrosopyrrolidine	*17*, 313 (1978); *Suppl. 7*, 68 (1987)
N-Nitrososarcosine	*17*, 327 (1978); *Suppl. 7*, 68 (1987)
Nitrosoureas, chloroethyl (see Chloroethyl nitrosoureas)	
5-Nitro-*ortho*-toluidine	*48*, 169 (1990)
Nitrous oxide (see Anaesthetics, volatile)	
Nitrovin	*31*, 185 (1983); *Suppl. 7*, 68 (1987)
NNA [see 4-(N-Nitrosomethylamino)-4-(3-pyridyl)-1-butanal]	
NNK [see 4-(N-Nitrosomethylamino)-1-(3-pyridyl)-1-butanone]	
Nonsteroidal oestrogens (see also Oestrogens, progestins and combinations)	*Suppl. 7*, 272 (1987)
Norethisterone (see also Progestins; Combined oral contraceptives)	*6*, 179 (1974); *21*, 461 (1979)
Norethynodrel (see also Progestins; Combined oral contraceptives	*6*, 191 (1974); *21*, 461 (1979) *(corr. 42*, 259)

CUMULATIVE CROSS INDEX

Norgestrel (see also Progestins, Combined oral contraceptives)	6, 201 (1974); 21, 479 (1979)
Nylon 6	19, 120 (1979); Suppl. 7, 68 (1987)

O

Ochratoxin A	10, 191 (1976); 31, 191 (1983) (corr. 42, 262); Suppl. 7, 271 (1987)
Oestradiol-17β (see also Steroidal oestrogens)	6, 99 (1974); 21, 279 (1979)
Oestradiol 3-benzoate (see Oestradiol-17β)	
Oestradiol dipropionate (see Oestradiol-17β)	
Oestradiol mustard	9, 217 (1975)
Oestradiol-17β-valerate (see Oestradiol-17β)	
Oestriol (see also Steroidal oestrogens)	6, 117 (1974); 21, 327 (1979)
Oestrogen–progestin combinations (see Oestrogens, progestins and combinations)	
Oestrogen–progestin replacement therapy (see also Oestrogens, progestins and combinations)	Suppl. 7, 308 (1987)
Oestrogen replacement therapy (see also Oestrogens, progestins and combinations)	Suppl. 7, 280 (1987)
Oestrogens (see Oestrogens, progestins and combinations)	
Oestrogens, conjugated (see Conjugated oestrogens)	
Oestrogens, nonsteroidal (see Nonsteroidal oestrogens)	
Oestrogens, progestins and combinations	6 (1974); 21 (1979); Suppl. 7, 272 (1987)
Oestrogens, steroidal (see Steroidal oestrogens)	
Oestrone (see also Steroidal oestrogens)	6, 123 (1974); 21, 343 (1979) (corr. 42, 259)
Oestrone benzoate (see Oestrone)	
Oil Orange SS	8, 165 (1975); Suppl. 7, 69 (1987)
Oral contraceptives, combined (see Combined oral contraceptives)	
Oral contraceptives, investigational (see Combined oral contraceptives)	
Oral contraceptives, sequential (see Sequential oral contraceptives)	
Orange I	8, 173 (1975); Suppl. 7, 69 (1987)
Orange G	8, 181 (1975); Suppl. 7, 69 (1987)
Organolead compounds (see also Lead and lead compounds)	Suppl. 7, 230 (1987)
Oxazepam	13, 58 (1977); Suppl. 7, 69 (1987)
Oxymetholone [see also Androgenic (anabolic) steroids]	13, 131 (1977)
Oxyphenbutazone	13, 185 (1977); Suppl. 7, 69 (1987)

P

Paint manufacture and painting (occupational exposures in)	47, 329 (1989)
Panfuran S (see also Dihydroxymethylfuratrizine)	24, 77 (1980); Suppl. 7, 69 (1987)
Paper manufacture (see Pulp and paper manufacture)	
Paracetamol	50, 307 (1990)
Parasorbic acid	10, 199 (1976) (corr. 42, 255); Suppl. 7, 69 (1987)
Parathion	30, 153 (1983); Suppl. 7, 69 (1987)
Patulin	10, 205 (1976); 40, 83 (1986); Suppl. 7, 69 (1987)
Penicillic acid	10, 211 (1976); Suppl. 7, 69 (1987)

Pentachloroethane	41, 99 (1986); Suppl. 7, 69 (1987)
Pentachloronitrobenzene (see Quintozene)	
Pentachlorophenol (see also Chlorophenols; Chlorophenols, occupational exposures to)	20, 303 (1979); 53, 371 (1991)
Permethrin	53, 329 (1991)
Perylene	32, 411 (1983); Suppl. 7, 69 (1987)
Petasitenine	31, 207 (1983); Suppl. 7, 69 (1987)
Petasites japonicus (see Pyrrolizidine alkaloids)	
Petroleum refining (occupational exposures in)	45, 39 (1989)
Some petroleum solvents	47, 43 (1989)
Phenacetin	13, 141 (1977); 24, 135 (1980); Suppl. 7, 310 (1987)
Phenanthrene	32, 419 (1983); Suppl. 7, 69 (1987)
Phenazopyridine hydrochloride	8, 117 (1975); 24, 163 (1980) (corr. 42, 260); Suppl. 7, 312 (1987)
Phenelzine sulfate	24, 175 (1980); Suppl. 7, 312 (1987)
Phenicarbazide	12, 177 (1976); Suppl. 7, 70 (1987)
Phenobarbital	13, 157 (1977); Suppl. 7, 313 (1987)
Phenol	47, 263 (1989) (corr. 50, 385)
Phenoxyacetic acid herbicides (see Chlorophenoxy herbicides)	
Phenoxybenzamine hydrochloride	9, 223 (1975); 24, 185 (1980); Suppl. 7, 70 (1987)
Phenylbutazone	13, 183 (1977); Suppl. 7, 316 (1987)
meta-Phenylenediamine	16, 111 (1978); Suppl. 7, 70 (1987)
para-Phenylenediamine	16, 125 (1978); Suppl. 7, 70 (1987)
Phenyl glycidyl ether (see Glycidyl ethers)	
N-Phenyl-2-naphthylamine	16, 325 (1978) (corr. 42, 257); Suppl. 7, 318 (1987)
ortho-Phenylphenol	30, 329 (1983); Suppl. 7, 70 (1987)
Phenytoin	13, 201 (1977); Suppl. 7, 319 (1987)
Picloram	53, 481 (1991)
Piperazine oestrone sulfate (see Conjugated oestrogens)	
Piperonyl butoxide	30, 183 (1983); Suppl. 7, 70 (1987)
Pitches, coal-tar (see Coal-tar pitches)	
Polyacrylic acid	19, 62 (1979); Suppl. 7, 70 (1987)
Polybrominated biphenyls	18, 107 (1978); 41, 261 (1986); Suppl. 7, 321 (1987)
Polychlorinated biphenyls	7, 261 (1974); 18, 43 (1978) (corr. 42, 258); Suppl. 7, 322 (1987)
Polychlorinated camphenes (see Toxaphene)	
Polychloroprene	19, 141 (1979); Suppl. 7, 70 (1987)
Polyethylene	19, 164 (1979); Suppl. 7, 70 (1987)
Polymethylene polyphenyl isocyanate	19, 314 (1979); Suppl. 7, 70 (1987)
Polymethyl methacrylate	19, 195 (1979); Suppl. 7, 70 (1987)
Polyoestradiol phosphate (see Oestradiol-17β)	
Polypropylene	19, 218 (1979); Suppl. 7, 70 (1987)
Polystyrene	19, 245 (1979); Suppl. 7, 70 (1987)
Polytetrafluoroethylene	19, 288 (1979); Suppl. 7, 70 (1987)
Polyurethane foams	19, 320 (1979); Suppl. 7, 70 (1987)
Polyvinyl acetate	19, 346 (1979); Suppl. 7, 70 (1987)
Polyvinyl alcohol	19, 351 (1979); Suppl. 7, 70 (1987)

Polyvinyl chloride	7, 306 (1974); *19*, 402 (1979); *Suppl. 7*, 70 (1987)
Polyvinyl pyrrolidone	*19*, 463 (1979); *Suppl. 7*, 70 (1987)
Ponceau MX	*8*, 189 (1975); *Suppl. 7*, 70 (1987)
Ponceau 3R	*8*, 199 (1975); *Suppl. 7*, 70 (1987)
Ponceau SX	*8*, 207 (1975); *Suppl. 7*, 70 (1987)
Potassium arsenate (*see* Arsenic and arsenic compounds)	
Potassium arsenite (*see* Arsenic and arsenic compounds)	
Potassium bis(2-hydroxyethyl)dithiocarbamate	*12*, 183 (1976); *Suppl. 7*, 70 (1987)
Potassium bromate	*40*, 207 (1986); *Suppl. 7*, 70 (1987)
Potassium chromate (*see* Chromium and chromium compounds)	
Potassium dichromate (*see* Chromium and chromium compounds)	
Prednimustine	*50*, 115 (1990)
Prednisone	*26*, 293 (1981); *Suppl. 7*, 326 (1987)
Procarbazine hydrochloride	*26*, 311 (1981); *Suppl. 7*, 327 (1987)
Proflavine salts	*24*, 195 (1980); *Suppl. 7*, 70 (1987)
Progesterone (*see also* Progestins; Combined oral contraceptives)	*6*, 135 (1974); *21*, 491 (1979) (*corr. 42*, 259)
Progestins (*see also* Oestrogens, progestins and combinations)	*Suppl. 7*, 289 (1987)
Pronetalol hydrochloride	*13*, 227 (1977) (*corr. 42*, 256); *Suppl. 7*, 70 (1987)
1,3-Propane sultone	*4*, 253 (1974) (*corr. 42*, 253); *Suppl. 7*, 70 (1987)
Propham	*12*, 189 (1976); *Suppl. 7*, 70 (1987)
β-Propiolactone	*4*, 259 (1974) (*corr. 42*, 253); *Suppl. 7*, 70 (1987)
n-Propyl carbamate	*12*, 201 (1976); *Suppl. 7*, 70 (1987)
Propylene	*19*, 213 (1979); *Suppl. 7*, 71 (1987)
Propylene oxide	*11*, 191 (1976); *36*, 227 (1985) (*corr. 42*, 263); *Suppl. 7*, 328 (1987)
Propylthiouracil	*7*, 67 (1974); *Suppl. 7*, 329 (1987)
Ptaquiloside (*see also* Bracken fern)	*40*, 55 (1986); *Suppl. 7*, 71 (1987)
Pulp and paper manufacture	*25*, 157 (1981); *Suppl. 7*, 385 (1987)
Pyrene	*32*, 431 (1983); *Suppl. 7*, 71 (1987)
Pyrido[3,4-c]psoralen	*40*, 349 (1986); *Suppl. 7*, 71 (1987)
Pyrimethamine	*13*, 233 (1977); *Suppl. 7*, 71 (1987)
Pyrrolizidine alkaloids (*see* Hydroxysenkirkine; Isatidine; Jacobine; Lasiocarpine; Monocrotaline; Retrorsine; Riddelliine; Seneciphylline; Senkirkine)	

Q

Quercetin (*see also* Bracken fern)	*31*, 213 (1983); *Suppl. 7*, 71 (1987)
para-Quinone	*15*, 255 (1977); *Suppl. 7*, 71 (1987)
Quintozene	*5*, 211 (1974); *Suppl. 7*, 71 (1987)

R

Radon	*43*, 173 (1988) (*corr. 45*, 283)
Reserpine	*10*, 217 (1976); *24*, 211 (1980) (*corr. 42*, 260); *Suppl. 7*, 330 (1987)
Resorcinol	*15*, 155 (1977); *Suppl. 7*, 71 (1987)

Retrorsine	10, 303 (1976); Suppl. 7, 71 (1987)
Rhodamine B	16, 221 (1978); Suppl. 7, 71 (1987)
Rhodamine 6G	16, 233 (1978); Suppl. 7, 71 (1987)
Riddelliine	10, 313 (1976); Suppl. 7, 71 (1987)
Rifampicin	24, 243 (1980); Suppl. 7, 71 (1987)
Rockwool (see Man-made mineral fibres)	
The rubber industry	28 (1982) (corr. 42, 261); Suppl. 7, 332 (1987)
Rugulosin	40, 99 (1986); Suppl. 7, 71 (1987)

S

Saccharated iron oxide	2, 161 (1973); Suppl. 7, 71 (1987)
Saccharin	22, 111 (1980) (corr. 42, 259); Suppl. 7, 334 (1987)
Safrole	1, 169 (1972); 10, 231 (1976); Suppl. 7, 71 (1987)
The sawmill industry (including logging) [see The lumber and sawmill industry (including logging)]	
Scarlet Red	8, 217 (1975); Suppl. 7, 71 (1987)
Selenium and selenium compounds	9, 245 (1975) (corr. 42, 255); Suppl. 7, 71 (1987)
Selenium dioxide (see Selenium and selenium compounds)	
Selenium oxide (see Selenium and selenium compounds)	
Semicarbazide hydrochloride	12, 209 (1976) (corr. 42, 256); Suppl. 7, 71 (1987)
Senecio jacobaea L. (see Pyrrolizidine alkaloids)	
Senecio longilobus (see Pyrrolizidine alkaloids)	
Seneciphylline	10, 319, 335 (1976); Suppl. 7, 71 (1987)
Senkirkine	10, 327 (1976); 31, 231 (1983); Suppl. 7, 71 (1987)
Sepiolite	42, 175 (1987); Suppl. 7, 71 (1987)
Sequential oral contraceptives (see also Oestrogens, progestins and combinations)	Suppl. 7, 296 (1987)
Shale-oils	35, 161 (1985); Suppl. 7, 339 (1987)
Shikimic acid (see also Bracken fern)	40, 55 (1986); Suppl. 7, 71 (1987)
Shoe manufacture and repair (see Boot and shoe manufacture and repair)	
Silica (see also Amorphous silica; Crystalline silica)	42, 39 (1987)
Simazine	53, 495 (1991)
Slagwool (see Man-made mineral fibres)	
Sodium arsenate (see Arsenic and arsenic compounds)	
Sodium arsenite (see Arsenic and arsenic compounds)	
Sodium cacodylate (see Arsenic and arsenic compounds)	
Sodium chlorite	52, 145 (1991)
Sodium chromate (see Chromium and chromium compounds)	
Sodium cyclamate (see Cyclamates)	
Sodium dichromate (see Chromium and chromium compounds)	
Sodium diethyldithiocarbamate	12, 217 (1976); Suppl. 7, 71 (1987)
Sodium equilin sulphate (see Conjugated oestrogens)	
Sodium fluoride (see Fluorides)	

Sodium monofluorophosphate (*see* Fluorides)
Sodium oestrone sulfate (*see* Conjugated oestrogens)
Sodium *ortho*-phenylphenate (*see also ortho*-Phenylphenol) 30, 329 (1983); *Suppl. 7*, 392 (1987)
Sodium saccharin (*see* Saccharin)
Sodium selenate (*see* Selenium and selenium compounds)
Sodium selenite (*see* Selenium and selenium compounds)
Sodium silicofluoride (*see* Fluorides)
Soots 3, 22 (1973); 35, 219 (1985); *Suppl. 7*, 343 (1987)

Spironolactone 24, 259 (1980); *Suppl. 7*, 344 (1987)
Stannous fluoride (*see* Fluorides)
Steel founding (*see* Iron and steel founding)
Sterigmatocystin 1, 175 (1972); 10, 245 (1976); *Suppl. 7*, 72 (1987)

Steroidal oestrogens (*see also* Oestrogens, progestins and combinations) *Suppl. 7*, 280 (1987)
Streptozotocin 4, 221 (1974); 17, 337 (1978); *Suppl. 7*, 72 (1987)

Strobane® (*see* Terpene polychlorinates)
Strontium chromate (*see* Chromium and chromium compounds)
Styrene 19, 231 (1979) (*corr.* 42, 258); *Suppl. 7*, 345 (1987)

Styrene-acrylonitrile copolymers 19, 97 (1979); *Suppl. 7*, 72 (1987)
Styrene-butadiene copolymers 19, 252 (1979); *Suppl. 7*, 72 (1987)
Styrene oxide 11, 201 (1976); 19, 275 (1979); 36, 245 (1985); *Suppl. 7*, 72 (1987)

Succinic anhydride 15, 265 (1977); *Suppl. 7*, 72 (1987)
Sudan I 8, 225 (1975); *Suppl. 7*, 72 (1987)
Sudan II 8, 233 (1975); *Suppl. 7*, 72 (1987)
Sudan III 8, 241 (1975); *Suppl. 7*, 72 (1987)
Sudan Brown RR 8, 249 (1975); *Suppl. 7*, 72 (1987)
Sudan Red 7B 8, 253 (1975); *Suppl. 7*, 72 (1987)
Sulfafurazole 24, 275 (1980); *Suppl. 7*, 347 (1987)
Sulfallate 30, 283 (1983); *Suppl. 7*, 72 (1987)
Sulfamethoxazole 24, 285 (1980); *Suppl. 7*, 348 (1987)
Sulfites (*see* Sulfur dioxide and some sulfites, bisulfites and metabisulfites)
Sulfur dioxide and some sulfites, bisulfites and metabisulfites 54, 131 (1992)
Sulfur mustard (*see* Mustard gas)
Sulfuric acid and other strong inorganic acids, occupational exposures to mist and vapours from 54, 41 (1992)
Sulphisoxazole (*see* Sulfafurazole)
Sunset Yellow FCF 8, 257 (1975); *Suppl. 7*, 72 (1987)
Symphytine 31, 239 (1983); *Suppl. 7*, 72 (1987)

T

2,4,5-T (*see also* Chlorophenoxy herbicides; Chlorophenoxy herbicides, occupational exposures to) 15, 273 (1977)

Talc 42, 185 (1987); *Suppl. 7*, 349 (1987)
Tannic acid 10, 253 (1976) (*corr.* 42, 255); *Suppl. 7*, 72 (1987)

Tannins (*see also* Tannic acid) 10, 254 (1976); *Suppl. 7*, 72 (1987)

TCDD (see 2,3,7,8-Tetrachlorodibenzo-*para*-dioxin)
TDE (see DDT)
Tea   51, 207 (1991)
Terpene polychlorinates   5, 219 (1974); *Suppl. 7*, 72 (1987)
Testosterone (see also Androgenic (anabolic) steroids)   6, 209 (1974); 21, 519 (1979)
Testosterone oenanthate (see Testosterone)
Testosterone propionate (see Testosterone)
2,2',5,5'-Tetrachlorobenzidine   27, 141 (1982); *Suppl. 7*, 72 (1987)
2,3,7,8-Tetrachlorodibenzo-*para*-dioxin   15, 41 (1977); *Suppl. 7*, 350 (1987)
1,1,1,2-Tetrachloroethane   41, 87 (1986); *Suppl. 7*, 72 (1987)
1,1,2,2-Tetrachloroethane   20, 477 (1979); *Suppl. 7*, 354 (1987)
Tetrachloroethylene   20, 491 (1979); *Suppl. 7*, 355 (1987)
2,3,4,6-Tetrachlorophenol (see Chlorophenols; Chlorophenols,
    occupational exposures to)
Tetrachlorvinphos   30, 197 (1983); *Suppl. 7*, 72 (1987)
Tetraethyllead (see Lead and lead compounds)
Tetrafluoroethylene   19, 285 (1979); *Suppl. 7*, 72 (1987)
Tetrakis(hydroxymethyl) phosphonium salts   48, 95 (1990)
Tetramethyllead (see Lead and lead compounds)
Textile manufacturing industry, exposures in   48, 215 (1990) (*corr.* 51, 483)
Theobromine   51, 421 (1991)
Theophylline   51, 391 (1991)
Thioacetamide   7, 77 (1974); *Suppl. 7*, 72 (1987)
4,4'-Thiodianiline   16, 343 (1978); 27, 147 (1982);
                                                                        Suppl. 7, 72 (1987)
Thiotepa   9, 85 (1975); *Suppl. 7*, 368 (1987);
                                                                        50, 123 (1990)
Thiouracil   7, 85 (1974); *Suppl. 7*, 72 (1987)
Thiourea   7, 95 (1974); *Suppl. 7*, 72 (1987)
Thiram   12, 225 (1976); *Suppl. 7*, 72 (1987);
                                                                        53, 403 (1991)
Titanium dioxide   47, 307 (1989)
Tobacco habits other than smoking (see Tobacco products,
    smokeless)
Tobacco products, smokeless   37 (1985) (*corr.* 42, 263; 52, 513);
                                                                        Suppl. 7, 357 (1987)
Tobacco smoke   38 (1986) (*corr.* 42, 263); *Suppl. 7*,
                                                                        357 (1987)
Tobacco smoking (see Tobacco smoke)
ortho-Tolidine (see 3,3'-Dimethylbenzidine)
2,4-Toluene diisocyanate (see also Toluene diisocyanates)   19, 303 (1979); 39, 287 (1986)
2,6-Toluene diisocyanate (see also Toluene diisocyanates)   19, 303 (1979); 39, 289 (1986)
Toluene   47, 79 (1989)
Toluene diisocyanates   39, 287 (1986) (*corr.* 42, 264);
                                                                        Suppl. 7, 72 (1987)
Toluenes, α-chlorinated (see α-Chlorinated toluenes)
ortho-Toluenesulfonamide (see Saccharin)
ortho-Toluidine   16, 349 (1978); 27, 155 (1982);
                                                                        Suppl. 7, 362 (1987)
Toxaphene   20, 327 (1979); *Suppl. 7*, 72 (1987)
Tremolite (see Asbestos)
Treosulfan   26, 341 (1981); *Suppl. 7*, 363 (1987)

Triaziquone [see Tris(aziridinyl)-para-benzoquinone]	
Trichlorfon	30, 207 (1983); Suppl. 7, 73 (1987)
Trichlormethine	9, 229 (1975); Suppl. 7, 73 (1987); 50, 143 (1990)
Trichloroacetonitrile (see Halogenated acetonitriles)	
1,1,1-Trichloroethane	20, 515 (1979); Suppl. 7, 73 (1987)
1,1,2-Trichloroethane	20, 533 (1979); Suppl. 7, 73 (1987); 52, 337 (1991)
Trichloroethylene	11, 263 (1976); 20, 545 (1979); Suppl. 7, 364 (1987)
2,4,5-Trichlorophenol (see also Chlorophenols; Chlorophenols occupational exposures to)	20, 349 (1979)
2,4,6-Trichlorophenol (see also Chlorophenols; Chlorophenols, occupational exposures to)	20, 349 (1979)
(2,4,5-Trichlorophenoxy)acetic acid (see 2,4,5-T)	
Trichlorotriethylamine hydrochloride (see Trichlormethine)	
T_2-Trichothecene	31, 265 (1983); Suppl. 7, 73 (1987)
Triethylene glycol diglycidyl ether	11, 209 (1976); Suppl. 7, 73 (1987)
Trifluralin	53, 515 (1991)
4,4',6-Trimethylangelicin plus ultraviolet radiation (see also Angelicin and some synthetic derivatives)	Suppl. 7, 57 (1987)
2,4,5-Trimethylaniline	27, 177 (1982); Suppl. 7, 73 (1987)
2,4,6-Trimethylaniline	27, 178 (1982); Suppl. 7, 73 (1987)
4,5',8-Trimethylpsoralen	40, 357 (1986); Suppl. 7, 366 (1987)
Trimustine hydrochloride (see Trichlormethine)	
Triphenylene	32, 447 (1983); Suppl. 7, 73 (1987)
Tris(aziridinyl)-para-benzoquinone	9, 67 (1975); Suppl. 7, 367 (1987)
Tris(1-aziridinyl)phosphine oxide	9, 75 (1975); Suppl. 7, 73 (1987)
Tris(1-aziridinyl)phosphine sulphide (see Thiotepa)	
2,4,6-Tris(1-aziridinyl)-s-triazine	9, 95 (1975); Suppl. 7, 73 (1987)
Tris(2-chloroethyl) phosphate	48, 109 (1990)
1,2,3-Tris(chloromethoxy)propane	15, 301 (1977); Suppl. 7, 73 (1987)
Tris(2,3-dibromopropyl)phosphate	20, 575 (1979); Suppl. 7, 369 (1987)
Tris(2-methyl-1-aziridinyl)phosphine oxide	9, 107 (1975); Suppl. 7, 73 (1987)
Trp-P-1	31, 247 (1983); Suppl. 7, 73 (1987)
Trp-P-2	31, 255 (1983); Suppl. 7, 73 (1987)
Trypan blue	8, 267 (1975); Suppl. 7, 73 (1987)
Tussilago farfara L. (see Pyrrolizidine alkaloids)	

U

Ultraviolet radiation	40, 379 (1986)
Underground haematite mining with exposure to radon	1, 29 (1972); Suppl. 7, 216 (1987)
Uracil mustard	9, 235 (1975); Suppl. 7, 370 (1987)
Urethane	7, 111 (1974); Suppl. 7, 73 (1987)

V

Vat Yellow 4	48, 161 (1990)
Vinblastine sulfate	26, 349 (1981) (corr. 42, 261); Suppl. 7, 371 (1987)
Vincristine sulfate	26, 365 (1981); Suppl. 7, 372 (1987)

Vinyl acetate	19, 341 (1979); 39, 113 (1986); Suppl. 7, 73 (1987)
Vinyl bromide	19, 367 (1979); 39, 133 (1986); Suppl. 7, 73 (1987)
Vinyl chloride	7, 291 (1974); 19, 377 (1979) (corr. 42, 258); Suppl. 7, 373 (1987)
Vinyl chloride–vinyl acetate copolymers	7, 311 (1976); 19, 412 (1979) (corr. 42, 258); Suppl. 7, 73 (1987)
4-Vinylcyclohexene	11, 277 (1976); 39, 181 (1986); Suppl. 7, 73 (1987)
Vinyl fluoride	39, 147 (1986); Suppl. 7, 73 (1987)
Vinylidene chloride	19, 439 (1979); 39, 195 (1986); Suppl. 7, 376 (1987)
Vinylidene chloride–vinyl chloride copolymers	19, 448 (1979) (corr. 42, 258); Suppl. 7, 73 (1987)
Vinylidene fluoride	39, 227 (1986); Suppl. 7, 73 (1987)
N-Vinyl-2-pyrrolidone	19, 461 (1979); Suppl. 7, 73 (1987)

W

Welding	49, 447 (1990) (corr. 52, 513)
Wollastonite	42, 145 (1987); Suppl. 7, 377 (1987)
Wood industries	25 (1981); Suppl. 7, 378 (1987)

X

Xylene	47, 125 (1989)
2,4-Xylidine	16, 367 (1978); Suppl. 7, 74 (1987)
2,5-Xylidine	16, 377 (1978); Suppl. 7, 74 (1987)

Y

Yellow AB	8, 279 (1975); Suppl. 7, 74 (1987)
Yellow OB	8, 287 (1975); Suppl. 7, 74 (1987)

Z

Zearalenone	31, 279 (1983); Suppl. 7, 74 (1987)
Zectran	12, 237 (1976); Suppl. 7, 74 (1987)
Zinc beryllium silicate (see Beryllium and beryllium compounds)	
Zinc chromate (see Chromium and chromium compounds)	
Zinc chromate hydroxide (see Chromium and chromium compounds)	
Zinc potassium chromate (see Chromium and chromium compounds)	
Zinc yellow (see Chromium and chromium compounds)	
Zineb	12, 245 (1976); Suppl. 7, 74 (1987)
Ziram	12, 259 (1976); Suppl. 7, 74 (1987); 53, 423 (1991)

PUBLICATIONS OF THE INTERNATIONAL AGENCY FOR RESEARCH ON CANCER

Scientific Publications Series

(Available from Oxford University Press through local bookshops)

No. 1 **Liver Cancer**
1971; 176 pages (*out of print*)

No. 2 **Oncogenesis and Herpesviruses**
Edited by P.M. Biggs, G. de-Thé and L.N. Payne
1972; 515 pages (*out of print*)

No. 3 **N-Nitroso Compounds: Analysis and Formation**
Edited by P. Bogovski, R. Preussman and E.A. Walker
1972; 140 pages (*out of print*)

No. 4 **Transplacental Carcinogenesis**
Edited by L. Tomatis and U. Mohr
1973; 181 pages (*out of print*)

No. 5/6 **Pathology of Tumours in Laboratory Animals, Volume 1, Tumours of the Rat**
Edited by V.S. Turusov
1973/1976; 533 pages (*out of print*)

No. 7 **Host Environment Interactions in the Etiology of Cancer in Man**
Edited by R. Doll and I. Vodopija
1973; 464 pages (*out of print*)

No. 8 **Biological Effects of Asbestos**
Edited by P. Bogovski, J.C. Gilson, V. Timbrell and J.C. Wagner
1973; 346 pages (*out of print*)

No. 9 **N-Nitroso Compounds in the Environment**
Edited by P. Bogovski and E.A. Walker
1974; 243 pages (*out of print*)

No. 10 **Chemical Carcinogenesis Essays**
Edited by R. Montesano and L. Tomatis
1974; 230 pages (*out of print*)

No. 11 **Oncogenesis and Herpesviruses II**
Edited by G. de-Thé, M.A. Epstein and H. zur Hausen
1975; Part I: 511 pages
Part II: 403 pages (*out of print*)

No. 12 **Screening Tests in Chemical Carcinogenesis**
Edited by R. Montesano, H. Bartsch and L. Tomatis
1976; 666 pages (*out of print*)

No. 13 **Environmental Pollution and Carcinogenic Risks**
Edited by C. Rosenfeld and W. Davis
1975; 441 pages (*out of print*)

No. 14 **Environmental N-Nitroso Compounds. Analysis and Formation**
Edited by E.A. Walker, P. Bogovski and L. Griciute
1976; 512 pages (*out of print*)

No. 15 **Cancer Incidence in Five Continents, Volume III**
Edited by J.A.H. Waterhouse, C. Muir, P. Correa and J. Powell
1976; 584 pages (*out of print*)

No. 16 **Air Pollution and Cancer in Man**
Edited by U. Mohr, D. Schmähl and L. Tomatis
1977; 328 pages (*out of print*)

No. 17 **Directory of On-going Research in Cancer Epidemiology 1977**
Edited by C.S. Muir and G. Wagner
1977; 599 pages (*out of print*)

No. 18 **Environmental Carcinogens. Selected Methods of Analysis. Volume 1: Analysis of Volatile Nitrosamines in Food**
Editor-in-Chief: H. Egan
1978; 212 pages (*out of print*)

No. 19 **Environmental Aspects of N-Nitroso Compounds**
Edited by E.A. Walker, M. Castegnaro, L. Griciute and R.E. Lyle
1978; 561 pages (*out of print*)

No. 20 **Nasopharyngeal Carcinoma: Etiology and Control**
Edited by G. de-Thé and Y. Ito
1978; 606 pages (*out of print*)

No. 21 **Cancer Registration and its Techniques**
Edited by R. MacLennan, C. Muir, R. Steinitz and A. Winkler
1978; 235 pages (*out of print*)

No. 22 **Environmental Carcinogens. Selected Methods of Analysis. Volume 2: Methods for the Measurement of Vinyl Chloride in Poly(vinyl chloride), Air, Water and Foodstuffs**
Editor-in-Chief: H. Egan
1978; 142 pages (*out of print*)

No. 23 **Pathology of Tumours in Laboratory Animals. Volume II: Tumours of the Mouse**
Editor-in-Chief: V.S. Turusov
1979; 669 pages (*out of print*)

No. 24 **Oncogenesis and Herpesviruses III**
Edited by G. de-Thé, W. Henle and F. Rapp
1978; Part I: 580 pages, Part II: 512 pages (*out of print*)

Prices, valid for July 1992, are subject to change without notice

List of IARC Publications

No. 25 Carcinogenic Risk. Strategies for Intervention
Edited by W. Davis and C. Rosenfeld
1979; 280 pages (*out of print*)

No. 26 Directory of On-going Research in Cancer Epidemiology 1978
Edited by C.S. Muir and G. Wagner
1978; 550 pages (*out of print*)

No. 27 Molecular and Cellular Aspects of Carcinogen Screening Tests
Edited by R. Montesano, H. Bartsch and L. Tomatis
1980; 372 pages £29.00

No. 28 Directory of On-going Research in Cancer Epidemiology 1979
Edited by C.S. Muir and G. Wagner
1979; 672 pages (*out of print*)

No. 29 Environmental Carcinogens. Selected Methods of Analysis. Volume 3: Analysis of Polycyclic Aromatic Hydrocarbons in Environmental Samples
Editor-in-Chief: H. Egan
1979; 240 pages (*out of print*)

No. 30 Biological Effects of Mineral Fibres
Editor-in-Chief: J.C. Wagner
1980; Volume 1: 494 pages Volume 2: 513 pages (*out of print*)

No. 31 N-Nitroso Compounds: Analysis, Formation and Occurrence
Edited by E.A. Walker, L. Griciute, M. Castegnaro and M. Börzsönyi
1980; 835 pages (*out of print*)

No. 32 Statistical Methods in Cancer Research. Volume 1. The Analysis of Case-control Studies
By N.E. Breslow and N.E. Day
1980; 338 pages £25.00

No. 33 Handling Chemical Carcinogens in the Laboratory
Edited by R. Montesano *et al.*
1979; 32 pages (*out of print*)

No. 34 Pathology of Tumours in Laboratory Animals. Volume III. Tumours of the Hamster
Editor-in-Chief: V.S. Turusov
1982; 461 pages (*out of print*)

No. 35 Directory of On-going Research in Cancer Epidemiology 1980
Edited by C.S. Muir and G. Wagner
1980; 660 pages (*out of print*)

No. 36 Cancer Mortality by Occupation and Social Class 1851-1971
Edited by W.P.D. Logan
1982; 253 pages (*out of print*)

No. 37 Laboratory Decontamination and Destruction of Aflatoxins B_1, B_2, G_1, G_2 in Laboratory Wastes
Edited by M. Castegnaro *et al.*
1980; 56 pages (*out of print*)

No. 38 Directory of On-going Research in Cancer Epidemiology 1981
Edited by C.S. Muir and G. Wagner
1981; 696 pages (*out of print*)

No. 39 Host Factors in Human Carcinogenesis
Edited by H. Bartsch and B. Armstrong
1982; 583 pages (*out of print*)

No. 40 Environmental Carcinogens. Selected Methods of Analysis. Volume 4: Some Aromatic Amines and Azo Dyes in the General and Industrial Environment
Edited by L. Fishbein, M. Castegnaro, I.K. O'Neill and H. Bartsch
1981; 347 pages (*out of print*)

No. 41 N-Nitroso Compounds: Occurrence and Biological Effects
Edited by H. Bartsch, I.K. O'Neill, M. Castegnaro and M. Okada
1982; 755 pages £50.00

No. 42 Cancer Incidence in Five Continents, Volume IV
Edited by J. Waterhouse, C. Muir, K. Shanmugaratnam and J. Powell
1982; 811 pages (*out of print*)

No. 43 Laboratory Decontamination and Destruction of Carcinogens in Laboratory Wastes: Some N-Nitrosamines
Edited by M. Castegnaro *et al.*
1982; 73 pages £7.50

No. 44 Environmental Carcinogens. Selected Methods of Analysis. Volume 5: Some Mycotoxins
Edited by L. Stoloff, M. Castegnaro, P. Scott, I.K. O'Neill and H. Bartsch
1983; 455 pages £32.50

No. 45 Environmental Carcinogens. Selected Methods of Analysis. Volume 6: N-Nitroso Compounds
Edited by R. Preussmann, I.K. O'Neill, G. Eisenbrand, B. Spiegelhalder and H. Bartsch
1983; 508 pages £32.50

No. 46 Directory of On-going Research in Cancer Epidemiology 1982
Edited by C.S. Muir and G. Wagner
1982; 722 pages (*out of print*)

No. 47 Cancer Incidence in Singapore 1968-1977
Edited by K. Shanmugaratnam, H.P. Lee and N.E. Day
1983; 171 pages (*out of print*)

No. 48 Cancer Incidence in the USSR (2nd Revised Edition)
Edited by N.P. Napalkov, G.F. Tserkovny, V.M. Merabishvili, D.M. Parkin, M. Smans and C.S. Muir
1983; 75 pages (*out of print*)

No. 49 Laboratory Decontamination and Destruction of Carcinogens in Laboratory Wastes: Some Polycyclic Aromatic Hydrocarbons
Edited by M. Castegnaro *et al.*
1983; 87 pages (*out of print*)

No. 50 Directory of On-going Research in Cancer Epidemiology 1983
Edited by C.S. Muir and G. Wagner
1983; 731 pages (*out of print*)

No. 51 Modulators of Experimental Carcinogenesis
Edited by V. Turusov and R. Montesano
1983; 307 pages (*out of print*)

List of IARC Publications

No. 52 Second Cancers in Relation to Radiation Treatment for Cervical Cancer: Results of a Cancer Registry Collaboration
Edited by N.E. Day and J.C. Boice, Jr
1984; 207 pages (*out of print*)

No. 53 Nickel in the Human Environment
Editor-in-Chief: F.W. Sunderman, Jr
1984; 529 pages (*out of print*)

No. 54 Laboratory Decontamination and Destruction of Carcinogens in Laboratory Wastes: Some Hydrazines
Edited by M. Castegnaro et al.
1983; 87 pages (*out of print*)

No. 55 Laboratory Decontamination and Destruction of Carcinogens in Laboratory Wastes: Some N-Nitrosamides
Edited by M. Castegnaro et al.
1984; 66 pages (*out of print*)

No. 56 Models, Mechanisms and Etiology of Tumour Promotion
Edited by M. Börzsönyi, N.E. Day, K. Lapis and H. Yamasaki
1984; 532 pages (*out of print*)

No. 57 N-Nitroso Compounds: Occurrence, Biological Effects and Relevance to Human Cancer
Edited by I.K. O'Neill, R.C. von Borstel, C.T. Miller, J. Long and H. Bartsch
1984; 1013 pages (*out of print*)

No. 58 Age-related Factors in Carcinogenesis
Edited by A. Likhachev, V. Anisimov and R. Montesano
1985; 288 pages (*out of print*)

No. 59 Monitoring Human Exposure to Carcinogenic and Mutagenic Agents
Edited by A. Berlin, M. Draper, K. Hemminki and H. Vainio
1984; 457 pages (*out of print*)

No. 60 Burkitt's Lymphoma: A Human Cancer Model
Edited by G. Lenoir, G. O'Conor and C.L.M. Olweny
1985; 484 pages (*out of print*)

No. 61 Laboratory Decontamination and Destruction of Carcinogens in Laboratory Wastes: Some Haloethers
Edited by M. Castegnaro et al.
1985; 55 pages (*out of print*)

No. 62 Directory of On-going Research in Cancer Epidemiology 1984
Edited by C.S. Muir and G. Wagner
1984; 717 pages (*out of print*)

No. 63 Virus-associated Cancers in Africa
Edited by A.O. Williams, G.T. O'Conor, G.B. de-Thé and C.A. Johnson
1984; 773 pages (*out of print*)

No. 64 Laboratory Decontamination and Destruction of Carcinogens in Laboratory Wastes: Some Aromatic Amines and 4-Nitrobiphenyl
Edited by M. Castegnaro et al.
1985; 84 pages (*out of print*)

No. 65 Interpretation of Negative Epidemiological Evidence for Carcinogenicity
Edited by N.J. Wald and R. Doll
1985; 232 pages (*out of print*)

No. 66 The Role of the Registry in Cancer Control
Edited by D.M. Parkin, G. Wagner and C.S. Muir
1985; 152 pages £10.00

No. 67 Transformation Assay of Established Cell Lines: Mechanisms and Application
Edited by T. Kakunaga and H. Yamasaki
1985; 225 pages (*out of print*)

No. 68 Environmental Carcinogens. Selected Methods of Analysis. Volume 7. Some Volatile Halogenated Hydrocarbons
Edited by L. Fishbein and I.K. O'Neill
1985; 479 pages (*out of print*)

No. 69 Directory of On-going Research in Cancer Epidemiology 1985
Edited by C.S. Muir and G. Wagner
1985; 745 pages (*out of print*)

No. 70 The Role of Cyclic Nucleic Acid Adducts in Carcinogenesis and Mutagenesis
Edited by B. Singer and H. Bartsch
1986; 467 pages (*out of print*)

No. 71 Environmental Carcinogens. Selected Methods of Analysis. Volume 8: Some Metals: As, Be, Cd, Cr, Ni, Pb, Se Zn
Edited by I.K. O'Neill, P. Schuller and L. Fishbein
1986; 485 pages (*out of print*)

No. 72 Atlas of Cancer in Scotland, 1975-1980. Incidence and Epidemiological Perspective
Edited by I. Kemp, P. Boyle, M. Smans and C.S. Muir
1985; 285 pages (*out of print*)

No. 73 Laboratory Decontamination and Destruction of Carcinogens in Laboratory Wastes: Some Antineoplastic Agents
Edited by M. Castegnaro et al.
1985; 163 pages £12.50

No. 74 Tobacco: A Major International Health Hazard
Edited by D. Zaridze and R. Peto
1986; 324 pages £22.50

No. 75 Cancer Occurrence in Developing Countries
Edited by D.M. Parkin
1986; 339 pages £22.50

No. 76 Screening for Cancer of the Uterine Cervix
Edited by M. Hakama, A.B. Miller and N.E. Day
1986; 315 pages £30.00

List of IARC Publications

No. 77 **Hexachlorobenzene: Proceedings of an International Symposium**
Edited by C.R. Morris and J.R.P. Cabral
1986; 668 pages (*out of print*)

No. 78 **Carcinogenicity of Alkylating Cytostatic Drugs**
Edited by D. Schmähl and J.M. Kaldor
1986; 337 pages (*out of print*)

No. 79 **Statistical Methods in Cancer Research. Volume III: The Design and Analysis of Long-term Animal Experiments**
By J.J. Gart, D. Krewski, P.N. Lee, R.E. Tarone and J. Wahrendorf
1986; 213 pages £22.00

No. 80 **Directory of On-going Research in Cancer Epidemiology 1986**
Edited by C.S. Muir and G. Wagner
1986; 805 pages (*out of print*)

No. 81 **Environmental Carcinogens: Methods of Analysis and Exposure Measurement. Volume 9: Passive Smoking**
Edited by I.K. O'Neill, K.D. Brunnemann, B. Dodet and D. Hoffmann
1987; 383 pages £35.00

No. 82 **Statistical Methods in Cancer Research. Volume II: The Design and Analysis of Cohort Studies**
By N.E. Breslow and N.E. Day
1987; 404 pages £35.00

No. 83 **Long-term and Short-term Assays for Carcinogens: A Critical Appraisal**
Edited by R. Montesano, H. Bartsch, H. Vainio, J. Wilbourn and H. Yamasaki
1986; 575 pages £35.00

No. 84 **The Relevance of N-Nitroso Compounds to Human Cancer: Exposure and Mechanisms**
Edited by H. Bartsch, I.K. O'Neill and R. Schulte-Hermann
1987; 671 pages (*out of print*)

No. 85 **Environmental Carcinogens: Methods of Analysis and Exposure Measurement. Volume 10: Benzene and Alkylated Benzenes**
Edited by L. Fishbein and I.K. O'Neill
1988; 327 pages £40.00

No. 86 **Directory of On-going Research in Cancer Epidemiology 1987**
Edited by D.M. Parkin and J. Wahrendorf
1987; 676 pages (*out of print*)

No. 87 **International Incidence of Childhood Cancer**
Edited by D.M. Parkin, C.A. Stiller, C.A. Bieber, G.J. Draper, B. Terracini and J.L. Young
1988; 401 pages £35.00

No. 88 **Cancer Incidence in Five Continents Volume V**
Edited by C. Muir, J. Waterhouse, T. Mack, J. Powell and S. Whelan
1987; 1004 pages £55.00

No. 89 **Method for Detecting DNA Damaging Agents in Humans: Applications in Cancer Epidemiology and Prevention**
Edited by H. Bartsch, K. Hemminki and I.K. O'Neill
1988; 518 pages £50.00

No. 90 **Non-occupational Exposure to Mineral Fibres**
Edited by J. Bignon, J. Peto and R. Saracci
1989; 500 pages £50.00

No. 91 **Trends in Cancer Incidence in Singapore 1968–1982**
Edited by H.P. Lee, N.E. Day and K. Shanmugaratnam
1988; 160 pages (*out of print*)

No. 92 **Cell Differentiation, Genes and Cancer**
Edited by T. Kakunaga, T. Sugimura, L. Tomatis and H. Yamasaki
1988; 204 pages £27.50

No. 93 **Directory of On-going Research in Cancer Epidemiology 1988**
Edited by M. Coleman and J. Wahrendorf
1988; 662 pages (*out of print*)

No. 94 **Human Papillomavirus and Cervical Cancer**
Edited by N. Muñoz, F.X. Bosch and O.M. Jensen
1989; 154 pages £22.50

No. 95 **Cancer Registration: Principles and Methods**
Edited by O.M. Jensen, D.M. Parkin, R. MacLennan, C.S. Muir and R. Skeet
1991; 288 pages £28.00

No. 96 **Perinatal and Multigeneration Carcinogenesis**
Edited by N.P. Napalkov, J.M. Rice, L. Tomatis and H. Yamasaki
1989; 436 pages £50.00

No. 97 **Occupational Exposure to Silica and Cancer Risk**
Edited by L. Simonato, A.C. Fletcher, R. Saracci and T. Thomas
1990; 124 pages £22.50

No. 98 **Cancer Incidence in Jewish Migrants to Israel, 1961–1981**
Edited by R. Steinitz, D.M. Parkin, J.L. Young, C.A. Bieber and L. Katz
1989; 320 pages £35.00

No. 99 **Pathology of Tumours in Laboratory Animals, Second Edition, Volume 1, Tumours of the Rat**
Edited by V.S. Turusov and U. Mohr
740 pages £85.00

No. 100 **Cancer: Causes, Occurrence and Control**
Editor-in-Chief L. Tomatis
1990; 352 pages £24.00

No. 101 **Directory of On-going Research in Cancer Epidemiology 1989/90**
Edited by M. Coleman and J. Wahrendorf
1989; 818 pages £36.00

List of IARC Publications

No. 102 Patterns of Cancer in Five Continents
Edited by S.L. Whelan and D.M. Parkin
1990; 162 pages £25.00

No. 103 Evaluating Effectiveness of Primary Prevention of Cancer
Edited by M. Hakama, V. Beral, J.W. Cullen and D.M. Parkin
1990; 250 pages £32.00

No. 104 Complex Mixtures and Cancer Risk
Edited by H. Vainio, M. Sorsa and A.J. McMichael
1990; 442 pages £38.00

No. 105 Relevance to Human Cancer of N-Nitroso Compounds, Tobacco Smoke and Mycotoxins
Edited by I.K. O'Neill, J. Chen and H. Bartsch
1991; 614 pages £70.00

No. 106 Atlas of Cancer Incidence in the German Democratic Republic
Edited by W.H. Mehnert, M. Smans and C.S. Muir
Publ. due 1992; c.328 pages £42.00

No. 107 Atlas of Cancer Mortality in the European Economic Community
Edited by M. Smans, C.S. Muir and P. Boyle
Publ. due 1992; approx. 230 pages £35.00

No. 108 Environmental Carcinogens: Methods of Analysis and Exposure Measurement. Volume 11: Polychlorinated Dioxins and Dibenzofurans
Edited by C. Rappe, H.R. Buser, B. Dodet and I.K. O'Neill
1991; 426 pages £45.00

No. 109 Environmental Carcinogens: Methods of Analysis and Exposure Measurement. Volume 12: Indoor Air Contaminants
Edited by B. Seifert, B. Dodet and I.K. O'Neill
Publ. due 1992; approx. 400 pages

No. 110 Directory of On-going Research in Cancer Epidemiology 1991
Edited by M. Coleman and J. Wahrendorf
1991; 753 pages £38.00

No. 111 Pathology of Tumours in Laboratory Animals, Second Edition, Volume 2, Tumours of the Mouse
Edited by V.S. Turusov and U. Mohr
Publ. due 1992; approx. 500 pages

No. 112 Autopsy in Epidemiology and Medical Research
Edited by E. Riboli and M. Delendi
1991; 288 pages £25.00

No. 113 Laboratory Decontamination and Destruction of Carcinogens in Laboratory Wastes: Some Mycotoxins
Edited by M. Castegnaro, J. Barek, J.-M. Frémy, M. Lafontaine, M. Miraglia, E.B. Sansone and G.M. Telling
1991; 64 pages £11.00

No. 114 Laboratory Decontamination and Destruction of Carcinogens in Laboratory Wastes: Some Polycyclic Heterocyclic Hydrocarbons
Edited by M. Castegnaro, J. Barek, J. Jacob, U. Kirso, M. Lafontaine, E.B. Sansone, G.M. Telling and T. Vu Duc
1991; 50 pages £8.00

No. 115 Mycotoxins, Endemic Nephropathy and Urinary Tract Tumours
Edited by M. Castegnaro, R. Plestina, G. Dirheimer, I.N. Chernozemsky and H Bartsch
1991; 340 pages £45.00

No. 116 Mechanisms of Carcinogenesis in Risk Identification
Edited by H. Vainio, P.N. Magee, D.B. McGregor & A.J. McMichael
1992; 616 pages £65.00

No. 117 Directory of On-going Research in Cancer Epidemiology 1991
Edited by M. Coleman, J. Wahrendorf & E. Démaret
1992; 773 pages £42.00

No. 119 The Epidemiology of Cervical Cancer and Human Papillomavirus
Edited by N. Muñoz, F.X. Bosch, K.V. Shah & A. Meheus
1992; 240 pages £28.00

List of IARC Publications

IARC MONOGRAPHS ON THE EVALUATION OF CARCINOGENIC RISKS TO HUMANS

(Available from booksellers through the network of WHO Sales Agents)

Volume 1 Some Inorganic Substances, Chlorinated Hydrocarbons, Aromatic Amines, *N*-Nitroso Compounds, and Natural Products
1972; 184 pages (*out of print*)

Volume 2 Some Inorganic and Organometallic Compounds
1973; 181 pages (*out of print*)

Volume 3 Certain Polycyclic Aromatic Hydrocarbons and Heterocyclic Compounds
1973; 271 pages (*out of print*)

Volume 4 Some Aromatic Amines, Hydrazine and Related Substances, *N*-Nitroso Compounds and Miscellaneous Alkylating Agents
1974; 286 pages Sw. fr. 18.

Volume 5 Some Organochlorine Pesticides
1974; 241 pages (*out of print*)

Volume 6 Sex Hormones
1974; 243 pages (*out of print*)

Volume 7 Some Anti-Thyroid and Related Substances, Nitrofurans and Industrial Chemicals
1974; 326 pages (*out of print*)

Volume 8 Some Aromatic Azo Compounds
1975; 357 pages Sw. fr. 36.

Volume 9 Some Aziridines, *N*-, *S*- and *O*-Mustards and Selenium
1975; 268 pages Sw.fr. 27.

Volume 10 Some Naturally Occurring Substances
1976; 353 pages (*out of print*)

Volume 11 Cadmium, Nickel, Some Epoxides, Miscellaneous Industrial Chemicals and General Considerations on Volatile Anaesthetics
1976; 306 pages (*out of print*)

Volume 12 Some Carbamates, Thiocarbamates and Carbazides
1976; 282 pages Sw. fr. 34.-

Volume 13 Some Miscellaneous Pharmaceutical Substances
1977; 255 pages Sw. fr. 30.

Volume 14 Asbestos
1977; 106 pages (*out of print*)

Volume 15 Some Fumigants, The Herbicides 2,4-D and 2,4,5-T, Chlorinated Dibenzodioxins and Miscellaneous Industrial Chemicals
1977; 354 pages Sw. fr. 50.

Volume 16 Some Aromatic Amines and Related Nitro Compounds - Hair Dyes, Colouring Agents and Miscellaneous Industrial Chemicals
1978; 400 pages Sw. fr. 50.

Volume 17 Some *N*-Nitroso Compounds
1978; 365 pages Sw. fr. 50.

Volume 18 Polychlorinated Biphenyls and Polybrominated Biphenyls
1978; 140 pages Sw. fr. 20.

Volume 19 Some Monomers, Plastics and Synthetic Elastomers, and Acrolein
1979; 513 pages (*out of print*)

Volume 20 Some Halogenated Hydrocarbons
1979; 609 pages (*out of print*)

Volume 21 Sex Hormones (II)
1979; 583 pages Sw. fr. 60.

Volume 22 Some Non-Nutritive Sweetening Agents
1980; 208 pages Sw. fr. 25.

Volume 23 Some Metals and Metallic Compounds
1980; 438 pages (*out of print*)

Volume 24 Some Pharmaceutical Drugs
1980; 337 pages Sw. fr. 40.

Volume 25 Wood, Leather and Some Associated Industries
1981; 412 pages Sw. fr. 60

Volume 26 Some Antineoplastic and Immunosuppressive Agents
1981; 411 pages Sw. fr. 62.

Volume 27 Some Aromatic Amines, Anthraquinones and Nitroso Compounds, and Inorganic Fluorides Used in Drinking Water and Dental Preparations
1982; 341 pages Sw. fr. 40.

Volume 28 The Rubber Industry
1982; 486 pages Sw. fr. 70.

Volume 29 Some Industrial Chemicals and Dyestuffs
1982; 416 pages Sw. fr. 60.

Volume 30 Miscellaneous Pesticides
1983; 424 pages Sw. fr. 60.

Volume 31 Some Food Additives, Feed Additives and Naturally Occurring Substances
1983; 314 pages Sw. fr. 60

Volume 32 Polynuclear Aromatic Compounds, Part 1: Chemical, Environmental and Experimental Data
1983; 477 pages Sw. fr. 60.

Volume 33 Polynuclear Aromatic Compounds, Part 2: Carbon Blacks, Mineral Oils and Some Nitroarenes
1984; 245 pages Sw. fr. 50.

Volume 34 Polynuclear Aromatic Compounds, Part 3: Industrial Exposures in Aluminium Production, Coal Gasification, Coke Production, and Iron and Steel Founding
1984; 219 pages Sw. fr. 48.

Volume 35 Polynuclear Aromatic Compounds, Part 4: Bitumens, Coal-tars and Derived Products, Shale-oils and Soots
1985; 271 pages Sw. fr. 70.

List of IARC Publications

Volume 36 Allyl Compounds, Aldehydes, Epoxides and Peroxides
1985; 369 pages Sw. fr. 70.

Volume 37 Tobacco Habits Other than Smoking: Betel-quid and Areca-nut Chewing; and some Related Nitrosamines
1985; 291 pages Sw. fr. 70.

Volume 38 Tobacco Smoking
1986; 421 pages Sw. fr. 75.

Volume 39 Some Chemicals Used in Plastics and Elastomers
1986; 403 pages Sw. fr. 60.

Volume 40 Some Naturally Occurring and Synthetic Food Components, Furocoumarins and Ultraviolet Radiation
1986; 444 pages Sw. fr. 65.

Volume 41 Some Halogenated Hydrocarbons and Pesticide Exposures
1986; 434 pages Sw. fr. 65.

Volume 42 Silica and Some Silicates
1987; 289 pages Sw. fr. 65.

Volume 43 Man-Made Mineral Fibres and Radon
1988; 300 pages Sw. fr. 65.

Volume 44 Alcohol Drinking
1988; 416 pages Sw. fr. 65.

Volume 45 Occupational Exposures in Petroleum Refining; Crude Oil and Major Petroleum Fuels
1989; 322 pages Sw. fr. 65.

Volume 46 Diesel and Gasoline Engine Exhausts and Some Nitroarenes
1989; 458 pages Sw. fr. 65.

Volume 47 Some Organic Solvents, Resin Monomers and Related Compounds, Pigments and Occupational Exposures in Paint Manufacture and Painting
1989; 536 pages Sw. fr. 85.

Volume 48 Some Flame Retardants and Textile Chemicals, and Exposures in the Textile Manufacturing Industry
1990; 345 pages Sw. fr. 65.

Volume 49 Chromium, Nickel and Welding
1990; 677 pages Sw. fr. 95.

Volume 50 Pharmaceutical Drugs
1990; 415 pages Sw. fr. 65.

Volume 51 Coffee, Tea, Mate, Methylxanthines and Methylglyoxal
1991; 513 pages Sw. fr. 80.

Volume 52 Chlorinated Drinking-water; Chlorination By-products; Some Other Halogenated Compounds; Cobalt and Cobalt Compounds
1991; 544 pages Sw. fr. 80.

Volume 53 Occupational Exposures in Insecticide Application and some Pesticides
1991; 612 pages Sw. fr. 95.

Volume 54 Occupational Exposures to Mists and Vapours from Strong Inorganic Acids; and Other Industrial Chemicals
1992; 336 pages Sw. fr. 65.-

Supplement No. 1
Chemicals and Industrial Processes Associated with Cancer in Humans (IARC Monographs, Volumes 1 to 20)
1979; 71 pages (*out of print*)

Supplement No. 2
Long-term and Short-term Screening Assays for Carcinogens: A Critical Appraisal
1980; 426 pages Sw. fr. 40.-

Supplement No. 3
Cross Index of Synonyms and Trade Names in Volumes 1 to 26
1982; 199 pages (*out of print*)

Supplement No. 4
Chemicals, Industrial Processes and Industries Associated with Cancer in Humans (IARC Monographs, Volumes 1 to 29)
1982; 292 pages (*out of print*)

Supplement No. 5
Cross Index of Synonyms and Trade Names in Volumes 1 to 36
1985; 259 pages (*out of print*)

Supplement No. 6
Genetic and Related Effects: An Updating of Selected IARC Monographs from Volumes 1 to 42
1987; 729 pages Sw. fr. 80.

Supplement No. 7
Overall Evaluations of Carcinogenicity: An Updating of IARC Monographs Volumes 1–42
1987; 440 pages Sw. fr. 65.

Supplement No. 8
Cross Index of Synonyms and Trade Names in Volumes 1 to 46
1990; 346 pages Sw. fr. 60.

List of IARC Publications

IARC TECHNICAL REPORTS*

No. 1 Cancer in Costa Rica
Edited by R. Sierra,
R. Barrantes, G. Muñoz Leiva, D.M. Parkin, C.A. Bieber and
N. Muñoz Calero
1988; 124 pages Sw. fr. 30.-

No. 2 SEARCH: A Computer Package to Assist the Statistical Analysis of Case-control Studies
Edited by G.J. Macfarlane,
P. Boyle and P. Maisonneuve
1991; 80 pages (out of print)

No. 3 Cancer Registration in the European Economic Community
Edited by M.P. Coleman and
E. Démaret
1988; 188 pages Sw. fr. 30.-

No. 4 Diet, Hormones and Cancer: Methodological Issues for Prospective Studies
Edited by E. Riboli and
R. Saracci
1988; 156 pages Sw. fr. 30.-

No. 5 Cancer in the Philippines
Edited by A.V. Laudico,
D. Esteban and D.M. Parkin
1989; 186 pages Sw. fr. 30.-

No. 6 La genèse du Centre International de Recherche sur le Cancer
Par R. Sohier et A.G.B. Sutherland
1990; 104 pages Sw. fr. 30.-

No. 7 Epidémiologie du cancer dans les pays de langue latine
1990; 310 pages Sw. fr. 30.-

No. 8 Comparative Study of Antismoking Legislation in Countries of the European Economic Community
Edited by A. Sasco, P. Dalla Vorgia and P. Van der Elst
1990; 82 pages Sw. fr. 30.-

No. 9 Epidémiologie du cancer dans les pays de langue latine
1991; 346 pages Sw. fr. 30.-

DIRECTORY OF AGENTS BEING TESTED FOR CARCINOGENICITY (Until Vol. 13 Information Bulletin on the Survey of Chemicals Being Tested for Carcinogenicity)*

No. 8 Edited by M.-J. Ghess,
H. Bartsch and L. Tomatis
1979; 604 pages Sw. fr. 40.-

No. 9 Edited by M.-J. Ghess,
J.D. Wilbourn, H. Bartsch and
L. Tomatis
1981; 294 pages Sw. fr. 41.-

No. 10 Edited by M.-J. Ghess,
J.D. Wilbourn and H. Bartsch
1982; 362 pages Sw. fr. 42.-

No. 11 Edited by M.-J. Ghess,
J.D. Wilbourn, H. Vainio and
H. Bartsch
1984; 362 pages Sw. fr. 50.-

No. 12 Edited by M.-J. Ghess,
J.D. Wilbourn, A. Tossavainen and
H. Vainio
1986; 385 pages Sw. fr. 50.-

No. 13 Edited by M.-J. Ghess,
J.D. Wilbourn and A. Aitio 1988;
404 pages Sw. fr. 43.-

No. 14 Edited by M.-J. Ghess,
J.D. Wilbourn and H. Vainio
1990; 370 pages Sw. fr. 45.-

No. 15 Edited by M.-J. Ghess, J.D. Wilbourn and H. Vainio
1992; 318 pages Sw. fr. 45.-

NON-SERIAL PUBLICATIONS †

Alcool et Cancer
By A. Tuyns (in French only)
1978; 42 pages Fr. fr. 35.-

Cancer Morbidity and Causes of Death Among Danish Brewery Workers
By O.M. Jensen
1980; 143 pages Fr. fr. 75.-

Directory of Computer Systems Used in Cancer Registries
By H.R. Menck and D.M. Parkin
1986; 236 pages Fr. fr. 50.-

---

* Available from booksellers through the network of WHO Sales agents.

† Available directly from IARC

www.ingramcontent.com/pod-product-compliance
Ingram Content Group UK Ltd.
Pitfield, Milton Keynes, MK11 3LW, UK
UKHW051258180426
11947UKWH00020B/1784